DOWN TO THE BARE BONES

DOWN TO THE BARE BONES

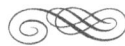

A Soulful Memoir Exposing the Unfiltered Truth of Being Human

DANIELLE LOUISE ROSA TOOLEY

Author

Divinity Bubbles of Love

Copyright © 2023 by Divinity Bubbles of Love
All rights reserved. No part of this book may be reproduced in any manner whatsoever without written permission except in the case of brief quotations embodied in critical articles and reviews.

First Printing, 2023 V2

www.downtothebarebones.com
www.divinitybubbles.love

Dedicated to Humanity

Contents

Dedication   v

1	It's Time to Wake Up	1
2	Tears of Joy	6
3	The Day Life Changed Forever	9
4	A Family United	21
5	Global Wave of Healing Energy	25
6	Back in the ICU	28
7	Childhood Flashbacks	33
8	A Re-Birth After 17 Years	41
9	Trauma that Morphined into Something Else	48
10	Transferred for Treatment	53
11	The debrideMEnt Process	61
12	Glass Windows of Hope	65
13	Cultivating a Commitment	69
14	Washed Away	77
15	Intentionally Defective	83

16	Truth Beyond the Pain	88
17	A Home Away From Home	92
18	Medium Care Yet Top Priority	110
19	These Legs Were Made for Walking	114
20	Finally!	122
21	Beyond Medical Expertise	128
22	The Grind	134
23	My Own Version of Senior Year	144
24	Mid-Year Exams	152
25	Let Your Light Shine	158
26	A Graduation Gift for Life	164
27	Summer SOULstice	174
28	Tested Faith	179
29	Who Am I?	188
30	Where Am I?	218
31	The Beautiful Life in Between	223
32	Deconstruct the Ego to Reconstruct the Heart	304
33	Trust in the Process	313
34	Finding My Soul's Light	317
35	Replacing My Heart's Fear with Love	325
36	Connecting to My Spiritual Senses	336
37	Fueling My Passionate Heart	361
38	Authentic Self-Love	382

39	Angels Amongst Us	404
40	Sacred Orchid of Divinity	411
41	Understanding Love, My Light Language	470
42	The Realms of Existence	484
43	The Scientific Truth of Spiritual Love	500
44	From My Heart to Yours	603

I

It's Time to Wake Up

"Open your big beautiful blue eyes...

...it's time to wake up."

Those were the words my parents desperately spoke only weeks after my seventeenth birthday. With only one person allowed in my room at a time, fully dressed in sterile garments, my Mom sat at my bedside and uttered those words over and over again. She spoke to me and kept telling me to open my big beautiful blue eyes, to wake up and look at her with my pretty blues. For days, she sat and spoke to me in my silence and continued to encourage me to wake up. Yet, every day, I had no response.

Each day, the visits came to an end, and my parents were forced to leave, only to try again the next. They had to leave me behind wondering if I would ever wake up, and if they would ever see my blue eyes again. At the close of each day, they went home in anticipation of the next, and to wonder if they would be able to reach me. As soon as visiting hours permitted, my Mom returned to my bedside and continued to speak words of encouragement to open my eyes. After days passed with no response, my Mom believed that I would respond to my Dad. She knew that we had a special father-daughter bond and suspected that I would respond to his voice. She left my room and asked him in to try and reach me.

My Dad entered my room and sat at my bedside. He began doing the same thing. He spoke words of encouragement to open my big beautiful blue eyes. Within his first visit to wake me, I slowly became conscious of the world around me. I was waking up, and in a hazy, blurry state of confusion, I saw my Dad sitting next to my bed. I examined everything within the confines of my isolation room. First, with my eyes, and then I tried to move my very stiff, bandaged wrapped body. I had no idea where I was or what was going on, but cognitively I was becoming more aware of the situation around me.

I saw my body wrapped in bandages from my neck to my toes. Then my eyes moved around the room to examine the IV poles with numerous medication bags, the multiple monitors, and then my eyes stopped once they were able to focus on my Dad. My Dad sat weeping beside me. He was sitting at my bedside, sobbing, behind the slightest glimpse of a smile. I was terrified and confused. I wanted to know what was going on. I tried to understand what was happening to me. Where was I? Why was I wrapped like this? It was apparent, even to me, that I was in a very critical state, but why? What was going on?

I instantly tried to speak, to ask my Dad the many questions that started swirling around in my confused and cloudy mind, but as I tried to project my voice, nothing came out. I could not speak. I could not get a single sound to come out. With this, I became increasingly more terrified. What was going on? My Dad saw the agitation and fear in my eyes and quickly explained that I had been on a ventilator, which had irritated my larynx, in essence causing laryngitis. He indicated that all I had to do was rest my throat for my voice to come back. But I had so many questions. Did he say that I was on a ventilator? Why did I need a ventilator? Why was I wrapped in bandages like a mummy? Why was I even in the hospital? I desperately wanted to understand what had happened.

My Dad began to tell me bits and pieces about what had happened. He started at the very beginning. He was slow and cautious of what he told me, as not to overwhelm or cause anxiousness. He would ask if I remembered anything along the way, with portions of the stories seeming vaguely familiar. It was very overwhelming, but the one thing I could not understand was why he was so happy.

My Dad continued to cry as he slowly told me small segments of the story, but I wanted to know more. I wanted to know faster. I had so many more questions, such as when was I going home? What about school? Were any of my friends also sick? When were we going shopping for Jr. Prom? When were we going to get a birthday present for my Sister? But it was not that easy. I could not talk. I did not have a voice.

It would be days before I would barely be able to get just a whisper to come out. So, my resourceful Dad found a dry erase board and wrote out the alphabet from A-Z. He held the board, and I would slowly extend my finger and point to each letter of every word I wanted to say. It became very tiring to hold my arm up long enough to point to every letter of every word, so I quickly learned to spell out keywords so my Dad could fill in the blanks. The image is still vivid of him sitting at my bedside and holding the board with tears in his eyes and a smile on his face.

He patiently waited and anticipated each question with tremendous caution. He would collect his thoughts in a way to not overwhelm me and slowly provide one answer at a time. He summarized eight weeks of my life. He started with the evening after school, the doctor's appointment the following morning, which resulted in the immediate admittance into the ER, and the three weeks that followed in the intensive care unit. He continued to explain that after the initial three weeks, I had been transferred to another hospital where a five-week coma was medically induced. All of which brought us to the very moment that he sat before me when I opened my pretty blues and woke up.

Although the limited visiting hours had been extended due to my awakening, few details were shared while addressing the more imminent questions and concerns. My Dad was conscientious not to convey the actual depths of the trauma. Instead, he carefully navigated through the story to focus the discussion on the five-week coma and to address my most pressing questions of why I was wrapped like a mummy. He explained that I had become very ill, and my body had been destroyed from the inside out. The extent of the damage on the inside was still unknown, but the exterior damage was so significant that it required surgical procedures to remove the damaged tissue. A coma was induced for five weeks while medical professionals performed surgical procedures and tended to my every need for survival while they repaired my body.

Through his words and behind his tears, he had the biggest smile.

Even the nurses and doctors who came into my room were excited and overjoyed. Why was everyone so happy? I remember thinking, "Did you hear the story you just told me? Look at me. I am about to die! I am not in a happy situation." There were so many things that I did not understand, especially why everyone was so happy. I knew in those moments I was not, and the more I learned of my condition, I wondered if I ever would be again.

The visit eventually came to an end. Upon my Dad's departure, I was left with the remnants of the story he had shared, the reality of my new being, and the uncertainty of who I would become. It did not take long for me to realize there was an unfiltered story behind the mummy-like bandages that clothed my body.

2

Tears of Joy

The next day when my parents returned, my Mom found herself explaining the joy I saw in those around me. The explanation she gave was as if I had woken up in the middle of a soap opera, and that the intense climatic uncertainty was already over. So much had already transpired over the eight weeks of my oblivion. There had been numerous moments that I had evaded death, which made my waking such a joyous event. Everyone kept saying the same thing, and each time the words were spoken, it resonated differently within me. The sadness within me was met by the joy everyone was expressing around me. It seemed and felt as if I was about to die, and somehow, I was still very much alive.

Through the drug-induced haze, I was still trying to make sense of what I had learned the day before. Five weeks? In a coma? Eight weeks had passed since I went to school? That's two months; sixty days. Had I been in the hospital that whole time? Doctors removed damaged tissue? What does that even mean? I almost died numerous times? Nothing made sense. I wanted to wake again, but this time from what I hoped was a false reality. I wanted to run out of the room, home, and to my safe place around the lake. I wanted to get back to my life, but I was unable. I was tired. I was drugged. I was bandaged. I was incapable of doing anything on my own. Even taking a breath felt questionable at times. I was tremendously broken — all parts of me.

Although my parents were allowed in my room, visiting hours were limited and restricted to one visitor. Many days, especially following surgeries, visits were only allowed through a glass window and phone, the only means by which I could see and hear my siblings and friends. I was very lonely and scared, yet quickly learned that I had to find a way to make it through the days. It was even challenging to engage the hospital staff. Hardly any of them spoke English, nor had the time to sit and really connect. I spent many hours alone, with myself and my new reality, within the isolate walls of my room.

As I was left alone in my isolated intensive care unit room, memories started to flood back. I had little control over the immediate reflections of my life before, and the uncertainty of what was to come. As each moment passed, my senses were forced to reckon with my reality. Engaging with my truth allowed the details of my journey to fall into place. I saw what had happened to my body. I could hear what was said about my condition. I could smell the sterilized environment around me. I could taste the medication as it was injected into my IV line. I could feel the pain throughout my entire body – physically, emotionally, psychologically, and spiritually. It was clear that I had to somehow cultivate a commitment to create the best life experience I could, for it was indeed my new reality. It was dreadful, but it was mine. While everyone cried tears of joy, when left alone, I cried my own, yet mine were tears of sadness, fear, uncertainty, and pain.

3

The Day Life Changed Forever

It was just another ordinary day at school. I was attending high school with students from all over the world, participating in after school sports practice, focused on school and homework, running to free my spirit, and spending as much time as I could with friends, my boyfriend, and my family. This was what ordinary turned out to be for me as a sixteen-year-old southern girl from Louisiana, transplanted into the International School in Brussels, Belgium, in Europe. Among many things, preparing for the weekend softball tournament in Germany was top on my list.

I played sports every season, but before the softball season began, I had decided to become more physically fit. Outside of sports activities, my exercise preference was running. I loved to run. In hindsight, I think it gave me a sense of going somewhere as if affirming that I was moving forward with intention. I would wake up at five o'clock in the morning, put on my running gear, and head out the door. A block away from our house was a human-made lake with a running track perimeter and a small park to the side. I would play my favorite tunes and run the track for at least an hour and a half. After a good run, I would head back home, get ready for school, and then head out the door for the day.

When the school day was over, I would stay after school for sports practice, come home via public transport or walk, eat dinner with the family, do homework, and then hit the pavement again for another run around the lake. My evening run usually lasted about an hour or so, or until I got tired. I ran for about three hours every day. It was never about distance, so I honestly don't know how many miles I ran around that lake, but I know it made a difference.

It was a Friday afternoon, and the softball team was about to travel to Germany for a two-day softball tournament with other participating European schools. When the school's sports teams traveled for overnight away games, the opponent team and their families opened their homes and housed teammates for the duration of the trip. This trip was no different.

We arrived in Germany on a Friday evening, and for this particular trip, I was housed by a girl named Penelope. I do not recall her nationality, nor personality, and I barely remember her appearance. I do not remember anything about who she was as a person, yet I remember her name and the room of her home within which I laid my head to rest.

Once settled in, we engaged in the usual events when away on sports trips. Usual events entailed eating with the opposing team's family, experiencing their cultural traditions, and then going out to the local bars to socialize with all the tournament team members; from my school, those from the housing team, and the other tournament participating teams. If you played a lot of sports, it was an opportunity to meet up with friends from around the world who shared the same experiences, transplanted into a foreign school as teenagers trying to navigate our unique life situations.

The following Saturday morning, our team was on the schedule for an early doubleheader. To make the weekend more interesting, it was snowing. We were a bunch of determined sports fanatics, and it was evident that the snow flurries were not going to slow us down. Everyone was determined to play, so we played ball. Game one was about to begin, and our team took to the field for warm-ups. Up to when it was time to start the game, the teams did a very minimal warm-up while bundled and shivering in the show.

I do not remember playing either of the two games that day. I do recall that I didn't feel well that night and stayed in bed while Penelope met up with the teams downtown. I remember that Sunday was an even more significant blur, with only the faint memory of leaving the tournament grounds, and somehow being present at school the next day. Long ago, I acknowledged the truth that I lack memories from these days. I have always been aware of this truth due to the rarity of such an absent recollection. I believe it is because of what was already happening inside my body.

On Monday afternoon, the day after our return from the sports tournament, I was sitting in history class, my last class of the day. I eagerly waited for the day to end as a headache began to set in. I could hear the teacher talk but could not understand what was said. His voice was just a muffled, monotone sound in the background. I was unable to concentrate, and my headache was getting more and more intense. To pass the time, I began doodling a bouquet of three rose buds with a new technique learned in art class, pointillism. As I waited for the class bell to ring, I focused on drawing roses as my Mom had taught me, with the new dot technique to get shading and depth.

At one moment, I turned my head to look out of the window. In doing so, I was startled by the experience that followed. When I rotated my head to the left, there was an unexpected stiffness and soreness in my neck. When I finally completed the uncomfortable turn of my head, there was a tremendous sensitivity to the brightness of the sun. It was the same bright sun, yet that day my eyes could not bear the intensity of its light rays. It was a light so bright that it blinded me to tears. Finally, the class bell rang.

When the bell rang, I knew I did not feel well enough for softball practice. I quickly collected my things to allow time to locate my softball coach before catching the bus home. He told me not to worry about missing practice, to go home and get some rest. He even mentioned he was likely going to cancel practice because others had also reported not feeling well. None of us thought anything more about it, and we all went our separate ways. I caught the school bus and went home to do just that, rest.

Meanwhile, while I was at school, close family friends from Louisiana had arrived at our house. Aunt Max and Uncle Gene were taking a European excursion, and our house was going to be their base between the various parts of their trip. Our families were extremely close, especially Aunt Max and my Mom. They were the closest of friends and remained present for each other in the complexities of life, and without expectation. A truly genuine friendship. They were so close that Aunt Max became the Godmother to my younger Sister, hence the reference as an Aunt. I always admired Aunt Max for her medical knowledge and her sincere, compassionate, and joyous heart. Aunt Max and Uncle Gene have always been and remain very special and dear to our family.

During their flight to Belgium, Aunt Max mysteriously lost her voice, and once arrived, she quickly scheduled an appointment with our American doctor. She felt fine, but her loss of voice was concerning, and she wanted to ensure she was healthy enough for their impending journey around Europe. She scheduled an appointment for 7:00am the next morning, Tuesday, March 30, 1993, which unbeknownst to me would become the most critical doctor visit in my life. It became the day my life changed forever. It became the first day of my new reality.

By the time I made it home from school, I felt terrible. After a very brief greeting, I headed up the stairs, made it to my bed, and found relief in the moment to finally rest. When I awoke an hour or so later, I knew something was wrong. I felt strange. There was an indescribable sensation throughout my body. I did not know what it was, but I knew it was not familiar in any way. I went downstairs to tell my Mom that I thought I needed to see a doctor. Reluctant due to the ever-evolving perception of hypochondria, she encouraged me to take action myself, and to schedule an appointment if I believed it was needed.

That was all I needed to hear to take matters into my own hands. I called Dr. Owen to request that I join Aunt Max during her pre-scheduled appointment the next morning. Dr. Owen agreed, so Aunt max and I would both see her at 7:00 am. I exchanged goodnight wishes with my family before I excused myself, headed back upstairs, and returned to my bed to succumb to the inescapable fatigue.

After several hours I was awoken in the middle of the night by unusual cramping in my legs. If my legs were straight, it felt like I needed to bend them. If they were bent, it felt like I needed to straighten them. For a while, I tried to get comfortable and connect with whatever it was that caused the discomfort. The more nothing made sense, the more I knew I needed my parents. Eager to get to my parents to find comfort, I pulled the covers back, stood up, and fell straight to the floor. Somewhat confused and in disbelief, I tried again to bear weight on my legs as they buckled in pain, sending me straight to the floor for a second time. I quickly became scared and desperate to reach my parents.

Unable to put weight on my legs, I found my only option was to army crawl my way out of my room, down the hall and to my Mom's side of the bed closest to the door. Although I was calling out to them along the way, muffled by the tears that had started to fall, it was only once I had arrived at their bedside that my voice awoke them from their slumber. My Dad assisted me onto the bed, and they began to discover my state of being. They found my pain, a high fever, the waves of chills, and dehydration sweeping over me. And quickly. They rushed to slow down the visual appearance of my body, slipping away from life.

When we were younger, my siblings and I used to get growing pains in our shins — especially me and my Sisters as our bodies tried to adjust to the rapid vertical growth endured. When requested, my Dad used to massage our legs, and it would ease the discomfort temporarily. This night, when I mentioned my legs were hurting, instinctively, my Dad grabbed my legs and started massaging them as he did in my younger years. This time the loving touch was different. When something that usually felt relieving instead felt excruciating, I knew something was terribly wrong.

In the moments of my screaming reaction, begging him to stop, my Mom gave me a muscle relaxer and acetaminophen to help with the cramping and pain. By this time, my fever had elevated to 106° F, and I was shivering and sweating at the same time while drinking liters of water. My Mom immediately called the doctor in the middle of the night for reassurance. Dr. Owen advised her to keep me covered, even though the fever was causing the sweats, ensure that I remained hydrated, and to try to hold out for a few more hours until the appointment.

I finally rested in my parent's bed. My Dad must have left and slept elsewhere while I stayed in their bed with my Mom. And honestly, I am not convinced that I slept. I believe it was the onset of my intermittent loss of consciousness. I do know that had I not been woken for the doctor's appointment several hours later, I would never have woken into this life again.

As I started to get ready for the doctor, my body felt stiff like my skin was too tight for my body. I do not remember it hurting, just that my body could not bend because my skin was not giving. I could barely sit up on the side of the bed. I definitely could not bend over to put on my shoes. My younger Sister, who was twelve at the time, helped me put on my sweatpants and shoes, and then helped me down the stairs. As I found stability with my arm around her neck, she guided me with her arms around my waist. Together, she guided me down the stairs, one step at a time. I remember the sensation of not feeling my legs, only the pressure throughout my body with every step I took.

Once I made it to the car, my Dad drove while Aunt Max was in the front passenger seat, and I was lying in the back seat. I do not remember much about that drive only that when I arrived, Aunt Max had to help me navigate a long, narrow flight of stairs to get to the doctor's office, which was inside her home. Upon our entrance, despite my 106° fever, Dr. Owen escorted me to her bed so that I could rest while examining Aunt Max first.

When it was my turn, Dr. Owen had to wake me and escort me through her house. Once I entered the exam room, she completed a couple of routine assessments, the first being a full-body scan of visible symptoms. The bruising that was noted around my knees, and my screaming discomfort when she touched them, led to her immediate recommendation to take me directly to the emergency room. Dr. Owen remarked that she was hopeful that it was only the flu, yet the bruising gave reason to believe it was much more severe. She feared it was bacterial meningitis, and if it was, time was of the essence.

Next, I was lying on the back seat, in and out of consciousness, and then strangely, something happened during the moments before I entered my new realm of existence. I encountered an out of body experience. My consciousness was found above, looking down upon myself as I tried to understand my situation. I was above myself, floating around to get a better view of reality. I was far above the car, yet it somehow did not obstruct my view of self. I examined my feeble body in the car's back seat and observed my fate in the unfolding. It seemed like it lasted an eternity when in actuality, it was only a matter of minutes, ending as we arrived at the hospital.

We made it to the ER, and I do not remember the intake process, how long it took, or any details except ending up in a bed within a room with five other beds, some of which were occupied. There were three beds on each side, and they all faced the center of the room. My bed was one of two near the windows. I recall seeing the trees outside of the window behind Aunt Max as she stayed in the room by my side while my Dad sought answers.

The pain intensified as my body began to deteriorate. My organs were failing, and delirium was setting in while confusion, anger, and despair began to surface. My body, the one I had worked so hard to get healthy, was falling apart. I pleaded with Aunt Max to make the pain stop. I begged her to do something. I begged her to do anything. She tried to explain that they had already begun to administer morphine and that it would soon relieve the pain. She tried to remind me that I had to be patient, as I fought her with claims that she didn't care enough to aid me. She stayed beside me and comforted me while time passed, and I slowly was relieved from the engulfing pain.

The bruises on my legs continued to get worse, they were running test after test, and the ER doctors were about to conduct a spinal tap to confirm a diagnosis. In those very moments, Dr. Jean Louis Vincent, the ER Chief Physician who had stopped by to retrieve something while on vacation, heard me screaming, came into my room, and examined my state of being. He immediately told his staff that they did not have time to do a spinal tap and wait for the results. He was confident that I had bacterial meningitis. He ordered an immediate transfer to intensive care and gave the orders to start specific treatments upon my arrival.

My miracle doctor. Not only did he cancel his vacation to ensure proper and sufficient administration of therapies, but he also personally balanced the perfectly portioned medical cocktails that kept me alive. Dr. Jean Louis Vincent delicately balanced his knowledge and the inherent truth of my prognosis in such a meticulous manner that it was ultimately his presence that saved my life. Medications that were good for my heart were bad for my kidneys. Treatments that were good for my kidneys were bad for my liver. The delicate balance was the scenario prevalent with every intervention that was required to sustain stability. It was a tremendous act of balance and accuracy to achieve effective treatments. I am forever grateful for his instinct, intellect, and precision.

Dr. Jean Louis Vincent returned to my Dad and Aunt Max, pulled my Dad to the side, and spoke words everyone dreads to hear; that the loss of a loved one was imminent. The doctor told him that I had bacterial meningitis and that I would likely not make it through the night. In utter disbelief, my Dad told Aunt Max, and together they called Uncle Gene to inform him of my situation. My Dad spoke to Uncle Gene, and not my Mom because he could not bear to tell her over the phone. He wanted her to hear the news face to face. He wanted her to be supported when receiving the news of her daughter. Although my Dad sincerely wished to be present with my Mom, so together they could navigate their grievances, he felt he had no other option but to ask Uncle Gene to bear that burden for him. Uncle Gene somberly accepted and agreed to tell my Mom of my condition, remain present in consolation, and support her while my Dad and Aunt Max stayed at the hospital.

As a parent, I cannot imagine what it must have been like to receive news that your child may not survive the night and to feel utterly helpless. How sad their hearts must have felt in those moments of uncertainty. How unaware I was that all this was happening to my family. How unaware I was to what was happening to me, and because of me. For most of my life that followed, my heart ached for the sadness and grief they must have felt as they watched me fight for my life. Once recovery was underway, I never allowed myself to connect to the truths of my own deeply felt sadness and grief as I navigated the newness of my reality. I felt more sadness for those around me than I ever allowed myself to feel for myself. I didn't have the energy nor time to do so. More importantly, I felt I had to focus on how I was going to make it through every unbelievably hard day of my new existence. And no matter what that would turn out to be, I knew that sadness and grief for self could not be a part of that experience.

Although I made it through the first night, each night that followed over the following two weeks was just as uncertain as the first. Many unknowns continued to present themselves, yet every day that I lived was merely just another day that I had not died. It took about two weeks for the medical cocktails to stabilize my condition. While working to sustain life within those two weeks, my body struggled tremendously and even went into cardiac arrest on two separate occasions, both of which required resuscitation and defibrillation. These initial two weeks began highlighting the sequence of unexplainable events that led up to the continuance of my breath in life. It was the meticulously timed and placed events that ultimately gave purpose to my continued survival, even when the odds were entirely against me.

It is still tremendously humbling to know that part of my life story is that I have been resuscitated twice. It is terrifying and gratifying within the same breath and thought. During those times, the truth of the medical dangers, and the fragility of my physical state made everything even more surreal. As everyone began spinning in the unfathomable uncertainty in everything, there was a great urgency for my family to reunite and be present together, and it needed to happen quickly. The family had to be together. My family had to be united. Our reality held the potential to be our last moments together as a nuclear family unit as a whole in this life.

4

A Family United

At age twelve, my family had the opportunity to move overseas to Brussels, Belgium. My Dad was the IT Administrator for a chemical company and was offered a two-to-three-year project abroad to build the datacenter for a new office. This meant leaving behind the only home, friends, and life I knew.

First, my Mom and Dad took a trip to visit the area, potential schools, and a sense of what life would be like abroad. Once they returned and presented us with information, videos, and discussions, the majority would rule. My hand was one of the first to go up. It was not a unanimous vote, but the majority did rule, and in the summer of 1989, our family of six packed up our lives and moved to Belgium.

I was thirteen by the time we moved at the end of my seventh-grade school year. I was ready for the adventure. I was excited about the possibilities. I welcomed the change. The excitement I felt outweighed any emotion that surfaced in the truth of leaving family, friends, and life as I knew it behind. My life was my family, and they were with me, so it felt like life would be the same just somewhere different. I remember looking out of the airplane window as we flew out of the New Orleans International Airport. There was a single tear that fell as the thought of "goodbye life as I know it" flooded my being.

Once we arrived in Belgium, every experience endured was an incredible gift in this life. I spent three years exploring, growing, and evolving by the diverse and unique experiences abroad. I felt extremely fortunate for what seemed like a rare and unusual life journey, especially in the early 1990s, and at my youthful age.

By the time of my impending medical experiences, it was me, my younger Sister, Diana, and my parents that still lived in Brussels. Doug, my older brother, did not want to move but promised my parents one full school year abroad. It was agreed that if he didn't like it, he could move back to his home. He completed one year as promised and decided he wanted to return to the place he called home. He returned to the boarding school he attended before moving overseas, which had him coming from Bay St. Louis, Mississippi. My older Sister, Dina, graduated from high school the year before and returned to the United States to attend Georgia Tech University in Atlanta, Georgia; she began her journey from there.

In a rush against time, my Dad called my siblings and told them of my condition. Then, he called his employer that moved us overseas, and they authorized him to call the corporate travel center to book the flights for my siblings. In was a gracious gift that my Dad's company paid for my family to reunite. The arrangements were made, and my parents waited for Doug and Dina to make it home to solidify our family reunited.

My Sister's journey was particularly challenging because she was booked on the first available flight, which turned out to be a ferry flight. That meant that the flight was solely for returning the aircraft and was not a regular passenger flight. These circumstances left her alone on the plane as she traveled halfway across the world to be present in my potential final hours. During a nine-hour flight, alone on a plane, with only the pilots and one stewardess, she anxiously sat in disbelief of her reality, which was merely a result of my own reality. What used to sadden my heart the most about the journey my Sister took is knowing the internal turmoil she was experiencing hinged on a childhood pact that we had made years prior.

When we were younger, before we had moved overseas, we were very, very close. We looked a lot alike, except I have blue eyes and hers are brown, just like everyone else in the family. She was always an inch or so taller than me, but otherwise, we could pass as twins. Everything about us was different but the same, from our clothes to our personalities. I must have been about 10, and she was about 12, and we were in the back seat of my Dad's red Chrysler Volare.

A song came on the radio, which interrupted our playfulness. As we listened to the words, we both thought it was such a beautiful song, and it described how we would feel should one of us die. It was not in a morbid sense; it was in a loving, connected sense because of how deeply we would miss each other if we did not have one another in this life. At that moment, in our young minds, we made a pact with each other. We promised each other that when one of us dies, the surviving sister shall sing the song at the memorial service. Not really understanding the gravity of what we had committed to do, we laughingly agreed and carried on in our youthfulness singing aloud from our hearts.

Little did we know that our youthful pact would be put to the test a short six years later. While Dina traveled on the ferry flight alone, she struggled and frantically tried to recall the song's name and lyrics because she thought she was going to be called upon to sing it as promised. Our reality was unfolding long before internet access was available on planes, and even longer before electronic devices. For a nine-hour flight, she thought about the song, the words, how she could not remember either and felt she needed to find both of them desperately.

She was only eighteen years old, flying across the world alone, trying to remember the words to a silly song that she feared would be needed at my memorial. She spent nine hours preparing for the death of her sister. It was an innocent childhood pact, unknowing of who would have to put it into action, and surely not expecting it to be so soon in life. Once the song lyrics were retrieved, they became etched in our minds forever. It is a pact that we will honor and uphold even more so after our strength was tested at such a young age.

With Doug and Dina's arrival, the family was reunited within two days of my hospital admittance. Everyone waited to hear what the doctors had to say with each passing moment. They waited to find out the results of the myriad of tests. They waited to see if I would survive another day. Every day they waited. They waited as a family united.

5

Global Wave of Healing Energy

While the family was reuniting and trying to grasp what was happening, the International School of Brussels (ISB) community was doing the same by obtaining updates from my parents, relaying it to the students, and uniting in support.

The day I was admitted to the ER, the doctors notified the school of my condition. The medical team was concerned about the source of the infection. They even reached out to Penelope's family in Germany to inform them and recommend precautionary treatment. The intent was to treat anyone in close contact with me throughout the days preceding my hospitalization. On that day, six of my closest friends were called into the principal's office, all unsure of the reason. The diverse group awaited in anticipation. They waited for news that would change the course of everything.

My friends learned that I had fallen fatally ill and that I may not survive through the night. Because I was so close to all of them, they were advised to take a prescribed prophylactic. The recommendation was to ensure that if they were the source, or if they had contracted it from me, that they would receive treatment immediately. I recall afterward when being told of the stories that my friends claimed the medicine turned their urine bright orange-yellow, and that they were slightly terrified of the whole idea of it all. Understandably so.

The school continued to inform the community, and it was those efforts that began what I have always called my Global Wave of Healing Energy. The high school students would gather to receive updates on my condition. Newsletters went out to students and their families. The school encouraged prayers and support from family and friends. As a community, they came together in support and waited for the next update in anticipation. And the next one. And the next one.

I was attending an international school. There were students from over sixty countries, creating diversity from different backgrounds and speaking different languages. Yet none of that mattered. The school community united and unknowingly fueled the global healing energy that I have always felt was a part of my survival.

As students and their families became aware of the situation, they relayed my condition to their families and friends in their homelands. In response, my name was added to prayer chains around the world. Just as my condition deteriorated quickly, I was lifted in prayer, love, and healing energy within every corner of the globe. Due to the love and support from the international community, I soon had a tribe of Global Prayer Warriors. I received cards and letters from students and families whom I did not know, from families in other countries, from churches and groups from all over the world. A couple of my favorites came from 1st graders and the class of my fourth-grade teacher. The children created posters and letters of healing support and encouragement. They even included photos of their sweet faces.

Prayers were said, and healing energy sent from around the world. The global energy accumulated and built momentum with every school announcement, with every update, and with every healing thought. It was the Butterfly Effect in action, setting ripples of energy in motion from every corner of the world, created in love and healing intention, directed solely at my being. The intense and powerful Global Wave of Healing Energy was instrumental in my survival. It altered my energetic signature within this universe. Although I felt it deeply during those times, it would take many years for me to understand the truths in the energetic shifts I experienced.

It was authentic spiritual energy in motion. The handwritten cards and letters poured in, and eventually, once out of intensive care, they were hung on the walls in my hospital room to remind me of my Global Pray Warriors. My wall of motivation often gave me the strength to push through the challenges. So many people were supporting me, so many people I didn't even know. I knew I had to survive and fight for myself, but it also felt like I needed to do it for everyone else. Perhaps it was also the truth in that my journey would somehow, in some way, help someone. Someday.

I desperately wanted to believe that Global Energy would carry me. I cried, prayed, and wanted to believe so deeply that it would be so. It felt like I needed to be carried on the ripples of strength, courage, and love that were sent towards me, for I felt I had none of my own.

6

Back in the ICU

There remains a blank space in my mind, not in the same sense as a forgotten memory. The two weeks when I was critical, being diagnosed, treated, resuscitated, and stabilized in the intensive care unit remain empty. My parents were not allowed to see me, and doctors reported one bad scenario after another. Every organ was failing, and every medication targeting one organ was adversely affecting the others. All of them were affecting my heart. It was during this time that the combination of the illness and the drugs caused my heart to stop on two separate occasions. It was during this time when my miracle doctor dedicated his time to monitor and stabilize the numerous events occurring inside of my body. It was during this time that my heart was changed forever, beyond its purpose as a functioning organ that sustains breath.

My parents were starting to receive specific details about my condition. It was confirmed that I had contracted meningococcal meningitis, which turned septic, causing fulminant meningococcemia with the onset of Waterhouse-Friderichsen Syndrome. To provide a basis for what was happening to my body, Table 1 presents the details of each illness, the cause, symptoms, treatments, and prognosis. They were all triggered by each other, and fatal if not treated within the first 24 hours, or sooner.

Table 1 – Medial Diagnoses, Causes, Symptoms, Treatments and Prognoses

Diagnosis 1 - Meningococcal Meningitis

Cause	The bacterium Neisseria meningitidis. About 1 in 10 people carry this bacterium in the back of their nose and throat with no signs of symptoms of the disease. These individuals are known as carriers. However, sometimes the bacteria invade the body ad cause certain illnesses, known as meningococcal disease.
Symptoms	General poor feeling * Sudden high fever * Severe, persistent headache * Neck stiffness * Nausea or vomiting * Discomfort to bright lights * Drowsiness * Shivering or cold hands and feet * Joint pain * Confusion or other mental changes * seizures * Petechiae – signs of septicemia (blood poising) and is a medical emergency
Treatment	Act quickly * Do not wait * Steroids * Supportive treatments for other symptoms * Breathing support * Wound care
Prognosis	Fatal if not treated within 24 hours. Even with treatment, 1 in 10 patients will die from complications, and 1 in 5 patients that survive will have long-term disabilities such as loss of limb, deafness, blindness, nervous system problems and/or brain damage

© 2022 World Health Organization

Diagnosis 2 – Fulminant Meningococcemia

Cause	The bacterium Neisseria meningitidis disseminated into the bloodstream; sepsis
Symptoms	Fever * Chills * Petechiae * Internal bleeding * Blood clots * Low blood pressure
Treatment	Act quickly * Antibiotics * Supportive treatments for other symptoms
Prognosis	Fatal if not treated within 2-6 hours. Can be one of the most dramatic and rapidly fatal of all infectious diseases. Damaged organs and leaking blood vessels cause large areas of skin, muscle, and internal organs to die from lack of oxygen and blood. A significant percentage of survivors will have tissue damage that requires surgical treatment (skin grafts and/or partial or full amputations).

© 2022 *Center for Disease Control*

Diagnosis 3 – Waterhouse – Friderichsen Syndrome

Cause	Severe infection with meningococcus bacteria, or from infections from several other sever bacterial infections. It us the failure if the adrenal glands to function normally which is a result of bleeding into the gland.
Symptoms	Sudden onset of symptoms * Fever and chills * Joint and muscle pain * Headache * Vomiting * Petechiae when septicemia is involved * Septic shock * Dizziness and weakness * Very low blood pressure * Very fast heart rate * Confusion or coma * Disseminated intravascular coagulation (small blood clots cutting off blood supply to organs)
Treatment	Act quickly * Antibiotics * Steroids * Supportive treatments for other symptoms
Prognosis	Fatal if not treated within 24 hours. Approx. 50% fatality rate in cases with a delay in diagnosis and treatment.

© 2022 *NIH National Library of Medicine*

All of my blood vessels were leaking. Some even busting, causing the oxygen and blood supply to my organs to cease. The swelling of my spinal cord and brain was likely to leave me brain dead and paralyzed. My organs were shutting down, which caused discussions centered around colostomy bags, dialysis, blindness, permanent hearing loss, brain damage, amputations, and death was still a very realistic outcome. Every day was full of more tests, more bad news, and more sadness within the family. I, on the other hand, remained completely unaware as my mind was unconscious, and my body fought to survive.

Then, after about two weeks, I finally stabilized. They had managed to get all the illnesses under control, filtered my blood with numerous transfusions, balanced the medications with precision, and my body was able to hold steady. I was weak and fragile, but stable. While doctors spent their time assessing and analyzing tests, I remained isolated in intensive care, heavily sedated on morphine, and many other life-saving medications. To give some perspective, I was on so much morphine for such an extended period, and this was only the beginning, that eventually, addiction would become a prevalent concern to also monitor.

I was still on a ventilator, but my body was fighting to hold on. After the initial two weeks passed, and I continued to show signs of very slight improvement, which only meant I had not yet died, it was recognized that the treatment plan needed to be much more extensive and would continue for many months to come.

In the second week, I was finally stable enough and breathing on my own to be removed from the ventilator. I was still extremely critical and monitored very closely in intensive care, but I was able to take my own breath. The doctors continued to plan and coordinate the next phase of treatment, factoring in every slight change in my condition. Everyone, including the doctors, tried to wrap their minds around what had and continued to transpire. Each day, everyone was left wondering what it really meant in terms of treatment and recovery. Nobody knew. Nobody could know. It had everything to do with me.

Once they took me off the ventilator, they allowed my family to start visiting. They had to dress in sterile garments from head to toe. Robes, gloves, face masks, hats, shoes, the whole sterile works. This was when I had to start identifying people by their eyes and their voice. At the time, I did not realize that it would be all I would see for the next six months. It was during this time when my Mom's childhood lesson about my eyes would begin to forge its path on the journey. Everyone became nothing more than a pair of eyes, a set of hands, and a voice. I could tell everyone by any one of these elements which represented who they were to me.

7

Childhood Flashbacks

When I was born, I had the most prominent blue eyes. They were bright and wide, and I always looked surprised. My eyes were especially unique because they were the only blue ones out of everyone in the family. The other five members of our family had brown eyes. I always thought it was neat that our family made for the perfect example of the genetic Punnett square when mapping dominant brown and recessive blue genes across four offspring. My parents were both brown eyed with recessive blue genes as carriers from their fathers, who both had blue eyes. When two recessive blue gene carriers have four offspring, one offspring will ultimately get the two recessive blue genes, one from each parent, causing blue eyes. That is me.

Although beautiful to the world, to me, they were always a very sensitive topic. My eyes were big and blue, unlike everyone else in the family. My Mom would even innocently joke and say that I was the milkman's daughter. And yet we never had a milkman, at least not at that point in our life.

There is one particular experience that holds the significance I placed on one's eyes even at an early age and encapsulates everything about how I viewed myself as a child. It had a significant influence on my ability to relate to the eyes of those that crossed my path.

I was about eight years old, and my family was sitting around our kitchen counter for dinner. We had my favorite meal that night, spaghetti. I filled my plate with as much as I could, sat at the end of the counter in my usual spot, and began to eat. I eventually became full and was unable to eat all that I had served. When I stated that I was finished, my Mom innocently stated, "somebody's eyes were bigger than her stomach."

Not knowing that the statement was a common gesture used to indicate that someone thought they were hungrier than they were, I instinctively jumped up, screamed, and cried my way to my room. I proceeded to slam and lock the door behind me. In complete disbelief, my Mom followed to figure out what had transpired. Refusing to let her in, I sobbed and proclaimed that I knew my eyes were ugly and desperately reminded her that she did not have to make fun of them. She remained close as she continued to try and piece everything together while consoling me through the door.

Through her thoughtful reflection, it all became clear as to how and why my reaction was as such. She then transformed it into a beautiful teaching opportunity, and through this one instance, managed to teach me a lifelong lesson.

She began to explain to me that ever since I was born, people would stop her and comment on my eyes. She said many, if not all, of the encounters were initiated with the phrase, "Ahhh...look at those eyes." Everyone always knew what that meant; that they were big, blue, and beautiful — everyone but me. Over the years of hearing these expressions about my eyes, coupled with how they caused me to feel separated from my family, I became very sensitive to the comments and reactions of others towards my eyes. So, in an effort to reverse the years of negativity that I associated with my eyes, my Mom came up with one simple task.

Every day when I came home from school, before I could do anything, even homework, I would have to sit across from her at the kitchen counter, look her in the eye and answer one simple question. She would ask the same question, and my response was to be the same every time. Every day after school for what seemed like an eternity, but was actually only a week, for about five minutes each day, my Mom would ask me, "Danielle, who has pretty eyes?" and my response was always, "Mom, I have pretty eyes." Over time, I began to love my eyes and all their unique characteristics. If I ever had any doubts, I would ask myself that exact question and responded accordingly.

Years passed, the experience faded, and the ability to love my eyes grew stronger. In time, we moved overseas. Once we moved to Belgium, we actually had a milkman. He delivered fresh milk and juice to our home once a week. When I experienced and witness this concept of a milkman, I remember falling into the awareness of what the childhood statement implied. The memories came flooding back of the not so funny joke that I was the milkman's daughter. I remember the slither of wonder if my Mom would ever do that; have an affair with a milkman and further conceal the paternity of a child, and that be me. I believed my Mom would not do that, while admittingly saddened by the use of the jokingly phrase. I remember watching the milkman and imagining what would have had to occur for that to be true. I recall even imagining what it would be like if it were true, and the milkman never knew, but I did.

We settled into our new life and were a couple of years into the experience abroad when my eyes, yet again, were brought to the forefront of my reality. The abundant and beautiful moments abroad are too vast to surmise within the parameters of this book. Still, there is one in particular that circles back to my eyes. It transpired about seven years after my spaghetti freak out moment, nearly three years after our move overseas, and a combined ten years of self-reminders that my eyes are unique and beautiful. This story takes place in the basement of the ISB high school building at age fifteen in a chemistry class under the instruction of an Italian Professor, Dr. Prozzi.

I always sat in the front row to take notes. Dr. Prozzi's lecture podium was on a raised platform so he could see everyone, and everyone could see him. There were about 20 students in the class, most of whom were slightly terrified of his stern teaching methods. He was a kind, smart man but often came across as arrogant. He seemed to fit the stereotype of an older Italian man, bald, with a short, stalky stature and small circular glasses that mimicked the circular structure of his face.

One day a student challenged him in front of the class, and his response was particularly interesting, especially for someone like me who had buried my sense of spirituality due to preconditioned dogma. I never thought that the student was disrespectful, but by the teacher's response, he must have been perceived as such.

Our professor proceeded to dive into a five-minute rant proclaiming that he was the God of Chemistry and that he should never be questioned. He declared that he was always right and that he never apologized for anything. Ever. He ended the declaration of his importance with his ritualistic smile as if that put his temperament back into balance. The class remained silent, the daily lesson continued, and once the hour had passed, the class was dismissed.

About two weeks of classes had passed, and we were back in class, preparing for yet another chemistry lecture. Class began, the professor started to lecture, and I was sitting in my usual seat up front taking notes.

As he continued to lecture, I continued to take notes. At one point, instead of lifting my head to look at him, I looked at him over the top rim of my glasses while I continued to write. Thinking nothing of it, I proceeded to listen and take notes. I looked over the rim of my glasses again, but this time the reaction to my note-focused mannerism stopped everything.

As I looked at the professor over the top of my glasses, he projects out into the room, "You, with the big eyes..." I do not even recall what he was asking me, or the class, all I could think about was that he just made a comment about my eyes, and I had worked very hard to be proud of them, and I was not going to let him minimize my efforts in front of the class. They may have been unbeknown to him, but they were very known to me.

At that moment, I put my pen on my notebook and sat up and looked straight at him; eye to eye from my chair, just like I did across the counter with my Mom many years prior. After I sat in silence for a moment, he could tell that his comment did not amuse me. He asked me what was wrong, and since he asked, I decided to tell him. I never moved, and I never took my eyes off of him, and our conversation unfolded:

> **Dr. P:** What's wrong with you?
>
> **Me:** You offended me.
>
> **Dr. P:** {looking at the rest of the class} Ha! I offended her.
>
> **Dr. P:** {looking back at me} What would you like for me to do?
>
> **Me:** {recalling the declaration of importance weeks prior and claiming never to apologize for anything, calmly stated} I would like for you to apologize.
>
> **Dr. P:** {looking at the rest of the class} Did you hear that? She wants me to apologize.
>
> **Dr. P:** {looking back at me} I apologize for offending you.
>
> **Me:** Thank you.

I proceeded to pick up my pen to finish the notes I was taking. The class resumed as if nothing happened until after dismissal when my friends informed me of how crazy I was to have done what I did. It was not crazy at all. It was truthful and honest about how his comment affected me. I knew of my inner struggles, and even though those around me did not, there was a need to stand up for something important to myself, about myself. That alone was a precious lesson. I didn't realize it then, but it didn't matter at all what he said or even how others would perceive it. What mattered was what was within, and in that moment, there was still sensitivity, and he tapped right into it. That moment reinforced everything I wanted to believe about my eyes, likely because I stood up for them. I stood up for myself. I don't recall ever doing anything like that before in my youth. It allowed me to trust myself to know that if I needed to, I could and would do it again.

These experiences with my eyes and all the other eye-related encounters that I had in my youth would hold tremendous weight while I was in the hospital. The eyes of everyone became the sole means by which I could identify and connect with those around me. My experience forced me to become comfortable with eye contact; to find comfort in the sometimes discomfort brought on by locked eyes and silence. It forced me to look people in the eye to know who they were and to let them see me. Eyes became the entry point for me to connect, and it revealed the truth in that the eyes are the entry point to the soul.

It did not take long for me to discover that everyone I encountered created an opportunity for my soul to dance. My body could not dance while limited by the aliments that attacked it. My mind could not dance while limited by the language of the natives. My heart could not dance as it remembered how to beat on its own. The only thing that could dance was my soul. It felt like everyone's eyes were healing me. The healing love within another may be seen from within their eyes. Eyes have the capacity to touch and heal another's soul in the absence of words. It was the eyes of the many mysterious hospital aids that ultimately touched my soul with love and compassion in a time and space when I needed to heal. It was the eyes of healers that healed me as my soul danced in the reflection of their love.

The eyes of everyone became my everything.

8

A Re-Birth After 17 Years

My family was finally allowed to see me for the first time in almost two weeks. The last day they saw me in person was the morning I left home to go to the doctor's office. It had been even longer for my siblings returning from the United States. Once stabilized in the intensive care unit, the first visitors allowed were my Mom and Dad. Then after a few days, they let my siblings visit. Then they allowed Aunt Max and Uncle Gene since they had postponed their trip to stay close.

My family had to travel an hour to get to the hospital, and always allowed extra time to ensure they were there for the rigorous 30 minutes of allowed visitation. Most days, they would make the trip twice a day. And many days they made the trip and were not allowed to see me. But they still showed up. They always showed up. They were there waiting for me to survive another day.

My seventeenth birthday was twelve days after I entered the

emergency room. It took decades for me to realize that from the day of my seventeenth birthday, there is a part of me that was rebirthed into the forefront of my existence. Even when my body was unconscious, drugged and cognitively incoherent, my energy lived on. I remember more than I think I should from this time frame, and I humbly acknowledge that there are significantly more details that I do not remember.

Everything felt delicate and surreal —even the slow integration process needed for what had transpired. There was a newness in who I was transforming into and an uncertainty in who I would become. It was all so quick and unexpected. There were four separate visits on my birthday that remain clear in my mind, while concurrently, my mind is baffled as to how it could be given my condition and medications that were needed to sustain my life. These four visits marked a re-birth since, in truth, I had died and then brought back to life twice.

The first encounter was with a nurse within the intensive care. It was the first time that she was managing my needs, and I remember talking to her as she entered my room. Because it was my birthday, my parents were allowed to be with me throughout the day, and they were present when the nurse entered my room. As she came into the room, she smiled as she declared that we shared the same name. Her name was Danielle, and we shared laughter in the similarity. During our discussions, while she replaced IV bags and administered medications, it was revealed that it was my birthday. We were all mystified and amused when the nurse subtly affirmed that it was also her birthday. Intrigued and bewildered, we exchanged birthday wishes as she departed from my room.

It seemed too coincidental. I remember asking my Dad if he could verify that what she said was true. I saw him open the door to the nurse's station, watch him stick his head out of the door while asking if she was truthful. My Dad had "that" look on his face. It is the look he gives when he finds himself in the space of no explanation. It is the look of acceptance of what is without any explanation for the mysticism. He confirmed that it was so. My nurse's name was Danielle, and she was born on the same day. There were two physical bodies in the same room, with the same name, born on the same day, holding the same energy of the passionate and self-determined Aries. One healthy and aiding in the healing of the other. It has always remained an interesting reflection and an example of the wonderment in the Universe.

The next two visits were from my math teacher and our family's maid, both surprisingly unexpected guests. Mr. Lerda was my favorite math teacher. One of the fondest memories of him is how he would always draw circles with a whistling hum. It was a combination of a whistle and a hum that he would make while drawing circles on the chalkboard as a way to entertain his students and keep their interest. For me, it worked. It always made me chuckle, and eventually, I figured out how he did it and can mimic the sound. It is my contribution to math entertainment today. The day he came to visit me, I recall seeing him in the doorway of my hospital room. My bed faced directly at the door entry so that I could see visitors that were not allowed to enter. This was how we visited. I could see him, and he could see me.

Because of my situation, wearing a hospital gown was pointless, so I was covered only by sheets and blankets. When Mr. Lerda came to my doorway, my Mom came close to cover my chest. Not concerned that my math teacher was before me, I quickly threw the covers off and stated I was hot. She tried to cover me again, and I continued to push the covers away. The only thing that mattered was that I was hot and did not want covers on me. I had no awareness of my modesty and the appropriateness in front of my high school math teacher. I acknowledge that the sentiments of the situation were sad and disheartening, but in my modesty, I remained slightly embarrassed in the after-knowing of my actions. There was a mindful disregard of emotion when I came face to face with him again many months later when I was in a much more coherent state. He likely thought I didn't remember. Little did I know at that moment that I was going to have to disregard every ounce of modesty in the months ahead.

Mr. Lerda brought me a birthday gift. It was a gift from the heart. He created a Birthday Math Test titled n^{th} Birthday Test. It contained six math problems that had to be solved for the value on n. Since it was my seventeenth birthday, the value of n for each equation was equal to seventeen. It was the perfect gift from him as my math teacher and was a math test that could not compute the measure of gratitude held for the compassionate gesture.

Francoise, our maid, was not allowed in my room either. As with my math teacher, we visited from a distance. What I remember most about the visit from Francoise was the love and compassion she brought with her. I saw it and felt it radiate from the doorway straight to me. She was a sweet woman from Nigeria that only spoke French. She stood in the doorway in tears, trying to smile while holding a gift. It was a silver pen and pencil set. She didn't have a lot of money, which made the gesture even more thoughtful. And although it would be months before I could use them, the gesture of her kindness was so much more meaningful to me than the gift itself.

The next set of visitors created one of the most vivid images that remain in my mind. The images are as clear and vivid almost thirty years later and have the potential to last forever. I could not see my visitor's faces, only their eyes over the brim of their face masks. Although I instantly knew who they were, I don't recall looking into their eyes. I hardly remember anything, but I do remember their hands. They were not wearing gloves, and their hands held mine. They stood at my bedside, side by side, as we all held hands. I laid in the hospital bed, still very critical and drugged, but stabilized. And they stood strong, courageous, and loving, beside me.

Julie was my closest and dearest friend. She was my pillar of strength. We did everything together. We shared laughter, tears, dreams, and fears. She was my teenage voice of reason. She was my stability when I felt lost. She was my best friend. I had many close friends while overseas, and they all hold a very special space in my heart, but around the time of my illness, Julie was the one that new the most evolved version of myself. She was the only one that I felt knew me. And there she was, without fail, there for me when I needed her most.

Ahmad was my boyfriend. This relationship remains very dear to me. We originally met when I first arrived at ISB three years prior. Within a few months of our meeting, he became my first boyfriend in this life. He was sweet, kind, and funny, and we enjoyed the simplicity of having a good time. We both played sports and shared the same large circle of friends. We all enjoyed making each other laugh, hanging out, and experiencing a sense of belonging.

Seven months later, our relationship was interrupted by his family's relocation to Texas. Upon his return two years later, we rekindled our relationship and had enjoyed five months of meeting the new, improved versions of each other. We were very much in young love. Then everything changed. I cannot recall the last day I saw him before I got sick. I am sure it was Monday at school when I wasn't feeling well. But there he was. The first moment the hospital allowed it, he was at my bedside, holding my hand while I fought for my life. He was there and loved me in the worse state of my existence. We were so young to have love burdened with such tragedy.

Julie and Ahmad were standing beside me, holding my hands together, on my 17th birthday, in my intensive care hospital room. Not the ideal party location but having my two best friends in my forbidden room meant everything to me. Given the images that remain in my mind, it is unimaginable for me when I ponder the images that may remain in their minds. For a long time, I was able to imagine what it must have been like for them. I knew what I saw when I looked at me and the horrid truth of my experiences. I used to wonder what images remained from those few short moments confined to the Intensive Care visiting hours. They had to see a disfigured physical body and to hear the voice of their drug-induced friend. They had to do that in the presence of me and my unawareness of my new reality.

The images that remain are sourced in the beautiful gift received that day. As we all held hands, I received a gift from Ahmad. He brought me an elegant, handcrafted picture frame and jewelry box set. It was a two-tone, dark, and blond wood, octagonal-shaped jewelry box, lined with a red velvet material, and a matching two-toned picture frame.

What captivated my eyes was the red velvet material that lined the jewelry box. It was so beautiful and radiant. I remember reaching to touch it, wanting to experience its softness. As I did, I discovered that I felt nothing. My hands were so damaged with hard and tight skin that I was unable to feel anything. I kept rubbing the red velvet as my mind processed the truth. I could not feel the softness. I remember being scared that I had lost the ability to feel. First, with my hands and later mindfully assessing how much I could feel within my body. I felt numb to everything.

9

Trauma that Morphined into Something Else

As my world went on within the confines of my hospital room, coupled with the high doses of morphine, I eventually began to hallucinate. Incorporating real experiences with my drug-induced mind seemed to bring laughter to those around me during the midst of a very tragic time. This is how my situation morphed into something more than just trauma.

I was told that almost every day that I had a different story or a different problem that I was navigating. Ironically, none of them were problems at all compared to my actual situation. Although sad and at times hard to comprehend, there were amusing events that I recall, with detailed precision, and are what I refer to as my morphine trips. There are several of them, some more humorous than others, but there are two that deeply impacted me. They came from a deep place within. A place I was unable to connect with during the time of their occurrence. It was as if the drugs disarmed my mind, and my heart was able to speak through these morphine trips. Speak my pain and sorrow and then left in the subconscious mind to be brought into awareness once my coherency returned for processing.

One day, my family made the usual trip to visit. They could only visit for the allotted 30 minutes, and I always managed to fill those minutes with heartache, or with a comical depiction of a morphine filled adventure, or both. One particular day, my Mom entered my room and approached the side of my bed. I started fussing at her the moment she walked into my room. I was complaining about the color of my shirt and how much I did not like it. It was a dark purple, almost black, and the material was stiff and very uncomfortable. I told her how much I hated it and that I wanted her to help me change into something different, more comfortable.

She would not do it.

I could not understand why she would not help me. All I wanted was a different shirt. I begged her to please help me change the hideous garment and aid in improving my comfort. I pleaded through tears for her to love me enough to change my shirt. It seemed pretty simple, but it was anything but simple.

The shirt I hated so much and wanted to change was not a shirt at all. The truth was that it was my skin. My skin was damaged beyond recognition. Hardened and completely discolored from the septicemia that had infiltrated my blood and engulfed my body. Unrecognizable even to my own eyes.

Unaware of the heaviness that rested upon my Mom's heart each day that she entered and left my hospital room, I poured my heart out to her in whichever means it exited my being, without a filter. Somedays, it was harsh and ugly, somedays it was vulnerable and sincere, and somedays it was distant and quiet. As with the first, the next encounter was in sadness and misunderstanding.

My Mom was entering my room, and I was steady fussing. But this time it was not directed at her, just towards her about what had been happening. I was feeling sad and lonely. I couldn't make sense of what was happening around me and I was frustrated. These were all feelings that would be expected given my situation. I had a lot to be sad, lonely, and frustrated about. My caring Mom patiently tried to get to the source of what had occurred. She knew it would be my version of my reality, but it was equally important because, for me, it was the only reality I knew.

I proceeded to tell her that I had made a friend and that she would visit me in my room. Surprised since non-family member visitors were not allowed, my Mom continued to listen. I further explained that I loved it when she would visit. She would listen to me talk about everything I was going through, and I felt like she really listened and understood.

My Mom couldn't understand why I would be so upset and frustrated when it sounded like a positive experience. She continued to engage in finding out more and even asked about her name. I expressed that the thing that upset me the most was that she would listen, and was a great listener, but never spoke a word. Never. Not one word. I couldn't understand why she would listen so intently and then never say anything. She did not even speak a greeting upon entering my room.

Through my sobs, I managed to tell my Mom that her name was Milka. My Mom thought that was an unusual name, but then again, we were in the Dutch-speaking communes in Belgium. Perhaps it was a mere mispronunciation. At this point, I started to get frustrated even more, but this time it was directed at my Mom. My Mom continued to ask questions about Milka. She wanted to know when Milka came to visit, what she did when she visited, and even wanted a description of what she looked like — so many questions. I felt like my Mom did not understand any of my sentiments. This was when my Mom realized I was on another drug-induced expression of my reality. It was a morphine trip.

As she desperately tried to reassess the situation and figure out how to navigate the experience with her drug-induced daughter, I finally pointed to the foot of my bed so my Mom would know where to look to find her. There she was. Milka was in my room. She had been there the whole time, doing what she did best, standing quietly, and listening.

As my Mom curiously looked around the room where she knew she stood alone, she quickly discovered that I was pointing to my IV pole at the end corner of my bed. During this time, I had four IV poles full of numerous medications – one at each corner of my bed. But this particular pole at the bottom right-hand corner of my bed contained a big bad of protein nutrients, which was my nourishment. The bag was clear and about the size of a piece of copy paper, and inside was a white-colored nutritional substance that was being fed to me intravenously.

The bag of nutrients was adorned with the numerous coiled IV bag tubings that hung from the top of the pole down to the waist-side of her IV pole body. Milka was beautiful in all her glory. Her milky white skin, her golden rubber locks of hair, and her straight, stern stature. All I wanted was for her to respond. I was just unable to understand in that moment that her inanimate being was incapable of doing such a thing. I interpret that moment much differently today now that I have integrated the totality of my experiences.

Even in the moments when I was describing Milka to my Mom, there was an elevated part of me that knew the truths. It felt as if I knew who and what Milka was, but the words, and the beliefs behind the words, were so much more powerful than the reality around me. I was as if I could not control the imagery and the words that formed within even though I knew neither were real. I was split during the moment and unable to integrate back into one, as I experienced existing within two spaces concurrently.

Milka will remain a friend for life, albeit only in the deep recesses of my mind. During that time and space, there wasn't much anyone could say to lighten my burdens. It was more about me being able to say what I needed to say in anger and fear. Milka allowed me to do that. She allowed me to be vulnerable without judgment or attempt to advise. Her silence is what healed my weeping heart and calmed my confused mind. Her silence allowed me to find my peace within. I am grateful that I had someone to talk to during that time, even if it was just an IV pole. It was Milka, and she meant everything.

10

Transferred for Treatment

The two-week period at the first hospital came to an end. The day after my 17th birthday, the medical team advised my parents there was nothing more they could do for me. They had stopped the infection and had stabilized me, and although there was still so much to be done, they did not have the means by which to treat me any further.

My skin was blackened and hard like rigid plastic. An estimated twenty-five percent of my body's surface was cracked, and in some places, still oozing with infection, yet the destruction went much deeper than the surface. They could not even believe I was still alive. They could not understand how I managed to survive through everything thus far.

It was identified that the only way for me to survive would be to debris the dead and infected tissue. This meant cutting off and getting rid of sixty percent on my body's muscle and skin mass. How would I recover from that? What did that even really mean? Were my organs dying too? How can someone live with only forty percent of their body? What kind of life would someone have? Time would tell.

The only chance of my survival would be to transfer to the civilian Burn Center within a Belgian military facility, Queen Astrid Military Hospital. The burn unit's Head Surgeon came to assess my situation at the first hospital, and he agreed to accept me for further treatment. I used to wonder what would have happened if he had declined. I would hope that there is not a decision-maker when it comes to life or death, yet only a commitment to try. Concurrently I must honor the truth in that everyone has choices.

My transfer was coordinated, which required a complete transition of treatment to a new care team. Arrangements were made, and I was transported to the Military Hospital by ambulance. Once I arrived, my existence became the focus of a repair team. Their goal was to repair my body before its brokenness killed me.

Along with my broken body, the new team received a letter from the prior hospital that relayed what they could from the two weeks prior. Once translated from French to English, my family too had a better understanding of what I had been through and what was still to come.

> **Dear Colleagues,**
>
> **Your patient has stayed in the Intensive Care Unit from March 31, 1993, to April 13, 1993, for severe meningococcemia.**

On March 30, 1993, the patient presented an influenza-like illness and she consulted her doctor for treatment on March 31st for aggravation of the influenza-like illness. She was immediately referred to the emergency department of the hospital, where the diagnosis of meningococcemia was made in the view of the flagrant appearance of purpura. The diagnosis was confirmed by hemocultures and vesicle puncture, all of which had meningococcal disease.

During the stay, the following problems have been identified:

1. Fulminant purpura with evolution towards cutaneous necrosis on the surface of approximately 25%, mainly at the level of the thighs and the buttocks but also at the level of the lateral face of the calves and the posterior face of the arms, necrosis also of the extremity of the index and middle finger on the left. The patient also presents primarily intermediate-level cutaneous lesions in the arms and legs for which the evolution is currently satisfactory but whose viability remains unresolved. There is currently no evidence of superinfection.
2. Over renal insufficiency characterized by hypoglycemia, hyponatremia, hypokalemia, and improved fluid lability by administration of Solu-Cortef. Synachten test should be done soon to assess the need for further treatment.
3. Major CVID (Common Variable Immunodeficiency) with D-dimer amounting up to 160,000, fibrinogen levels falling to 80 and platelets to 6,000. This CVID will be resolutive in 72 hours.

Heparin treatment will be tried at very low doses, but this will cause the platelets to fall again. Heparin will be discontinued and later low molecular weight heparin will be started to prevent secondary venous thrombosis.

4. Significant Rhabdomyolysis with CPK culminating at 20,000 and significant edema of the 2 calves without signs of extreme tension or vascular pain. It should be noted, however, that the patient will develop pain in the 2 external sciatic nerves, but Dr. Dereume, a vascular surgeon, confirmed that there was no need of fasciotomy in the absence of tension in the calf.

5. Fluctuating intellectual disorders, currently characterized by the difficulty to perform intellectual acts such as mathematical calculations. A non-contract cerebral CT scan was performed and showed no hemorrhage and there was no evidence of hydrocephalus. No necrosis could be demonstrated.

6. The patient had circulatory insufficiency. Initially it was characterized by a large vasoplegia requiring administration of significant fluid infusions and dopamine. After a few days, the patient developed a right-sided heart failure demonstrated at Swan-Ganz catheterization and also at cardiac unltrasonography. After administration of dobutamine and PGE1 and fluid restriction, a rapid improvement of the hemodynamic state was observed, all of which could be progressively sewn. The control ultrasound carried out on April 9th showed a normal right

ventricle, a slightly hypertrophic left ventricle with impaired contractility and slight dilation of the cavities. The appearance of the valvular is strictly normal, but a discreet tricuspid leak persists.
7. Acute renal insufficiency related to shock and Crush Syndrome and which is slowly resolutive.
8. Leukocytosis and inflammatory syndrome without presently no infectious center could be shown. It is likely that this inflammatory syndrome is related to the presence of necrotic wounds.
9. Iatrogenic right pneumothorax requiring pleural drainage for 48 hours.
10. Depression and tendency to agitation which is very quickly calmed by an important presence of the family or nursing staff.

The patient's current problem being that of necrotic wounds on a large body surface with paucity of donor sites, it was decided in agreement with Dr. Goldschmidt, plastic surgeon, to transfer the patient to the Intensive Care Service at the hospital of large burns and Dr. Vanderkelen will take care of this patent.

<u>Treatment at the exit:</u>

- Paranteral nutrition with 2000 Kcal. And 9.5 g of nitrogen
- Maintenance infusion consisting of 1 L of saline and KC1 supply adapted to the ionogram
- Zantac 1 mg / H in continuous IV

- Solu-Cortef 100 mg daily IV
- Lexotan 1.5 mg in the morning and in the afternoon and 3 mg in the evening
- Lasix 2 x 40 mg daily IV
- Clexane 20 mg subcutaneously daily
- Normal rate and liquid contributions limited to 2000 cc

By remaining at your disposal for any additional information, please accept, Dear Colleague, our deepest sentiments.

Cordially signed by two tending physicians.

Once the team was situated with my arrival, I was brought into the operating room for a full assessment. Afterward, the head surgeon came out to meet with my parents. He started telling them in French, that he would have to amputate both of my legs at the waist. He proceeded to say to them that he had inserted a scapula straight through both calves, all the way to the bone, and there was no blood. All of the tissue in my legs was dead.

My Dad then had to translate this to English for my Mom. He had to become the one to tell the news to my Mom. He had to repeat what the surgeon had said while concurrently trying to process the information himself, as my Dad. Her immediate response was NO! She said, "Absolutely Not!" She told them that one day she would have to explain to me why she let them amputate my legs, and she better have a damn good reason. She demanded a second opinion. She demanded a damn good reason.

I started dancing when I was four years old, took gymnastics, played multiple sports every year, skied, and I was running for hours every day. I was the most athletic of everyone in our family. She couldn't bear the thought of having to tell me that she let them remove my legs. She knew how much peace and joy I got from my legs, especially from running and dancing.

The head surgeon finally agreed to a second opinion. He decided that he wanted to seek the advice of his mentor and have him review my case for a recommendation. The head surgeon's mentor was the Head of the American Burn Association and was considered an ideal candidate for the needed expertise.

Once his employer approved the financing for the second opinion, my Dad was persistent in his efforts to contact the doctor that may yield a different life outcome for me. He eventually learned that the doctor was on a special project in South Africa and was temporarily out of touch. Desperate to get a credible second opinion, my Dad tried to find someone, anyone that would be qualified. Someone would surely see hope for my legs.

My Dad eventually called upon one of his doctors, an orthopedist. This doctor had previously treated a torn ligament that had rolled up and formed a bump on my Dad's thigh. My Dad felt comfortable discussing my case with him, given his area of specialty and the dire straits of my condition.

After the consult with my Dad, the orthopedist had one recommendation to give the head surgeon at the burn unit. His only advice was for him to think of me as his daughter. He acknowledged the magnitude of the situation and honored the truth in the very unpredictable outcomes. He empathized with the hard decision of taking the risk while holding the commitment, sworn to by oath, to protect and heal the sick to the best of their ability. Since it was known the surgeon had a daughter close in age, he was challenged to fight for me as he would for his daughter if she was in my situation. It was the only thing that could ground the hope amidst the grave uncertainties.

In the end, all I know is that the head surgeon agreed. He made a choice. He chose to care for me as if I were his daughter. He knew he would risk everything for her. He would risk gangrene and death to save her legs. He would risk losing her while fighting for the very parts she loved most about herself. He agreed to take the same risk on me. He decided to fight for my legs. He chose to fight for me. Unbeknown to him, when he chose to fight for me, he was fighting for all me - even the silent and deep connection that my soul holds within the forever changed body he was saving.

11

The debrideMEnt Process

Every day while in the intensive care unit, the head surgeon chose to fight with, and beyond medical expertise to save me. Every part of me. He chose, despite knowing the challenges before him and his team. Collectively, they all knew that treating me like a burn patient was the best chance for survival, but the actual work had to begin. Since it was their area of specialty, they also knew that it would be an excruciating and very traumatic process.

Although contingent on my responses, the medical team had to develop a plan to navigate the very fragile and life-threatening process. The plan was to remove sixty percent of my body's muscle and tissue mass through a debridement process, which is simply the removal of dead tissue. The intention was to complete the process in one operation. The remaining forty percent of unaffected skin would then be used to repair my body. Doctors planned to remove the dead parts of me and then use my alive parts to mend me back into wholeness.

This would leave me open and exposed. I would be a female, teenage body-sized open wound. If it were not from where my tissue was removed, it would be from my abdomen and back that became donor sites. The doctors were highly concerned about the intensity of the pain that I was about to endure. They knew that it was a medical marvel that I was still alive. They also knew that if I had not died already from the illnesses themselves, my fragile body, coupled with the physical pain, would likely not survive the treatment process. To increase my chances of survival, the decision was made to put me in a medically induced coma. Everyone prepared for the five and a half week medical coma, medical teams and family alike, while I was at the mercy of the choices of others.

To protect my conscious mind from the trauma, and all that follows from the myriad of physiological processes it triggers, the medical team guided me into a coma. It was the same process that we undergo for any surgery. The only difference is that it lasted five weeks. This alone was an extremely rare duration for a medically induced coma. But I had a team that had chosen to fight for me, and this is how they could do that.

I was pumped with barbiturates for five weeks to keep me in a deep state of unconsciousness while relying on a ventilator to keep me alive, again. Five weeks of my life unknown. Five weeks of my life a mystery. Five weeks of my life when a team of medical professionals worked non-stop while monitoring, repairing, cleaning, treating, and taking care of my every need. Five weeks of family, friends, and Global Prayer Warriors watching, praying, and waiting in anticipation, and from afar.

The standard medical practice is to cut and remove all tissue until you get to pink, healthy tissue. The doctor's assessment had already revealed that there was no healthy tissue in my calves. It was all dead and gray. This meant that when they were debriding, there would be no pink tissue. They couldn't remove everything down to the bone. Or could they? They had to leave something. Didn't they? If they removed everything but bone, wouldn't that make amputation the only option? They had already set aside amputation while knowing the absence of healthy tissue. They had a plan they were relying upon would work.

Once the medical team began the debridement process, while in the coma, I laid naked on an operating table while numerous doctors cut off and removed the dead parts of my body with a scapula. They began in my right thigh, and once they penetrated the surface, a mass infection was revealed as it spewed from my leg. The doctors were forced to continue through the amazement of how I was still alive. The infection they had exposed alone should have killed me. Not to mention all the other events that I managed to fight through. The doctors debrided all that they could from my arms and legs and wrapped my body in cadaver skin until they were ready to begin the next phase, the skin grafting.

That's right, take that in for a moment. I was wrapped in cadaver skin. That is skin removed from a deceased being. How many people have ever needed to be covered in the skin from a deceased body for survival and live to tell the story? My heart fills with heaviness when the thought comes to awareness. The material idea of it is frightful, scary, disgusting, and makes my unscarred skin crawl. Yet the harmonious earthly energy and the resounding balance within my life journey overpowers, and I have nothing but a profound and humbling sense of gratitude.

It was clear that leaving gray tissue was part of the intention behind the head surgeon's commitment to the fight for my legs. Contrary to what is generally practiced, his team did not remove all the dead tissue. They left gray tissue and remained optimistic that the treatment plan would prevail. The team trusted that my tissue, all remaining tissue, including the gray tissue, would rejuvenate and return to a healthy state, and do so before gangrene could set in.

The way the head surgeon intended to do this was for me to receive hyperbaric oxygen therapy twice a day for up to five hours. This was how the medical team maximized the rejuvenation process of the already dead tissue; the same tissue that had to heal before receiving a graft. It would also expedite the healing of the donor sites between surgeries since they needed to occur as frequently as possible. There was a lot of me to cover.

Hyperbaric therapy enhances the body's natural healing process through the inhalation of 100% oxygen. In my situation, it was from within a full-body chamber. Unconscious and on a ventilator, I rested up to five hours a day in the hyperbaric chamber. My body was one big open wound. There were a lot of entry points for saturation. The hope was that the oxygenation would penetrate, saturate, and stimulate growth within each cell, and have life restored into my body. Even if it only boosted a small percentage of growth, it was that much more than I had. Every cell mattered. Somehow, my tissue had to grow and cover my body again. Somehow this had to work. Somehow it would.

12

Glass Windows of Hope

My limbs were the areas impacted the most: my arms, my legs, and my butt. The skin on my torso remained intact and had somehow recovered from the toughened textures from the septic infection. It was my arms, legs, and butt that remained damaged from the rigid, plastic-like condition. I felt fortunate that my face remained unscathed. There is one spot about the diameter of a sweet pea, above my left cheekbone, where a tiny scar remains. This scar would become very insignificant when compared to the physical scars that, in time, would adorn my body.

Due to the mysterious stopping point of the damaged skin, outlining the position where my limbs attached to my torso, my torso became the optimal donor sight for all the skin used to mend my body. While in the drug-induced coma, they would bring me to the operating room, take skin from my back and abdomen, and graft it to as many places as they could over my open wound body. They returned me to the sand bed in my isolation room, took care of every survival need until shuffled around again for the next repair.

The medical team waited for my back and abdomen to heal enough with a thin layer of skin regrown, and then they would start the process again. There was a lot of my body that needed covering. There was a lot of me that was opened and exposed. Just as quickly as I healed from the surgery to take the skin, they were wheeling me back in to do it again. And again. And again. It continued until my body was covered in my skin once again.

During this time of treatment, I was in strict isolation. I laid seemingly asleep, in a sand bed designed to relieve pressure points, for five weeks while my body healed. There were betadine antiseptic solution trays all over my room to further sterilize the space. Only the medical staff were allowed in my room. My family could not even enter beyond the intensive care unit doors. Instead, they could only look at me through a glass window that lined one side of my room. And this only occurred when it was visiting hours, and the nurse would open the blinds. When permitted, they stood gazing through the glass window with the hope that I would make it through another night.

There were also daily baths. I wasn't aware of the process until after I was awake, but it was the same process during the five weeks. Four nurses would carefully unwrap my fragile body, clean and disinfect every inch of me, carefully re-wrap me like a mummy and return me to my sand bed. During the baths, when I was completely unconscious, I was told that staff would speak to me in French, making requests to roll to one side, and I would respond in action. How is that even possible? To be saturated with pharmaceuticals, unconscious, on a ventilator and still respond in action? My life journey is evidence that anything is possible.

This took place for five weeks: surgeries, daily baths, bandage changing, hyperbaric chambers, glass windows, and hope. My family and friends would look through the glass windows and hold hope that I would come out of the coma; hope that this process would not kill me; hope that I would somehow, someday, be able to recover from all this.

The five weeks of debridement and skin grafting had come to an end. During the five weeks, there were many moments of uncertainty, yet in the presence of uncertainty remained a growing sense of hope. With every passing day, every successful surgery, every medical update, and every day I survived, there was an expansion of hope. The more I fought, the more hope grew within everyone around me. Everyone's sense of hope fueled the energy behind my Global Prayer Warriors, eventually evidenced in the continued decrease in the likelihood of amputation.

Although there were several more skin graft surgeries that I would need, it was time to wake me up. It was time to stop the medication, take me off the ventilator, and bring me back to conscious awareness. It was time for me to face my new reality after eight weeks of oblivion. It was time to meet the new me.

When I woke up from the coma and learned the story behind the scenes of the hospital room, it felt like the parts of me, lost on the operating table, were the same parts that created space for the potentiality of creation; the creation of a new, very different life for me. It was hard to remain sad when miracles continued to unfold towards the best possible outcome given the circumstances. The silent discomfort came from existing among the evolving sense of loss while concurrently feeling joy as I witnessed growth in its place. My being had been stripped to its bare essence and presented with a choice. To live or to die. It was clear that I kept choosing to live, so it was more about the quality of life I would be willing to accept for myself. It was about the choices I would make in honor of the parts of me left behind. And just as importantly, the parts of me that remained.

The prognosis started with full amputation of both legs at the waist. As time passed and my body continued to heal in ways that extended beyond the expertise of modern medicine, the doctors began to believe that anything was possible. The marvel continued to incrementally unfold until they were able to avoid any amputations of either leg. My legs. I was able to keep my legs.

Dr. Vanderkelen did it! He fought to save my legs, and he did it!

We did it!

I did it!

13

Cultivating a Commitment

The most important lesson my parents taught me in my youth was that life is about choices. There is abundant truth in this lesson. The choices I had to make were a matter of life or death. I had to choose between faith and fear. Love and hate. Joy and sadness. Hope and despair. Beginning and end. Life and death. I had to make these choices within all parts of me, and daily.

We always had choices growing up. Those choices always came with consequences. I had experimented with this truth in my own way, but this time was different. The choices I had to make had very real consequences. Every single choice held consequences, intentional and unintentional alike, all which held the infinite potential to change every aspect of my life. As it always does yet every choice felt critical to my continued survival. It felt so serious for my youthful spirit. It was serious. My life depended on it.

First and for most within my body, but also within the psychological, emotional, and spiritual parts of me - body, mind, heart, and soul. I never felt ill-prepared to make such critical decisions, yet I recall a sense of sadness that it was at such a young age and through such life-altering ways. I would sit quietly with the mystery of the great universal power by acknowledging the truth of my own, which I knew would require something equally powerful and life-altering to experience a balance to the forces I felt continuously up against.

Early on, I remember feeling fortunate that some of my prior life choices held serious consequences. I felt somewhat prepped for what I was enduring and what was yet to come. It felt in rhythm and could feel every aspect of me experience a fast-tracked maturity, especially into a mental state capable of processing my reality. It was indeed overwhelming on all levels. I found that the simplest element in the complexity of it all was a single choice. A single choice held the potential to change everything.

Making choices with clear intention became instrumental in my mindset while the rest of me tried to sort through the truths within every experience. It took over twenty-five years for it to become grounded into the truths of my reality. However, during my illness, my beliefs and mindful focus had everything to do with strength of body and the physical experience, and nothing to do with strength of heart and soul in the spiritual experience.

The lessons my parents taught in my youth echoed within as they encouraged me, with great emphasis, that it was my choice to believe in whatever it was at the source of my beliefs. They told me to pay no mind to the opinions of others. They reiterated that my beliefs were all that mattered, and I should focus on those intently.

At the time, all I could come up with was infinite potentiality. I believed that there were infinite possible outcomes in the very new reality I was forced to navigate. Anything could happen. Anything did happen, and it happened to me. I thought surely the unthinkable could happen again.

Their encouragement in self-belief was likely rooted more in their own religious experiences and accompanying prayers that I would find solace in God. I had never been challenged to believe so deeply and intimately in something. Anything. I had been spoon-fed religious beliefs up to our move overseas and then co-existed and loved within over sixty religions and belief systems, all by the age of thirteen. I was bewildered, with a new unexpected and confusing sense of betrayal, regarding my faith, beliefs, and truth in God. A betrayal by sixty-one Gods.

Nevertheless, the message I heard was to believe in myself. To me, that meant to follow where I was led, for I did believe in a greater power that would guide the way since I had apparently been guided thus far. I did not know the source of this mystical force, but I knew of its existence. It felt as though I was being challenged to believe in myself, not a God.

By this point, I held a stronger belief that none of those concepts had protected me, and somewhat disheartened by the abundance of Gods around the world that would let it be so. Knowing I needed to believe in something, and since the situation was centered around my physical body, choosing to believe in myself, primarily in body and mind, felt most natural.

In truth, I always found it difficult to disconnect from myself in a way to believe in something outside of me. Somehow, I would have to figure out a way to recover and heal. I chose to trust in me and allow my beliefs to guide my choices. My life depended on me. As I focused on healing my physical body and the lessons the experiences were teaching.

I focused on physical recovery and believed that anything is possible. I knew in time that me and my God would exchange words about it all. Even I knew that it was most definitely not the time for words. There was only time and space for strength of character, courage for self, and a dream of love to give me hope.

Throughout my youth my parents also taught me that in every outcome, there is always something positive to gain. Always. Something. There is always a positive consequence, and finding it is merely a matter of perspective. This has proven to hold true, even in the darkest moments of despair, when a desire, need, or even a prayer goes seemingly unfulfilled. There is a message within them all. When one door closes, another door opens was a gentle reminder that often echoed while siphoning my reality through the very truths trying to gain balance.

I held everything closely and privately as I chose to search for joy in everything. Even within the smallest and darkest of spaces. All I needed was one tiny perspective of positivity. That was all it took. Just one, and size was irrelevant, albeit the bigger the better for that meant more joy. A perceived positive is still a positive, and I was determined to celebrate them with gratitude. My devotion to the positives was often driven by the immense negativity and uncertainty around me, mainly when presumed my ears could not hear. I heard. I heard all of it. More-so my heart heard and felt it. Acutely hearing and further quieting the external noise became a practiced skill acquired.

Celebrating the positives, in turn, kept my hope alive. Hope had to be present if I were going to believe I would get through the unbeknown path before me. It became the purpose of each day. The daily quest to find the positives. To stay in joy as much as possible, which was difficult because there was nothing joyous about my reality. Except for maybe that I was alive. I admittedly already began to wonder if it was worth it. My deep desire to be aware of the positives, even in the seemingly insignificant moments, over time, developed into a core trait of my personality — sometimes perceived as the overzealous optimist or the lofty, irrational dreamer.

With the implications of a choice, I could find the positives that would then yield joy which gave me hope. It was a cycle that deepened in resonance with another message from my Mom during my early teenage years abroad. Our relationship had already become jaded by the time I became ill. I cannot even remember the source of our disagreements. What I do remember is that it would end with me getting frustrated with her calmness, firmness, and patience. In hindsight, it was the most absurd thing. Who gets angry at love and patience?

I did. As a young teenage girl who did not understand unconditional love. I would eventually get so frustrated and tell her how angry she would make me. When I raged in my juvenile egoism, she always responded the same. She would react to my nonsense in a calm and patient voice, and state that nobody can make me feel anything I do not want to feel, including her.

My Mom was so resounding and graceful in her way of teaching me these fundamental lessons. My Dad too. They were lessons that would not fully develop into my character until much later in life, however, with the rudimentary understanding of finding positives and having emotional control, I was able to more fully nurture that I could control my experiences through the choices I make. I found comfort in knowing that I had control over how I was going to let the experience make me feel. I was determined to live and be happy. The dream was to be extraordinary. Even so, this was a tremendous act of faith from within.

At times it felt like my mind had the most challenging journey of recovery to be endured, keeping my whole state of existence in check and at bay, protected and safe, nurtured and loved, healthy, and strong. My mind was unavoidably put to the ultimate challenge during my illness, and beyond. Mind over matter became a very real exercise.

It was the same jargon that we hear all the time about choices. But everything shifted, and everything was vastly different. The situation was real. My life depended on my ability to transform the same overused words into more than just words being spoken, or thoughts and reflections. The time was before me, and it was so very real. I had to trust that the choices I was making were the ones that would heal me. I often doubted my own readiness. Life did not.

In the moment of making critical choices, there are always very real consequences, good or bad, good and bad. It is all relative and a matter of perspective. It was up to me to choose wisely so that the consequences were perceived as pleasantly as possible by me, lovely, and enjoyable even. The only way I knew how to do that was to align my choices with my beliefs.

I also deeply believed that this Greater Power was being funneled to me through the Global Wave of Healing Energy that was continuously gaining quiet momentum. I always felt it, but never knew I could, nor how to connect more fully to it. The rest is up to me. It was the wonderment of the unknown, with a faith more profound than I even realized that cultivated the commitment to believe in something greater than me yet inside of me.

I could feel that force was greater than humanity. Greater than the horrific and hasty change in the reality I was living. Even though I did not know, nor believe in anything about the force behind my survival, I knew that it existed, and did so in harmony with the purest, and most amazing versions of life. My new life had to be part of that beauty. It had to be. I needed to focus on creating the best version of self that could possibly come from the horrific truths I continued to learn about my body.

I was given some pretty tough armor going into the intense experience. With these lessons embedded into my being, it felt natural. It felt easy. Everything seemed relatively clear among the chaos. There was only one choice to make - to live and move on. I was in control of my emotions, and I would not, could not, allow myself to feel something that I did not want to feel. I had to believe in myself, and there would be good in everything that happens. Most of all, the outcome of all those begin with a choice in each breath. These would become my anchors throughout my recovery.

The style and manner in which these lessons were tried and tested can never fully be explained, but at the end of the day, no matter how hard, no matter how painful, no matter how unfortunate it all was, I had to choose to live. I had to find a way to be happy. I had to always believe in all good things to come. And always, always celebrate successes. In every moment. I was already living. Now it was making the most out of every situation. Every unbelievable, heart-wrenching situation that challenged my will, challenged my determination, challenged my strength to continue.

Somehow, someway, I knew I had to remain determined to prevail. I am not even sure I know where or how I found the inner strength to hold such perseverance. Nor the wisdom to believe that I would prevail. Regardless of the mindful bewilderment, I honor that I was able to cultivate the commitment within my core to always to honor the choice to live.

Uncertain, scared, and alone, I was ready to face the journey. I did not like it one bit, but I trusted that I was as ready as I could possibly be. I had to be ready. The timing was one choice I did not have, but my response was. I had to trust that my responses would come from the readiness within, and I deeply trusted that I would be ready and would prevail over anything, and everything, that was before me. It felt like I was my only hope.

14

Washed Away

The main event of my day was the bath. I hated the bath. During the first five weeks of the bath, I was unconscious. Once I was awake, they would medicate me prior to the process beginning. The intention was to minimize the pain and to relax me, but I know those actions protected me from much more than just the physical pain.

Every day was the same in the intensive care unit. They would wake me up at around four-thirty every morning to start the almost four-hour bath and bandage changing process. Then I would sleep because it was so draining, followed by a restricted afternoon visit with family. I received a lot of visits from doctors and nurses taking vitals, resetting machines, changing medications, administering medications, and assessing anything and everything that needed attention.

In the beginning, my body was so fragile that they had to use a gurney suspended from a crane stand to weigh and transport me to the bath. They would roll me from one side, and then to the other side in my bed, positioning one vertical half of the gurney underneath me at a time, then securing them together. It was incredibly painful because, in the process, they had to peel off the metallic bed pad stuck to my back. It protected the surgically stitched gauze pads that covered my back like a jigsaw puzzle while the skin donor sights healed. I was severely traumatized by this process. Although I never associated it as stress from the trauma, the memory of pain, and vivid imagery replayed in my mind for several years that followed.

Only once I was separated from my bed, and on the gurney, I was securely strapped, lifted, weighed, and then rolled down the hall to the bath. The actual bath process took about two and a half hours, but there was a lot of pre and post work that was required. It was quite an extensive process to endure every day.

It was not like an ordinary bath. It was for burn patients. It meant unwrapping, cleaning, sometimes even scrubbing skin grafted tissue and donor site areas, medicating and re-wrapping ninety percent of my body. The bathtub itself was a chest-high, giant-sized stainless-steel tub with a suspended gurney in the middle where the patient laid. It had handrails and was wide enough to lay down on one's back, enough room to roll on one's side, and plenty of room near the feet. In the center of the tub underneath the gurney were faucets with three different hoses that were used - sterilized water, a medicated cleanser, and a medicated rinse. They had a pink color, and even though I cannot describe the smell, I know if I were to smell it, I would recognize it right away.

There were always at least four people giving the bath. Usually, three were nurses, and one was a physical therapist who would work in exercises to minimize muscle atrophy while the others bathed me. They would talk to me and tell me stories, sometimes in English, and sometimes in French. They tried to keep my attention anywhere and everywhere, except right there.

Once the crane gurney positioned me on the bathtub gurney and removed, the four aids removed every mummy-like bandage, peeled away every gauze pad stuck to my wounds, cleaned every inch of my body, and wrapped my entire body back up, hidden. The only time my body was fully exposed and could breathe air was during the bath. It was a long and excruciating process. At times it was so painful I would beg them all the way to the bathing room to just let me skip the bath for one day. Just one day. Please!

In desperation, one day, I asked the nurse if she would call my Dad before the bath. At first, she didn't know why I wanted to call him. She was very resistant and convinced that my Dad was not up that early. He probably wasn't. I knew he got up early, but I also knew that it was not at four-thirty in the morning. She finally agreed, dialed the phone, and held it by my ear since I could not bend my arms to hold the phone myself. My Dad answered. After saying good morning, he asked what was going on. I told him that it was bath time and that I was calling to get him to say to the nurse that it was ok to skip the bath, just for that one day. They would not listen to me, so I thought by calling him, he could tell them.

He sadly had to tell me that he could not do that. Part of my treatment plan was the daily bath, and I really had to do it to get better. I understood that, but it just felt like it was too much sometimes. As if my essence was being washed away with every bath. I cried and pleaded for just a small break, just one day to take a break from it all. It was so incredibly painful and uncomfortable on so many levels. I was a vulnerable seventeen-year-old girl.

I called my Dad many mornings, and they always ended the same. I called knowing that I had to do it and I would only be getting the needed support and encouragement from my Dad, hearing him believe that I could do it, and it would be ok. We would hang up, and I would go to the bath believing I could do it yet crying the whole way there.

Other than the brutal reality of my physical condition, one of the things I remember most about these daily baths was that every nurse and physical therapist was so kind and gentle. I could only see their eyes. They dressed from head to toe in sterile garments. The only skin I could see was the vertical strip across the face that contained their eyes, lined by the edges of the face mask and hat. While their hands unwrapped my body, all I could see were their eyes. I told of the importance of one's eyes, but this was when eye contact had the most significant impact on my journey.

They would stare into my eyes as my tears silently fell as they tended to my fragile body. Their eyes, locked onto mine, looked tired, sad, and empathetic yet fueled me with strength. I never thought that they were tired, sad, and empathetic for me, although likely for me too. I saw it more because of the work that they performed so selflessly, helping others in such tremendous pain and need.

They had seen trauma. They had healed trauma. They had lost to trauma. When they saw me raw and exposed in the bath, they knew the degree of what was before them. They knew what I was up against even though I did not. Along with the doctors and other medical professionals, they too, could not believe that I was still alive.

Since the bath was required every day, and I could never get out of it, I was forced to reconcile with the trauma. The strength and love I saw reflected in the eyes of the nurses who cleaned me, ultimately gave me the courage to face my truths. With compassion in their eyes and love in their touch, many days, I was consoled while I cried naked and exposed. It felt like they were holding me is their strength while I found my own as tears fell over the loss of my body. Every part of me cried as I met myself on the gurney. I cried over what was left of my body, and I cried over what was lost of my body and cried for the parts of me that still had to process the experience that created my new body. I knew there would be many days ahead when I would have to learn my new body.

The bath forced me to see myself. I was forced to see the trauma. I was forced to feel the trauma. I was forced to embrace it for all that it was. For the horrific and scary truth that it was. I would look at my naked body on the bathtub gurney and see that there was hardly anything remaining of my physically fit body and strong muscles. All I could see where legs with so much muscle and tissue loss that the shin bones were exposed. Raw skin and bare bones. Literally.

Were these really my legs? I could see how everyone would think I would have a poor quality of life, or that I may not ever walk again. I was beginning to understand why they may have thought the way they did. How was my body going to walk again when it looked like this? How were the bones on my shins going to get covered back up? What else did this mean? Nobody knew, and we all had to take every day as it came. One day at a time. For me, it felt like one breath at a time. During the bath, it felt like one bandage at a time.

It was the truth of my reality. It was the truth behind the mummy-like bandages that hardly anyone saw, but the nurses who bathed me and me. It was the truth that my body would never be the same, and there was nothing that could be done to reverse my circumstances. It was the truth that what I saw before me was indeed my truth. It was my truth that highlighted how critical it was to make choices that aligned with my commitment. I had to choose to remain committed to a belief in a sacred plan much greater than me. I held doubt, but I had to commit anyway.

With every sense of self that was washed away in the bath, a deeper sense of faith anchored within my core. The more I lost, the more faith I needed. Although ridden with fear and doubt, I knew staying committed to the belief that my body would heal, all of me - body, mind, heart, and soul. I believed that if I remained committed then the greater plan would be revealed in time. I knew in those moments that my life would become a journey of learning the greater purpose. To be at peace with my suffering was the deepest of my prayers.

15

Intentionally Defective

Although several impactful events transpired while I was in intensive care within the burn unit, it was within the days of complete isolation that paved the way for the unwavering determination and focus throughout my plight. Within the two months after I awoke from the coma, and before I transferred out of the intensive care unit, there was a lot of alone time. A lot.

I can vaguely recall my Mom and Dad, telling me what the doctors would say about my future. That I would never walk again, I may be in a wheelchair, and there was still the possibility of amputation if the skin grafts didn't heal as expected. Every time they would tell me what the doctor's claimed about my future limitations, all I would say was, "oh...I am going to walk again!"

My Dad encouraged me to not worry about what others thought, and if I believed I would walk again, then I would walk again. He was not even sure if I would walk again, but he knew I needed to believe that I would, even if the outcome was different. He knew it would motivate me to do everything I needed to do as if it would happen.

During my many hours alone, I remember it turning into a game in my mind. I would say it to nurses, doctors, technicians alike, anyone, and everyone who entered my room as if part of the greeting. At first, it was mainly to see how they would respond, how nervous they were in their response, how confident they were in the treatment plan, and how supportive they were in me and my statement.

I would tell everyone who came into my room...

"You know...I am going to walk again!"

Although hopeful that I would hear encouraging and optimistic words in response, I would only hear their broken English make spirit breaking statements such as:

I don't think so. Your legs have been very traumatized.

No, baby, you will never walk again.

I am not sure; you will need to discuss that with the doctor.

It may not work out that way, but we certainly hope for the best.

That's good that you think that, but I doubt it will happen.

And my response was always the same,

"I was not asking you; I was telling you. I am going to walk again."

I would usually get a short response back coupled with a look of despair or pity for me, for believing in something they had already deemed as impossible. They turned out to be a tough crowd. But that did not stop me. I was determined to let everyone know my intentions. Despite receiving laughter, doubt, disbelief, and extreme uncertainty, I stayed committed to the belief that I would walk again. Everything continued to unfold as though it were possible. Doctors held the belief that chances were slim, and I held the belief that anything was possible. I was determined to give my recovery everything I had. It became the focus. It became my everything. Learning how to walk again became the focal point of my thoughts and visions. It had to happen.

Every day was the same thing, and every day I kept improving. The skin graphs were attaching and forming new skin, the donor sites were healing, and things were looking promising. Then one day, the doctor tells my parents that he was confused about something. He explained that he was unsure as to why my right foot was still alive since they had to remove so much muscle, and thereby exposing bone on my right leg. He had expected my foot to die not long after the debridement operation because it would have no longer received the blood supply from the artery lost in the front of my shin during the process. It did not make sense to him when compared to his experiences and expertise.

To figure out what was going on, I was scheduled for an arteriogram test at another hospital. On the day of the test, I was transported by ambulance to the other facility, and they conducted the test. An arteriogram is an imaging test that uses x-ray and a special dye to see the insides of arteries. They wanted to see what was happening in my right leg and what was feeding my right foot, keeping it alive. After completing the test, they uncovered another astounding unexplainable truth within my body.

The main artery in my right leg was not where it was supposed to be. The anterior tibial artery commonly runs in the front of the shin to the foot. It is what supplies blood to the foot. The arteriogram revealed that my left leg was as expected, and the artery was in the front of my shin where it expected. However, my right leg revealed that at birth, my foot feeding artery grew down the backside of my leg and not the front, where I had lost so much tissue and muscle mass. So, in truth, when the doctor thought he was cutting out the major artery, he was not. The dead tissue and lack of blood flow must have camouflaged his knowledge. Instead, my artery remained intact on the backside of my leg, keeping my foot alive. Everyone was astonished by this finding.

This birth defect was the very thing saving my foot. It was as if my leg was intentionally defective. It was another opportunity to celebrate a miracle. Everyone was amazed, but I do not remember experiencing the same great sense of surprise and fascination that everyone else seemed to have. Their reactions gave a sense that miracles do not happen this frequently in one event for one person. It was clearly happening to me.

For me, I slowly realized that for some unbeknown reason, I was a living miracle, a living expression of divine intervention and Divine Intention. I did not feel divine. In fact, I felt everything but divine. In retrospect, I did not feel divine because divinity is not a feeling. It is a state of being. All I knew was that I always carried a hint of unexpected impossibilities in my spirit, and I expected nothing less since my focus was on walking. I needed MY legs and feet to walk.

It appeared everything was just as it needed to be; strangely perfect amongst the tragic truth I was living.

16

Truth Beyond the Pain

There was an unavoidable routine that I spent many heart and soul hours practicing during the days alone in the intensive care unit. The time and space allowed me to see my body as a machine, the mechanical system of sub-systems that it is. In the indescribable state of my being, I rested in the space detached from my body as I experienced what happened to it. There was an unexplainable comfort found in the truths uncovered within as I listened to my body and the voice within that guided me through.

During the healing process after the coma, I became very aware of my state of existence, especially my body, and the sensations felt throughout. This sense of awareness is the space of my existence that became profoundly present from the onset of the illness. It is the part of me that was present during the initial weeks when experiencing the morphine trips. It is the same awareness that responded in action even when unconscious and on a ventilator. It is the same sensations that only seemed to evolve and expand throughout my recovery and beyond.

I never saw it in the light that I see it now as a state of soul detachment. Instead, I saw it as a heightened internal awareness to overcompensate for the vast loss of sensation to the external world around me. All I knew to do was harness the awareness into my recovery. I was in an extensive amount of pain, yet everything about my state of existence was serene. I may have been sad, scared, and in pain, but deep within, I believed I would be ok. I believed my strength of body and mind would make the rest of it ok. I prayed so very deeply that I would be right.

When I gained control over the request for pain medication, I pushed the limits of my physical tolerance. Mainly, my tolerance for pain. I did not like all the medication being pumped into my body. I could feel the molecular changes it was causing within. I felt the medicine as it entered the IV and began to circulate throughout my body. I felt the warmth that blanketed my body to dissipate the pain. I felt the way it altered my mind and accompanying thoughts. I felt the pain disappear and then resurface over time. It made me aware of the most painful areas. It made me aware of how long the pain medication lasted. It made me aware of my tolerance. Not just for pain, but of many things.

The overwhelming state of awareness became part of how I passed the time. It was the same awareness of everyone's reactions as they witnessed my acclimations, which further fueled my motivation to prove them wrong about walking. Most prevalent was of the divide between my inner state and physical states of existence. I was aware of everything, and thereby everything became a part of my mission.

One day, probably weeks after I woke up, I requested some pain medication. The nurse came in and administered the medicine and then left my room. An action that caught my eye was that the nurse left all the administering supplies on the rolling bed table beside me. Due to prior experiences, it was noted and recorded in my mind. By the age of sixteen, I had experienced medical treatments enough to be educated on proper disposal guidelines. Leaving the supplies on the table beside the patient was surely not in accordance with best practices.

About forty-five minutes had passed, and I was still in a significant amount of pain. Just as I began questioning the effectiveness of the medicine, my parents arrived. It was through my Dad that I connected with the truths beyond the pain.

I asked my Dad if the doctors would ever give me something in lieu of pain medication. I recall him asking why I posed the question, and I told him what had transpired. We discussed the medical advice to manage the pain and not wait until it is too intense. I was very mindful of this advice, for the last thing I wanted was to experience continued physical pain if unnecessary. The truth was that the medication never eradicated the pain. It merely dulled it enough so that it did not overpower my mind. I felt proud that I was doing well with managing the pain and the need for medication. Frankly, I was proud of how well I was managing everything.

I was already hurting when the request was made, and due to my own attempts to manage the need, my request came at the brink of my own perceived limitations. After forty-five minutes, the pain became intense, pushing my tolerance even further beyond limits of comfort. I remember my Dad looked shocked by my question and laughed when he told me, "Yes, it's called a placebo." It was a term

I had not yet heard before, but I did know what I had experienced. The truth was that I had not received anything to ease the pain.

My Dad was determined to go find out if that was indeed what transpired. He went out into the hall, found the doctor, and discussed what I had stated. When my Dad came back into my room, he said, "Sure enough!" He said they wanted to ensure that I was not becoming addicted to morphine and that dependency had not set in. The doctors confirmed that a placebo had been administered in an effort to gauge my response and assess the possibility of addiction.

When I was able to identify what happened immediately after the first attempt, the doctor quickly ordered morphine administration. They were all a little surprised with my awareness, and it also lessened their concern about addiction. I did not want to take it any more than they wanted to keep giving it to me. But the truth was that it was an excruciating physical experience. I knew I was lengthening the intervals, and I knew that I would no longer need the medication in time. And eventually, that is what happened. Just like that. No need, no withdrawals, no issue.

I recall trying to reconcile the state of my existence - seemingly above my traumatized body. In those times, I was unable to rationalize anything about the most physically painful moments of my life. It was when I was left alone, with my awareness and visual mind, for the endless soul and heart hours that I filtered through every aspect of my reality like a record playing on repeat. I was unable to move. I was left seemingly paralyzed in my bed, open in trauma on the outside while peacefully relaxed on the inside with only the remains of my physical body to separate my worlds. It was a profound realization, even then, of the state of my existence and the sense of separation.

17

A Home Away From Home

After three and a half months into my illness, I was on the move again. This time, I was transferred to the medium care unit within the same hospital. The move meant that I no longer needed life-sustaining medication and equipment, nor did I require sterile isolation. It was only once I was in the medium care unit that I became aware of the extensive recovery ahead. It was a move that became the catalyst for the rest of me to wake up. It was time for me to start preparing for my re-entry into the world.

Before I arrived to my new room, the staff and my parents did what they could to prepare my new space. Nobody knew how long I would be there until three months later when I was discharged. In their kindness without knowing, the staff swapped TVs and gave me the one from the nurse's lounge. It was larger, and they said it would be easier to see from the bed, since that was where I would pass my days.

Once the bed and TV were in place, my parents decorated the walls with the cards received from around the world. The cards were a visual reminder of the prayers, love, and support that were being held in my name. The cards on the walls that surrounded me anchored the power of the Global Wave of Healing Energy directed at my body. This room became the sacred space that would grow me into my new sense of self and into the world around me.

It felt like I was being carried by the love energy being emitted from the walls. The wall of cards held a presence and sensation that I could never fully explain and felt too grand to contain within my fragile body. I was grateful that life circumstances placed me internationally and further yielded a global network before me on my walls. Even then, I saw and felt the connectivity but had no awareness of the truth in what I was experiencing. Many times, it felt like my body was in a traumatized state of healing and evolution, while my soul was carried in the words of truth that hung on my wall as I waited out the experience. I trusted that the forces would be joined in time, that of the Global Wave of Healing Energy and that which was inside of me. I trusted there would be time when they would meet.

As I began to settle into a space that felt like a home away from home, I was immediately introduced to what would become the ever-evolving presence and reminder of human anguish and mortality. In the silence of the day, there were sharp interruptions brought on by a humbling moan of agony. It was unbeknown as to when they would surface, and the timing relied solely upon the lips of another. Day or night, pain knows no time.

It was a sound I instantly knew for it was one I had experienced deep within, yet never gave a voice. It was the sound of my own heart echoing throughout the hallways from patients enduring some level of similarity. The reality of where I was, a burn unit, sunk to a deeper level as I imagined the truth in that fire could result in the same outcome as mine if in contact with the body. The process of disfigurement was different, but the outcome and its treatment were the same. I then knew I was not alone in my anguish. I sent prayers to their unbeknown faces that I knew their pain. It even feels like I asked my nurses to send them prayers of compassion and empathy from my room. I don't know if I did, but it is something I would most definitely do. I held the faith that they would know they were not alone just as I searched deeply to know that truth within myself.

I found a sense of relief not long after I moved into my new room when my parents brought and hooked up a VCR player, as well as my PC from home. Once I was in my new space, I was ready to start exercising my brain muscle beyond the realms of my own interactions. I watched movies to fill the quiet and ease the mind, and I was able to catch up on the two months of school assignments since school had already ended shortly after my transfer.

There was still plenty of quiet time for introspection since the days and nights were long. I needed them to be long. I needed a tremendous amount of time to process everything. But I also wanted to return to life in whichever way I was able. Schoolwork to complete junior year credits became a welcomed distraction. Often, I redirected in ways to focus, stimulate, and mold a sound mind. I needed my mind to be strong. I welcomed any opportunity to strengthen my mind, fill the silence and muffle the moans of despair. The ones within the hallways and the ones from within.

Staff were in and out throughout the day, and they always brought a smile and a warm heart. Even though there were language differences, it never imposed a barrier in our ability to connect. Their interactions always lifted my spirits, in every sense of the meaning. I always tried to reciprocate with a smile as the sense of isolation drifted away, even if only for a moment.

My interactions with the staff extended beyond keeping my physical body alive and thriving. They were the ones that kept my spirit alive. They somehow managed to keep me focused on the goals of recovery when there were so many less favorable options. They were the ones who helped me find joy in the presence of adversity. They helped me remember how to laugh when there were so many things to cry over. It was the many hours they spent hanging out in my room, even when they had the choice not to. Those were the moments that I needed. Those were the moments that mattered. It was during those moments that preserved my spirit, which fueled my reason to smile.

I recall the staff would get in trouble because they were often found in my room during their shifts. There were a few that were always in my room. We joked around, played a lot of games, and watched movies while passing the time. It felt like passing the time with new friends, weird work-patient friends, but friends that were supporting me during the most pivotal experience of my youthful life. I am sure there were many reasons why, but my room quickly became the most popular room in the unit. It was very meaningful and refreshing, given the circumstances. Fun in the midst of the chaos. Smiles in the midst of the tears. Meaning in the seemingly meaningless.

Through it all, I had to learn how to socially interact. I struggled to connect with people when I was struggling to connect within myself. It was me, but I was a different me. I was different yet the same. All along, I had to reconcile the truth that the changes in my physical body changed every other aspect of my existence. It was as if an instant filter had been constructed in the trauma that assessed every part of my existence for purpose and meaning before allowing it through to the next moment of breath. I was assessed in my totality for adaptability to change and self-sustainment for my best interest. Every single aspect of my existence was impacted and became filtered through my experience. I became very commanding and expecting of self.

It was difficult to hear others state that my experience did not change who I am. It most certainly changed who I am. I found it interesting that the statement generally came from those that knew me before. It was confusing to hear everyone state that my scars meant nothing, and that beauty comes from within. My scars most certainly meant something. My scars were my skin that came from my back, or maybe my stomach. I lived through making these scars. It most certainly meant something. It was mostly confusing because I knew that beauty comes from within and that my scars did not define me, yet I was now faced with holding faith as it was put into action through the example of my life. It felt extremely overwhelming that I would never again be able to escape practicing that truth, seeing beauty beyond the covers in life. Nor would I be able to escape the experience of another's ability to practice the same, with me and my covers.

Believing in the truth of love and beauty within myself was extremely hard. I remained nervous in my trust. Not just with my family and friends, but with the world. I felt strange and uncomfortable yet refreshed and optimistic. There was a profound awareness that I was re-entering into everything. There was newness in the ordinary. The ordinary became extraordinary. It became easy to get excited because everything became an accomplishment, an achievement, a glorious moment of joy. Even within the small ordinary acts of before, such as wiggling a toe.

I also found it extremely difficult to realize I held no autonomy. It became difficult for myself to experience me. There was no space to learn myself before others were brought into my experience. It was as if we were all learning me together, collectively. It felt like my moments alone were brief when compared to the rapid newness evolving with and within my body. When alone I felt proud and accomplished, when present with others, I felt as though my triumphs were menial.

I felt vulnerable and insecure. Everyone was out in the world living. My friends were preparing for summer vacations, making plans for senior year events, and preparing for their entrance into the rest of their lives. I was also doing the same, yet I was in the hospital, surviving death with a severely damaged body, incapable of walking, and years of physical therapy ahead of me. I could not relate to them. It was hard for them to relate to me. I could not even relate to myself. I had nothing of myself to give to anyone. I barely had anything to give to myself. Everything I did felt rudimentary in life. I felt like a child playing catch up to those who knew me and their memories of me.

I had no idea how to navigate the very real moments in discovery. All I knew to do was to be real and authentic in whatever unfolded. I was like a newborn with an awareness of mine. As I experienced the conflicting world of acceptance around me, my discoveries of strength and courage remained cherished closely within. A life of celebration and joy on the inside, and one of unexpected evolution through trauma on the outside. It felt like a dance between two worlds that played distinctly different music that could not sustain a shared rhythm nor beat. My evolving gratitude and celebration felt incapable of harmonizing with the world around me that felt heavy and sad. I felt confused as to which world was really mine. I saw a joint world I desperately wanted to return to as it slipped off into the distance.

I became accustomed to processing the truths of these sentiments while alone, but suddenly there were people always around reminding me of the comparisons. People I knew, and ones that I did not. I had moved from isolation in the intensive care unit to a never-ending flow of human presence surrounding me. The past, present, and future versions of self were constantly trying to find their space in what was evolving into a sense of constant change.

It was oftentimes easier to be with those who did not know me as I was before. I could relax into them knowing me as I would forever be, without the gauge of who I was. Simultaneously, it was frightening because, as I did so, I knew I was leaving parts of me behind. I feared that those who knew me before would never understand the implications my experience was having within the depths of me, and how it would inevitably change me, forever.

I feared abandonment, pity, and shame, even though it was not my fault. I felt dirty and scarred and doubted my worthiness of anything. It all felt silly in my youthful state while doubt clinched where it could. My new hospital staff friends, on the other hand, seemed to understand me better than I understood myself. They only knew me as they saw me, and I saw them as the ones that were growing me into my new body and into my new life.

Family and friends kept my room buzzing with their presence, stocked with movies, games, activities, and snacks. There was always plenty to do, something to eat, and someone to engage. With the many changes underway, I sensed it was time for the real work to begin. I knew my focus had to shift.

I saw the move as a progressive step towards returning home, while doctors saw it differently. As I left behind isolation and fragility, the doctors left behind concerns of death and amputation. As I approached goals and a road to recovery, the doctors approached concerns of muscle atrophy and mental health. I remember feeling grateful that I had made it to where I was because it felt like we held different perspectives and objectives. For the first time, I was able to shift from surviving to thriving. My focus shifted to physical recovery and life intentions. It was when the commitment cultivated in the intensive care unit would naturally take its course, only now through action.

It was also a time when my beliefs, my determination, and my resolve were challenged beyond measure. I was pushed to my limits every moment along the way. I wept in hopes that my cries would be heard, by someone, something in the ethers of my faith. I pleaded that I would always do my best to learn whatever it was I was to learn, just please, get me through this, and with a sound mind. I trusted that if I learned the lessons, I would be blessed beyond my imagination with blissful balance to the trauma. The only hope I had was to believe as I rebuilt my dreams. As I rebuilt my life.

I shielded and braced myself with nervous trust as I settled into my home away from home. I still had exposed bone on my shins, and almost all the skin grafts had healed and were ready for the next phase in the treatment plan. The main goals were to build strength in my thighs and upper body, skin graft scar massages, and most importantly, learning how to walk again.

I had to focus on how I was going to make it through eight hours of painful scar massaging and intense physical therapy a day. I had to figure out how I was going to endure the pain from more surgeries, bear weight on my traumatized legs, and what I could possibly do to make them walk again. I had to focus intently, especially since everyone tried to keep me in check with reminders of the possibilities. To them that meant possible limitations. All I had the capacity to care about was figuring out my masterful mechanical body and how I was going to get it walking home. I just wanted to walk and to go home. Not this home, my true home. But I was there, and so it was time for complete and utter focus. I believe it was my relentless focus that grounded my mental wellness. That, and my stubborn determination.

Somehow, I continued on, almost in a superhuman kind of way. Back then, I did not have a choice. Well, at least it didn't seem like I did. It was just part of who I am. It was only after many years that it became evident of how many choices were really available. As in life as we chose who we want to become. I am grateful for my stubborn determination.

Being stubborn had already caused some very unfavorable situations in my life, but this time was different. It was as if my many years of practice had led me to the ultimate situation when this characteristic alone would be the very thing that saved me. Not just with continued awareness and continued survival, but with a continued breath of meaning and purpose.

Even though I was in a new space, one thing stayed the same.

Although they required less time and were no longer the focal point of the day, the days still began with the bath. Before physical therapy could begin and consume the hours of my days, my wounds had to be assessed and cleaned. Even though they continued every day, they had changed. The exposed bone was less painful. The bathwater and gentle washing felt soothing, almost relaxing against the healing skin that repaired my body. As long as I closed my eyes.

When they were open, the emotional and psychological pain became prevalent at that moment. The baths would become increasingly more unpleasant and awkward to experience. It seemed like the further along in my recovery, the harder it became for me to swallow my pride and lay naked on the bath gurney. The dignity lost was unbearable at times while numerous nurses unbandaged me, piece by piece, stripping me down to nothing. The same nurses that I passed the time with by playing video games and watching movies. The same males that shared laughter and made me smile. The same healers that removed every protective layer from my being, exposing me naked and afraid. My heart prayed for peace when I kept my eyes open.

There was a new awareness that my senses were slowly returning. During the baths, I could feel the inner parts of me waking up. My modesty, my self-respect, my self-worth, all the human parts of my being, collectively, were waking up to my experience. My humanity was triggered by the world around me.

During the bath, the usual banter would take place to minimize the intensity, awkwardness, and disheartened truth of the reality. As I laid humbled and at their mercy, they gently washed and then re-bandaged my broken body. I felt vulnerable in my shame and embarrassment while fully exposed before them. At times I became angry that all I could see were their eyes, while I had no choice in the boundaries of my own exposure. I was even aware of the balance in the seemingly unjust circumstance - the healers standing fully clothed while I lay naked, broken, and exposed - in the literal and metaphorical sense of expression.

All the while, no one knew the difference because their touch was always with respect and held healing intention. It was not an easy situation for anyone. No matter how many times I had taken a bath, for me, every time seemed like the first.

I could sense that I was truly waking up. My sense of modesty and pride were returning with an overwhelming desire to build everything back up. That meant self-esteem, self-worth, and everything else I felt slipping away the more I woke up. Every moment became a lesson for a future encounter to become stronger, more courageous, and more loving of self.

At one point, I requested that my Mom bring underwear so that I could begin covering the private parts of me. Although it became a comical part of the bath for the young males who tried to orient female underwear, it was a silent and shameful experience to endure day in and day out at the vulnerable age of seventeen. I often chuckled on the outside while I wept on the inside. I felt very uncomfortable, always being so exposed. I hated how I did not have a choice in my own level of modesty. It left me feeling violated and betrayed in a way I never expected. Not just by the nurses who bathed me, but by life. And it was not in a negative, heavy way, but in a matter of fact in harsh acceptance.

As every minute passed, I evolved back into my humanity and tried to restore a sense of autonomy and privacy through whichever means I could. Underwear fulfilled a youthful sense of both. It was little and went unnoticed to everyone but me, but it was the honoring of self that slowly restored the broken parts of me beyond my physical body.

Somehow, despite the vulnerability during the baths, and the humility in my nakedness, it all dissipated when bandages and a hospital gown hid my body. I allowed my sentiments of despair within the shameful walls of the bath, yet there was a bareness of my soul unable to hide behind clothes. It was a bareness that followed beyond the doors of the bath.

I was grounded by my humanness beyond the doors of the bath. My body was clothed, and the nurses were less clothed. I was able to see the faces that framed their eyes. The faces that held the eyes that stared into mine. The eyes that watched my tears fall with every bandage they removed. I was able to see their hands. I saw the hands that gently unwrapped me, bathed my wounds, and wrapped me back in protection. I saw the strength in the arms that picked me up and moved me around from bed to gurney, to table to chair. For the first time in my treatment, I was able to see my team of healers for who they were beyond my shameful nakedness. Beyond the doors of the bath, they were able to see me for more than just a vulnerable and traumatized body.

I found peace that I was able to be in all my brokenness while I lived at the hospital. The broken physical parts that were healing, and the parts within that I felt breaking along the way. In a sense, it felt that the more my body healed, the more I broke on the inside by the doubt and fear in the life ahead. I felt mentally prepared for the moments before me but doubted the strength for a lifetime. I could not imagine my mind spending a lifetime trying to keep up and processing each passing moment. It felt as though there was so much potential to lose grasp of healing.

There were many mornings that I would wake up in anticipation of what I may find within myself. I tried to allow space to experience whatever needed to be experienced. It often felt like I was monitoring my vessel and allowing it to play out as it needed. I tried to use my self-monitoring as an indicator of the daily inner workload that awaited my attention. The self-checks felt critical for my future ability to live inside my body, and more so, inside my mind. There were no explanations as to why I was still alive, but I was. And there was no means to predict how my body would recover and adjust. All I knew was that I remained, and for a purpose greater than me. My prayer was that I too would someday be privileged to know.

There was never any indication that I was depressed nor mal adjusting. Even so, the hospital staff and doctors were convinced that I should be. Everything I was experiencing most definitely had the potential to make someone mentally unstable. What they did not know was that ever since I woke from the coma, I had prayed deeply that I would have the mental strength to endure my journey. As time passed, the prayers grew deeper as more strength was needed. I recall wondering back then if believing so firmly in my mental wellness was in itself evidence that I had crossed the brink, incapable of seeing my own demise, or my stubborn unwillingness to do so. Decades later, I realized it was an unwavering faith that shielded my intellect with resounding peace of mind.

Doctors were clear in their opinion that it is uncommon that one would not struggle with the circumstances that I had endured. They believed it so much so that they insisted that a psychiatrist visit and conduct a full evaluation, with the readiness to prescribe assistive medications if needed. It was a consultation that felt like it was more for the doctors than it was for me, but I welcomed the opinion of an expert. I was curious if we held the same perspective.

One unannounced afternoon, the Psychiatrist entered my room. While knocking, and with a team of individuals in white coats, a crowd entered my space. I remember having to quickly adjust to the uninvited attendance of a team of doctors with the sole intention to judge my sanity. As introductions took place, the group inspected the walls filled with cards, a PC on the dining tray, a VHS player, and a cabinet full of videos, games, and activities to keep me busy. Meanwhile, I pushed the table tray with the PC aside and paused the schoolwork I was doing to complete my history class credits.

We engaged in conversation for a while as I shared my state of mind. Among many things, I explained I was believing in what felt like a hollow faith and the reasons why it was so. I recall even telling them that I was unable to change anything about what had happened, and all I could do was choose how I would respond. And for me it was easy. I wanted to get better, walk, go home, and get on with life. So, that is what I was doing, and I was going to be happy while doing it.

They asked a few questions about how I passed the time, about visits from family and friends, and gauged their opinions of me. I felt very judged in the moment as they stood with their white coats of expertise and critical minds inferring what they could from my few spoken words. It was interesting that their assessment held the potential to change my path to recovery. It felt like a moment when my path could have easily become theirs.

After our visit, but before departing the room, the Psychiatrist turned to my doctor and provided his assessment. He claimed that there was absolutely nothing to be concerned about. He affirmed that my acknowledgments and processing of everything was being done in a healthy way. The most important piece of advice was that they should let me be.

It was of their opinion that in those moments I was fine and that I would continue to be fine as long as I continued to do what I was doing. Finally, someone believed that I would be fine. I believed I would be. I felt validated in my belief that I would have the mental strength to endure whatever came my way. I remained uncertain as to exactly what it was that I was doing, but I remained committed to doing and being the best that I could within every moment. I hoped that would be enough. I felt as though I was as ready as I could be.

While my external world was infusing me of love, healing energy, and support, my perspectives left me feeling defenseless, unguarded, and incredibly alone. Physically I knew I was not alone, but as a soul, I felt abandoned and betrayed within an illogical world. Behind the smile was a silence that felt so incredibly alone. I was aware of my mind's inability to rationalize my reality, while simultaneously at peace in the uncertainty. I was aware of the fear and doubt that muffled the voice of reassurance within while knowing it was a voice of truth that I needed to hear. I had to acknowledge the sense of split self that, at times, felt as though it was taking over my existence.

To counter the sentiments, and to balance into the faith that I would make it through the journey, I had to reconnect my inner and outer worlds. I desperately needed to reconcile the state of my body that divided them. I did not know how to do that in my unevolved youthful state of existence. I surely could not understand it, nor explain it. It was all very confusing. Overwhelming.

I could not make sense of many things, but I knowingly needed to draw upon the love and faith of others, as well as my own. As if I needed to balance the forces from those around me, and that within me. There was tremendous trust in the love and prayers being directed towards me. The choice was to trust in my own sense of love and faith within. I turned to my Mom for assistance, as a grounding force in my life experience.

During the many days alone, I recalled a popular poem that I often read for its metaphysical implications, yet not from the space of a grounded faith. However, it seemed prudent that I bring it into my experience given the circumstances, especially with the heightened sense of aloneness.

I asked my Mom to acquire copies of the poem so that I could read it throughout the hours of uncertainty. And she did. My Mom brought posters, bookmarks, printouts, and anything she could find that held the words of the poem. This poem was a significant anchor to the hope I held deep within. It fueled a much deeper trust in my faith than I even realized. At the time, my mind felt riddled in doubt as my soul rested in the truths of what I read.

Footprints In The Sand
- Authorship disputed so claiming Unknown

One night a man had a dream.
He dreamed he was walking
along the beach with the Lord.
Across the sky flashed scenes from his life.
For each scene, he noticed
two sets of footprints in the sand;
one belonging to him,
and the other set to the Lord.
When the last scene of his life flashed before him,
he looked back at the footprints in the sand.
He noticed that many times
along the path of his life
there was only one set of footprints.
He also noticed that it happened at the very
lowest and saddest times in his life.
This really bothered him
and he questioned the Lord about it.
"Lord you said that once I decided to follow You,
You'd walk with me all the way.
But I have noticed that during
the most troublesome times in my life,
there is only one set of footprints.
I don't understand why when
I needed you most you would leave me."
The Lord replied, "My precious, precious child,
I love you and would never leave you.
During your times of trial and suffering,
when you see only one set of footprints...
It was then that I carried you."

Everyone had been doing everything for me and it was apparent that it was time for me to step up. It was up to me to make all changes as positive as I could. There was tremendous support around me, and I continuously had to choose my nervous and doubtful faith. It felt as though I would now be living a life of healing and growing into peace. I became committed to my effort to forever meet the world in the fullness of who I am and from within whichever space of healing I have achieved. All I knew is that I would go forth in faith because I deeply needed to hold peace. It was time to put me into action and act on all that had been accumulating within and around me, and supported with a sound mind. It felt easy to rest in the truth that this home would grow me into the world beyond the walls of a hospital. Furthermore, beyond the walls of my body.

18

Medium Care Yet Top Priority

Some other, less dramatic events occurred in the medium care unit. Two were deemed a priority in their own time and space; and both occurred before I started walking again. The first one involved a visit from the doctor that sent me to the ER at the beginning of the illness. She came to check on me, and while visiting she noticed that I had a tanned color to my complexion. She asked if I had been sitting outside, which I thought was comical because they would never let me leave the unit. Of course, I was not sitting outside. And there was definitely not any way to capture the warmth of the sun on my face from the small window hidden in the corner. Intrigued, she left to research what could be happening.

I had been treated with steroids at the initial hospital due to the trauma that Waterhouse-Fredrickson had on my adrenal glands. When I was transferred to the burn unit, they continued to administer the steroids, but it morphed into part of my treatment protocol while treated like a burn patient. The adrenal steroids are often given to assist in the body's natural mechanism to fight through a stressful event. Therefore, by default, it became a part of my treatment plan. Before moving me into the medium care unit, doctors were steadily reducing and eliminating medicines when they could. Somewhere along the way, they had stopped the adrenal steroid medication. By the time I was in the medium care unit enough time had passed for symptoms to start setting in.

Once they stopped the medication, I began to show signs of one of the most common side effects of adrenal insufficiency, the darkening of the skin. It was concluded that there was still adrenal gland damage and malfunction as a result of everything and was added to the list of things to investigate further down the road in my recovery.

Appropriate diagnosis and treatment would require a week- long hospital study, and although I was already in the hospital, the facility could not perform the test and I was unable to endure a week-long test at another one. Not because of the testing itself, but because of the extensive wound care treatment I was still undergoing - the specialized baths, bandage dressings, scar massaging - it was too much too coordinate at another facility. Therefore, it was decided to re-administer the steroid supplements until further testing could be completed. It was a priority for another time.

Another priority surfaced while in the medium care unit. During the physical therapy and walking focused days, I was introduced to the concept of pressure garments as part of the skin graft treatment process. Massaging my skin grafts was a ritual that occurred no less than twice a day for two years. It was long, usually painful, yet instrumental in the healing process. In addition to the massaging, once they were finished healing, the pressure garments would need to be worn over all my scars for about two years to minimize scar tissue. The purpose of the garments was to fit very tightly and apply constant direct pressure while the scars matured. It takes anywhere between nine months to two or three years for skin grafts like mine to mature. The sooner I was fitted for the garments and started wearing them, the sooner I could stop wearing them.

About a month after arriving in the medium care unit, I was fitted for special ordered pressure garments to cover as many of my scars as possible. The only areas not covered were the sides of my hips and my butt. There was no real way to cover those areas when they had to consider the feasibility of me getting them on. I could not point nor flex my feet as they were basically stuck in a ninety-degree angle which made pulling the garments on extremely difficult. I ended up with a separate piece for each extremity. There were four in total, plus a glove.

Each leg was covered from the tips of my toes, up to the highest point on my thigh. The toes were not covered, and there was a built in heal. It was kind of like the tight circulation stockings used in hospitals, but much thicker and much tighter and all over my arms and legs. The back of the lower leg garments opened and closed with velcro, allowing for my foot to slip into the top opening and then extend out of the opening in the back, in order to slip my foot into the tight foot section. Each leg garment had fastening straps that would secure around my waist after they were pulled up as high as they would go.

The arm garments would pull up from my wrist, extending all the way up my arm to my shoulder, with straps that would cross around my back, under the opposite arm and fasten in the front of my torso, crisscrossing across my chest. Two straps across my back and torso, two straps around my waist, and extremely tight, non-breathing garments, and a glove on my right hand; fingerless but covered the thumb because of a scar that extended onto the back of my hand. My body could barely breathe. It felt like every cell of my being was trying to breathe air through the experiences.

They were tan in color, so it looked closer to skin color, and eventually I would add clothes on top of them. They were tight and sometimes very hot. But that was irrelevant. It was something that needed to be done. So, I did it. There was one element that I did like about the pressure garments…it hid my scars. I didn't have to look at them all the time. In a sense I could escape that small portion of the overwhelming reality.

Even though I sometimes liked it when they were covered, it was always such a great feeling to take them off. I did not have sensation on the scars, and still don't, but the small normal areas around the scars on my arms could feel the fresh air penetrating through the skin. Then they would get massaged with oily lotion, and once again hidden underneath the garments. These garments became a part of my existence for two years, day and night, as I continued to transformed beneath their covers. I knew one day my scars would be mature enough to leave the garments in my wake, however, I just wondered how long it would take to mature from the trauma. I had to remind myself that I had to keep on going until I could stop, and it was not that time.

19

These Legs Were Made for Walking

I remained in the medium care unit from the time of transfer from the intensive care unit until discharge, which came almost three months later. A lot can happen in three months. I made sure to make the most of it. For me, the main focus was walking again. So, for the first month, it was about strength building and working with my primary physical therapist to really understand the mobility and functionality of what remained of my lower legs. What were we really dealing with? What were the possibilities? This is what made my physical therapist the ideal participant in my recovery.

He understood the trauma. He understood the physical changes and the impact every loss had on a seemingly simple movement. He analyzed every functionality of my body and worked to help me achieve my goals. They became his goals too, but everyone knew it had to start with me.

Recovery was not easy, and it was a very drawn-out process. I remember having to get around in a wheelchair for a while. Using it to go down the hall to the physical therapy room, and on Sundays my parents would bring me to the hospital chapel for services. I had to go to physical therapy several times a day, whereas I only went to chapel service when I was unable to walk. I never resisted going to either, even though I never truly wanted to participate. It was strange. I wanted to voluntarily do both, yet I was angry that I felt forced. I felt forced that physical therapy was part of what I needed to want to do. I always went to physical therapy because it was important to me, and I always went to the chapel because it was important to my parents who thought it was important for me. I was very confused about both; physical therapy and whether the choice was really mine; and my faith and how it all related to my illness. All of which I was unable to explore until much later.

There was also a time when the staff found another wheelchair for my Sister, and they let us go on a closed floor of the hospital just to wheel around. She sat in the spare wheelchair, and together we raced up and down the abandoned hospital floor. I was coming to terms with the idea that if the doctors were right, this is what my life would be like. While my Sister was supporting and encouraging me with her actions that it would be ok if it did turn out to be my journey. I remember being even more determined after that day. More determined to walk. More determined to eliminate the wheelchair from my future life. It was not going to be that way. There were too many things I wanted to do in life, and a wheelchair would only get in the way. I had already told them that I was going to walk and demonstrated that it did not matter that they did not believe I would. I believed I would. I knew I would.

My physical therapist and I continued to prepare my legs and feet to support the task of walking. I could not move my feet at all. I had lost either all, or the majority of the muscles that control my feet. I could not point nor flex. I could not rotate nor move them from side to side. I could not even wiggle my toes. If there was movement it was very slight. My feet were just there, in a ninety-degree angle. Yet, they were there, serving as feet, to the legs that we just fought so hard to save. Somehow, they had to work together in harmony again.

I had always been very interested in human anatomy. Before I got sick, I had acquired anatomy coloring books from one of my high school teachers so that I could learn all about the body. This was another sign of a life intended that in a way prepared me for this journey. I had already studied the muscles of the body. I did not know them by name, but I knew where they were, where they started and ended, and what they controlled. I had even done weird muscle control exercises just to see if I could hone into the focus needed to isolate movement of a muscle, or subset of muscles. I recall sitting on my bed and picking different muscles on my arms and legs and then trying to isolate and contract only that muscle. Little did I know that these quirky characteristics were teaching me how to do something that would be critical in my recovery and my ability to walk again.

My physical therapist and I examined every fragment of muscle in my shins and feet. We did exactly what I had already practiced doing throughout the years before my illness. He would point to an area, tell me what muscle it was a part of, and the movement that would use that muscle. I would concentrate and visualize the movement, flex the muscles in my leg, even though there was not noticeable movement, and we would observe whether or not the muscle fragments would move from cell memory, or twitch. If they did, that meant that there were fragments intact throughout the length of the muscle, and we would repeat the exercise to build up strength in the portion that remained. We continued to discuss and focus on the muscle contractions, or until it was determined that the muscle was damaged so much, that they were no longer functional other than serving the purpose of covering my bones. By doing these exercises, we also learned which muscles remained and how they may be able to aid in the ongoing process. It was humbling each time a muscle revealed it was too damaged to assist further.

When it seemed like I was getting closer to actually trying to walk, we had to first ensure that I would be able to handle the vertical positioning needed to do so. I had been laying in a bed for four months. I had sat up in the bed, and in chairs, but I had not been standing upright on my feet in over four months. This meant my body needed to be acclimated back into the vertical standing position. Plus, the vascular system and my body's circulation had drastically been altered with the tissue loss and skin grafts. Everything needs to adjust, and slowly.

For a couple of weeks, every day, I had to spend several hours on a tilt table. The tilt table was a flat, thin, and narrow bed which was adjusted by any desired degree between the horizontal and vertical axes. When appropriate, the degree would increase further from the horizontal position, until I was vertical and symptom free. There were several straps that held me on the table, and I would usually just watch a movie to pass the time. Some days the increase was too drastic, and I would feel light-headed and nauseated. Other days it was exhilarating to feel the blood flow throughout the new paths in my new legs. It felt hopeful.

Once I was able to support the standing position, we began testing different braces and supports, and what would be needed for my unique situation. We also discovered that when standing, if I picked up my leg as if to take a step, my foot had just enough mobility to drop downward, with my toes dropping towards the ground, however, I did not have the muscle capacity to contract and pick my foot back up.

As one could imagine, this is slightly problematic with the concept of walking. If my foot dropped with every step, and I could not pick it up, I would not be able to clear the step, and I would trip over my own feet. I would have to walk in almost a marching walk with my knees pulled upward in order to clear my steps. That did not seem practical for long term walking. We would come up with a unique solution to address this later on, once walking became something to improve upon and not just achieve.

To get us through the immediate goal of walking, my physical therapist came up with customized braces that would support my legs and feet. The braces would keep my feet at a ninety-degree angle so that my foot would clear when I walk. We called these braces etelles. It was basically a piece of molded plastic that was shaped like the shin and foot of a leg, open in the front so my leg and foot would slide in and rest inside the open mold. There were four velcro straps, two around the shin, one at the top and one at the bottom, one on my foot close to my ankle and the other near my toes. Eventually we lined the inside and rigged certain areas with foam padding for added comfort. They surely were not the prettiest, but they were serving a very important purpose.

Then one day, I was sitting in the chair in my room, and my physical therapist and the unit chief were examining the mobility of my ankles. Switching between French and Flemish, they exchanged dialogue while fitting me with adjusted etelles, and going through ideas. Amidst the foreign spoken words, suddenly, broken English words filled my ears. Almost in sync, they asked me, "Do you want to try and walk?"

Stunned and uncertain about the seriousness of the question, I started to cry. Absolutely I wanted to try and walk. That had been the goal. I was overwhelmed with excitement and fear. Was it a good idea? Was it time? Could I do it? What if I couldn't? What if my legs give out on me like they did the last time I tried to walk the night I was became so sick? That was the last time I had walked. Or at least tried to walk. The trauma since the last would perhaps have been too much. I was so overwhelmed with the reality of what had been proposed that I didn't even recall my Sister being present on this day. More nervous and more apprehensive than I had ever been, I trusted that they would not subject me to harm and agreed to try. In that moment, it was the moment; the moment to do it.

My physical therapist rounded the troops to help him support me, found thick foam blocks to tape to the bottoms of the etelles to provide a softer, more giving surface, grabbed a walker and stood me up. For the first time in almost four and a half months, I took my first steps. With a walker, four staff members, etelles on both legs, exposed shin bones behind sterile bandages, and all the hours of hard work. I took five very uncoordinated and unsure steps to the door in my room, and then the same steps back to the chair. It was the most unbelievable steps I recall ever taking. The distance was short, yet I had come so far. The steps were unsecure, yet they were strong from the journey. It was sloppy and embarrassing but it was amazing. Amazingly hard. Amazingly scary. And I felt amazingly proud. We did it. I did it! I knew I could do it!

We practiced a couple more times before we brought it to the corridor. It was probably several days later, but it was an even bigger ordeal. We were going a farther distance. I made it to the hall, and this time with six staff members, a walker, and braces, I walked down the hall. Step by step. With each step, the therapists would support my gait, support my feet, and support the walker. Holding each in place while I prepared for the next step. It was a slow, uncomfortable, scary, and even a shameful process. Somehow it was easily countered with the commitment, support and encouragement of the entire unit staff cheering and watching from the side lines. We were all so excited and everyone was completely astonished at what they had witnessed. Even if they had never worked with me, everyone in the unit knew me. It seemed like nobody believed I would walk again. Even if they were hopeful, I don't think they ever really believed that it could or would happen. They finally were able to integrate the truth that I held, and that my legs were made for waking.

I understand their uncertainty now more than ever. They knew what I was up against. They worked in a hospital treating people who have been disfigured by burns from any source. I was comparable to a patient with fourth degree burns over sixty percent of my body, albeit never impacting my bones and only the muscles that exposed their bareness. They had seen this type of trauma. If they had not seen trauma like mine, they at least knew it was worse than anything they had seen. They had watched patients, tended to patients, and helped patients on their recovery journeys. They believed they had a better idea of what was to come and become of me. I showed them that my idea was better, and who I really am.

As I walked towards the end of the hall, I will never forget what

I saw when I looked up. My doctor, the head surgeon that fought for my legs as if I was his own daughter. He was standing there watching me and crying. Crying tears of happiness and joy. Crying tears of amazement. And possibly crying tears of relief. He had made a commitment to me, without knowing who I was or what would become of me, and I had just showed him that it was worth every ounce of doubt and wonder. Every morsel of himself that he selflessly gave to me, was most definitely worth it. Because of him, I was there, walking in the hall, face to face with him and his crystal-clear blue eyes. There were no words then, and there are no words now for the sentiments of compassion and gratitude that I hold for this surgeon. I owe so much of this life experience to him and his moments of choice. I hold deep gratitude with every step my legs make upon this Earth.

20

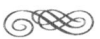

Finally!

Finally! After the hard work and healing, I was finally allowed to go home. I was not completely discharged, but after almost six months in hospitals, I was allowed to go home for short periods of time. When I was told I could go home, I remember feeling differently than I thought I would have. It was such a big goal filled with excitement and joy yet played out very differently in reality.

In reality, I was terrified. I was nervous. I was uncomfortable with the truths that being home really meant. I wondered who would care for me while knowing it would depend on my family, my Mom, Dad, and little Sister, Diana. I was terrified in the unknown of how that would be, and how well they would do; how well I would do. I was terrified for all of us.

I also remember the moment when I realized that I would never walk out of the hospital. By the time I was visiting home, I was walking, but not well nor a lot. In fact, even when fully discharged,

I was not permitted to walk out. I would have walked out of the hospital each and every time I went home if they had allowed it. I wanted to walk out of there just to stay true to what I always said, and that I was going to walk out of here. Eventually I did a time or two with a huge smile within my entire being.

When home visits began, they were short and over the weekends. Since I was still very stiff from the scaring, and riding in the car was not optimal, I was transported to and fro by ambulance. I was rolled into the house on a stretcher and transferred gently to a bed that had been moved into the TV room. The TV Room became the room within which I lived. I lived there along with everyone else flowing in and out, and who found comfort in that space while watching TV. It became the space where I rested my body while at home the best I was able. I did everything in the TV room for the first six months until I was able to climb stairs again and return to my room, and my bed.

In order for home visits to occur, I had to agree to the contingency that physical therapy would continue. Of course, that was ok. I was finally back home and walking. I still required sterile bandages on my exposed bones, I still used a walker and braces on my legs, and I never took more than a step or two around my bed outside of physical therapy. It was all still very unstable and new. But I was home and walking. I was willing to do whatever I needed to continue the progress in my recovery, especially now that I was home. I did not want to go back to the hospital, especially due to an inability to progress.

When I was going home for the weekend, my physical therapist came to the house for my therapy. We all knew it was on his days off from the hospital. There was a strange acceptance in gratitude that he was committed to my recovery even when he could have chosen otherwise. We also accepted that once I was fully discharged, a stable long-term arrangement would be needed.

After numerous weekend visits, and as full discharge approached, the hospital arranged for a new physical therapist to come to the house. This therapist was selected to fulfill my therapeutic requirements and the arrangement needed ahead. He lived near our house, and the six to eight hours of therapy a day worked within his schedule. This physical therapist came to the house one time. That was all it took for me to know that he was not going to be a part of my recovery.

I knew the minute he asked me to elevate onto the balls of my feet; to stand on my tippy toes. I gave him the benefit of the doubt, in that perhaps he was unable to read my file completely before arriving. It is rather long and extensive. So, I calmly advised him that I could not do the requested exercise. He immediately insisted that I was lazy and that I was not trying. He claimed that surely, I could complete the exercise, provided I tried. He was confident that everyone could, provided they tried.

I proceeded to explain that I had just recovered from a serious illness that had destroyed over sixty percent of my body's muscle mass, primarily in my legs, and I literally do not have the muscles any longer to complete the exercise. As he proceeded to minimize my experience and attack my character, I excused myself from the session, declined future appointments, and made sure to let him know he was no longer welcome. It felt right to awkwardly walk a few steps of the TV Room, the space where I lived, and walk away from such limited beliefs. I left him behind to collect his belongings, called for my parents to escort him out, and comprised a game plan.

My intention was to speak to the medical staff at the hospital upon my return the next day and arrange for something different. My request was simple. I wanted a different physical therapist. I wanted my physical therapist. I wanted Quentin. To my satisfaction, I never saw that man again. As to whether or not Quentin would continue the work remained to be known.

Once back at the hospital, I explained the situation and my doctor asked me who I wanted as my physical therapist. I told them that I wanted the same physical therapist that I had when in the hospital, since the beginning in intensive care. I wanted Quentin. They were not sure how to make that happen since I still required so much therapy. Once fully discharged, therapy had to continue every day, and he had his job at the hospital. Realistically he could not do both.

They eventually came back and agreed to an arrangement. The reassignment was made, and Quentin was approved to continue the work we had begun, now at home. Instead of reporting to work at the hospital, he reported to work at my house. Somehow the hospital managed the arrangement for when I was discharged, and he was officially the one, for however long I needed. Everything was back on track.

He had already been on the recovery journey with me for over six months. He already knew and had helped me through so much. I knew what I had already achieved with his assistance. It only made sense that he would be the one to continue the journey with me. This was when our relationship took on another level of authenticity.

Eventually, hospital life with weekend home visits flipped and became home life with hospital visits. When I was first allowed to stay home for longer than a weekend, I had to check-in at the hospital every other day. There was never an official discharge day to celebrate; over time, my check-ins reduced until one day I just stopped going. I was cleared to stop going, but it just happened. It slipped by in the passing of a day.

Once the new physical therapy schedule was in place, and I was home, Quentin and I spent hours upon hours together. He was always at the house. In the morning, the afternoons, the evenings. He took care of the baths that transformed into sponge baths. He changed the bandages that still covered my exposed shin bones. He massaged my scars and guided me through the physical therapy exercises. He did everything as it related to me, except change my bedpan when he was not around. My younger Sister, at times, was tasked with that.

As days passed, as I became stronger, and as walking became easier, it seemed like we were always doing something. Everywhere we could find space. I was doing squats against the walls in the dining room, leg exercises on the floor in the TV room, walking outside while swinging broomsticks to get my arms to swing naturally again. There was always something to be done, remembered, or to learn.

Plus, school started in less than a month, and it was my senior year. I really wanted to go back to school even though the excitement was tempered by my nerves. By the time I was home, everyone else started to believe that anything was possible. In a sense, everyone backed off and let me achieve whatever it was I wanted to do. I really wanted to go back to school. Since we were all witness to what I had overcome, everyone accepted that if I wanted to go back to school, then I would likely go back to school. I had a lot of work to do. We had a lot of physical therapy to do. This would naturally yield a lot of time spent together.

21

Beyond Medical Expertise

There were so many unexplainable occurrences that the medical team began documenting and journaling what they were experiencing in me. There was an emphasis on using my case as a real-life example in the medical educational arena. Photographs did not come into my awareness until I was home and returning for consultation visits throughout the weeks. During these visits there was a new and greater emphasis on teaching beyond medical expertise.

Although I was some-what discharged from the hospital, there was a very real truth that still required medical attention. My shin bones were still exposed. It was a part of my reality that was not easy to slip into a conversation, and thereby was very rarely discussed. Even so, everyone knew that something had to be done.

Part of the skin grafting process is that skin can only be grafted to muscle tissue. It cannot be grafted to bone. I often wondered what could then be done since both of my shins lacked their muscular covers. Although it seemed as though no one knew the plan, something would have to be done.

The first part of the process to cover my shin bones actually transpired while I was still in the intensive care unit. The doctors determined that the right shin was significantly more exposed; therefore, it became the priority. They concluded that the best way to cover my right shin bone was to attach a muscle flap over the exposed area. In order to do this, they removed a portion of a back muscle, the latissimus dorsi, which is a large muscle that wraps under the arm on the side of the body and around to the back. They used a piece of this muscle and reattached it to my shin to cover the bone.

During recovery while in the intensive care unit, a section at the top of the muscle transfer did not heal as expected, while the remaining seventy-five percent had healed nicely. By the time I was transferred into the medium care unit, the majority of my right shin bone was covered, leaving a one-inch long by a half-inch width exposure at the very top part of my shin. As for my left shin, there was a three-inch long by a half-inch width bone exposure straight down the front of my leg. More than half of the length of my shin bone was exposed on my left leg. And to think my left shin was better than my right shin before the muscle transfer.

I lived with my bare bones exposed for the entirety of my five-and-a-half-month hospital stay, and for almost four months after discharge. My bones touched the air I breathe for nearly nine months of my existence. That is the same amount of time it takes to grow a human body inside a Mother's womb.

It was important for life to go on even with shin bones exposed, so that is what I did. I kept them wrapped in sterile bandages and safeguarded while trying to return to as much of a normal life as possible. Seeing my bones, sterilizing them, and changing bandages were part of the daily self-care in my reality.

Once I was home, this was one of the main reasons I had to continue with consultation visits with my doctor three times a week. It was critical to monitor the exposed bone to confirm the absence of infections. It was during one of these consultation visits when the unthinkable, the never before seen, amazing wonder of the healing body took over.

The shin bone creates an angle as it approaches the front of the leg, forming a more rounded angle or edge. You can feel it if you run your fingers down the front of your shin. Bones also have a thin, tough, and protective covering called the periosteum. You may also feel indents or grooves in this protective layer when you run your fingers down your shin. Those grooves are caused by nicks in the periosteum. The portion of the bone that was exposed was this pointed angular strip down the front of the bone.

When assessing my legs during consultation visits, it was evident where the muscle and skin stopped at the base of the boney peak. Many visits had passed, just as the days in the hospital, when there was no change. The medical staff unwrapped, cleaned, assessed, and rebandaged my exposed shin bones many times over the months.

Then, one day we all noticed something was different. Initially, we were not even sure of what was different, we simply agreed that my shins looked different. We debated the perception that the exposed area seemed less than the days prior. We scrutinized the bones and tissue and contemplated the possibilities that there was less bone exposed. Collectively we knew that there was indeed less bone showing in one area, yet there were no explanations of how it could be so. The medical staff eventually decided on a means by which to track potential changes.

The closer we paid attention, the more we witnessed the changes in the unfolding. We noticed that the skin was expanding, and the space it outlined was changing. The edges were moving inward and beginning to close. Not only the skin, but the flesh was expanding too. As if the muscle and flesh were growing, with the skin riding on top, on a mission to close the gap. My body was covering my shin bone by itself.

Over the course of weeks, during the consultation visits, the medical staff continued to huddle around to witness the growth. Every visit contained expressions of amazement in what they were seeing. It was pretty fascinating to witness. None of us could believe that all a sudden, after months of bone exposure, that growth started to occur. My body was naturally and organically healing itself.

As we continued to watch over many more weeks, we noticed a point in time when things were no longer changing. The tissue was not expanding up the peak walls as it had before. It was as if the skin and tissue had traveled uphill as far as it could, and then tired and weary could not make it to the top. We were already shocked by what had transpired thus far, so collectively we decided to continue to observe and await what could possibly happen next. If anything. According to the projected timelines, I was already ahead of schedule in my overall recovery, and now there was less bone exposed than before. We patiently waited and continued to watch.

During a consultation visit, we noticed that there was greater instability in the bone that remained exposed on my left shin. We observed that there was a slight movement when enough pressure was applied. There was something on my bone that would give way and move when pushed with a delicate touch of a finger. Eventually, it was discovered that when we thought that the growth had stopped and nothing more was happening, well, we were wrong. Something was definitely happening.

The skin and tissue that was pushing its way up the boney peak decided to take an alternate route; one that was seemingly shorter. The path of the skin and tissue went straight into my bone, forcing its way through my bone. As if ascending the peak was too much effort. Somehow, the growth took a path of least resistance, and cut right through the protective layer of my shin bone in order to reach to the other side. The skin had grown between the inner bone and the periosteum protective layer on a mission to cover my body.

Eventually, the skin and tissue grew through and over my exposed bone, until it could no longer push through the bone. I later had a small operation to brake off the bone covering that proved to be too thick to pass through and remained attached to one edge of my bone. Prior to the surgery, I requested that they save the bone fragments, which they did and gave to me afterwards. I held on to them for a while, and at some point, someone, possibly Quentin, convinced me to get rid of them because they thought it was disgusting. A part of me that honors the experience wishes I would have preserved the pieces of my bones that my eyes once saw instead of listening to the voice of another.

While this took place on my left shin, the same thing was happening on my right shin. My body was working to close the remaining area of exposed bone on its own. My skin and flesh grew and expanded until I was completely covered again. Alas! I was completely closed and covered as a physical body is intended to be.

It was really quite amazing to watch what my skin and tissue were capable of doing, the reactions of the doctors, and the progress of my recovery. I was beating the odds within every experience. Somehow it all continued to work out, in its weird, terrifying, and uncertain way just as it needed to.

I was discharged from the hospital with exposed bones, returned to school with exposed bones, and went out in public with exposed bones, all the while my traumatized nervous system ultimately protected me from feeling any magnitude of pain. I recall it being tender and sore where the remaining muscle and new skin grafts butted up to the bone, but not a debilitating pain worthy of medication to mask it. A blessing among the tragedy.

Have you ever been able to look at your own bones? And feel them? It is strange, and yet I am oddly grateful to be able to reflect on how I watched my miraculous body do what it needed to do to heal. I was able to see and touch my bones, and then watch my body heal and re-cover them before my very eyes. I too was fascinated along with the medical minds as we watched, yet somehow I knew I stood alone in the intense mix of terror, pride, fear, and excitement. I was a mixed bag of unexpected emotions as the miraculous and unexpected events continued to unfold before my eyes. My big beautiful blue eyes.

22

The Grind

The summer was coming to an end, and amidst the hard work and dedication, I was able to walk without a walker. Somewhere along the way while at home, I ceased needing its support. I was still wearing newer versions of the same etelles, but I was able to maneuver around the house on my own. As long as there were no stairs, I was fine. Slow and awkward, but fine. I had no idea how I was going to do it, but school was about to start, and I was determined to be there.

When that day finally came, I was there. There I was, on the first day of my senior year, alongside my friends and fellow classmates. I made it and was actually there. I received a standing ovation at the high school's morning assembly. It was overwhelming, humbling, embarrassing, and even seemed a little silly. I did not feel like I had done anything extraordinary. I believed that everyone would have done the same had they been in a similar situation. I did, however, feel tremendously grateful and loved.

Somehow, I had taken enough credits in prior years, which meant that I was only required to take two courses during my senior year. I am still unsure how I managed to accomplish that since I always took what I thought was required. Even through the uncertainty, I accredited it to a greater force, as it was the perfect amount of time needed to slowly re-enter into a social life and expand the layer of unfamiliarity. It was considerably different from when friends had visited in the hospital and at home. Even so, I felt acceptance within the commonality of our school despite the global diversity amongst us.

A routine naturally began to take shape, and the events seamlessly fell into place. I woke up in the mornings, sometimes due to Quentin's arrival, to begin each day anew. Each day started with eating breakfast and then bandage changing. Once those were complete, physical therapy followed and took place for a couple of hours until it was time to go to school. My Mom generally brought me to school and then picked me up when it was time to return home, but I believe many days she just waited in the parking lot. She was known to do that for much longer durations and under vastly different circumstances. I was only there for a couple of hours, and it was just enough to gain a sense of normalcy and stay within my limited stamina range.

Once back home, physical therapy resumed for about three hours, which was primarily getting my scars massaged; the entirety of both arms and legs. The scar massaging occurred after school because all I had to do was sit there. It was not always enjoyable, but it did feel good on my scars that itched more and more as they continued to heal and mature. It also provided time for me to relax and process the school experiences from right before. After the massages were done, I rested or completed homework until it was time to do more physical therapy and to get ready for dinner. Everything was moving and progressing as I remastered basic survival skills.

Even though I was home and going to school, I was still extremely limited in my self-care, especially wound care. Although I likely could have physically done it, the emotional and psychological wounds it would have left may have become too much to bear. Seeing the wounds was traumatizing enough. Thankfully, it was never expected for me to tend to my own wounds, but I would have if I absolutely needed to, especially before allowing a family member to do it.

I had seen it done more times than desired. I knew how to do what needed to be done. It was all still very overwhelming, even for my family when they accidentally were present during any reveal. It was such a vulnerable and uncomfortable reality that it was never even considered to ask my family to care for my wounds. It was the doctor's decision, but there was a big part of me that didn't want them to be that involved. I never even wanted to allow them in the room, yet often times my experience was approached as though it was everyone's situation especially when I lived in the family room.

There was always a shameful awareness that I continued to be stripped from any autonomy and sovereignty over my body and experience, while I concurrently tried to rebuild a boundary. It was hard to ignore the feeling of powerlessness in my exposure while also trying to give it a voice. Changing a bedpan was as far as it needed to go, and trust me, that was far enough. Quentin became the one to tend to the more intimate, delicate needs as he fulfilled a double roll as a nurse and physical therapist.

By this time, Quentin had become a new member of the family. He was always at the house, always with the family, and joined us for meals if he was around. He had become commonplace within my home and within my family, not to mention the spaces already occupied within me as I healed with his support. He slowly and organically became part of my everything.

The way life was unfolding felt natural, and the path was always pretty clear before me. I knew the journey would be full of hard work and strength and not a physical strength, although that was needed too. I needed the strength of spirit, character, will, and heart. I could sense his presence was rebuilding all those within me. I welcomed his presence. I longed for my growth.

He eventually even took trips with our family since I could not sustain long periods without physical therapy. If too much time passed without physical therapy, my muscles and scars would tighten and become painful. I still had exposed bones on my shins, and I was not in a position to take care of that myself. Being that Quentin was caring for those needs, it made sense to my parents to bring him along on family trips.

Within a month after school started, our family was planning for the school's Fall Break vacation. The family decided to visit home in Louisiana. I think more than anything, my parents, mainly my Mom, needed to be in the presence of their support network from home. They were overcoming their own version of the traumatic experience. In a sense, we all needed a change in scenery and space to recharge. The preparations for the trip also included arrangements for Quentin. He was offered and agreed to travel to Baton Rouge, Louisiana, with my family for a two-week visit. He had never been to the United States before that trip. It was the first of two trips that he joined the family during vacation travels.

On the first trip to Louisiana, I clearly remember the flight over from Belgium. I sat in first-class because it had considerably more legroom. It was decided for me, and unbeknown to me, as a thoughtful surprise. My scars were still very stiff, and my body did not bend comfortably, so I was grateful for the extra space to extend my legs. It was a seven-hour flight, so for optimal comfort, I sat in first class, and the rest of the family, including Quentin, sat in coach.

As I settled into my seat by the window, a well-proportioned man that smelled of alcohol sat in the chair beside me. I quickly put in my earphones and gazed out the window. We had not even taken off, and he had already ordered his first cocktail on the plane. There was no way to know how many hours prior, and how many drinks since the first, but it was obvious that the most recent was just before boarding from the smell of his breath. The moment he sat down, and I smelt the alcohol, I knew it was going to be a long flight.

It did not take long for him to try and strike up small talk. As we taxied down the runway and prepared for take-off, we greeted each other, yet I was not interested in engaging. I was still learning how to engage in my vulnerability and had no interest in learning with this man. Therefore, my replies were short and sweet. Kind and respectful yet very brief and guarded.

I was still wearing the customized braces, and they did not fit into any shoes at the time. On this particular flight, I was wearing Birkenstock sandals over the braces, which could only be fastened with shoestrings connecting the buckles. It was a hideous sight, but I did not care.

Actually, I did care. I cared a lot. I just sucked it up because I didn't have a choice in the matter, only in my response, so I had to not care. I made myself not care. But I cared. I cared deeply. It even mattered that I had to choose to not care so much. Caring is what builds empathy and compassion. I grew up with Care Bears. I most certainly cared. I did not want to bring attention to my attention-grabbing feet.

My pants covered most of my feet, and plus, I was walking. I always reminded myself of the road I had traveled. With that, I tried my best to disregard spoken words, stares or actions that incited anything negative within. I had a younger version of knowing that it was my burden to carry, not someone else's. That alone made me sensitive to social interactions. I had more important things to focus on, and to expend my energy on, other than the looks of my so-called shoes, that housed the braces protecting my feet and attached to legs that have bones exposed. Indeed, I had more important things to focus on. I could sense my shield being slowly constructed around the perimeters of my heart, protecting my emotions as I re-entered into society.

All the while, this man knew nothing of my journey and navigated life differently. Instead of socially engaging and allowing us to meet each other where we were in life, I felt invaded while he pried for personal information. I felt defensive while he assumed I sat open to share. I felt vulnerable while he disregarded my attempts to remain silent. I felt unguarded while I sat alone in first class away from my family. He wanted to ask about my feet and the braces, and I wanted to retreat in shame and embarrassment. Of all things to talk about in life, I definitely did not want to talk about that. He seemed indifferent in my vulnerability and took no consideration to my disinterested expressions, empathized by his drunken mannerisms and what was perceived to be disingenuous curiosity.

After his repeated attempts to engage in conversation regarding my feet, I thought that if I engaged briefly and told him something, it would end the conversation. Too vulnerable and untrusting to expose myself, I replied to the questions he posed by reiterating what he asked. When he posed his first question by asking if I was in a car accident, I told him yes. I quickly slipped my earphones back into my ears and looked out the window in hopes it would end the inquiries.

A little while later, I felt a tap on my shoulder. I looked over, and he was staring at me, waiting for me to remove my earphones. When I did, he followed up on his curiosity with more questions. It was not over. I felt a pause of apprehension as I waited to hear what the next question would be.

He wanted to know who was driving when the car accident occurred. Surprised, and even more uncomfortable that he kept asking questions, it oddly felt safer to continue the fabricated story. Before proceeding with the lie, I even considered the likelihood of ever seeing this man again. With little delay to his inquiry as to who was driving, I told him it was my Dad. Just as astonished as anyone, I once again tried to quickly escape the conversation with my earbuds.

To no avail, he would not let it go. Next thing I knew, I had co-fabricated a dreadful story about my Dad driving when a car accident occurred. He was ejected from the car, and I was not. I suffered from severe burns, and my Dad did not. He feels horrible, and I am now like this. It was awful. Part of the story was brought on by what his nosey inquiries implied. The way he would ask the questions allowed me to play right into the story he expected to hear. I remember him saying, "Wow, I bet your Dad feels horrible about it all." I just played into it each time and agreed with his leading questions, "Yes, he feels absolutely horrible."

The flight was finally over, and when exiting the plane, a stewardess that was greeting passengers upon their eager departures noticed my feet and asked what had happened. In the steadily moving exit line, the length of the actual story did not allow for the truth. Her inquiry also felt disingenuous just by asking such a personal question in the hasty movement of everyone's departure. It felt very inconsiderate. Caught off guard by my own comical disregard of my true sentiments, I said the first thing that came out of my mouth. Since the car accident story did not go as planned, I went with a new one. This time, I told the woman as I shuffled by that I had fallen out of a tree. She looked surprised and tried to get one more question in before too many people divided us and asked what happened to my feet. I tried not to laugh and cry, as I told her that I broke both of them as I tried to break my fall. I walked off the plane, made my way to the gate, and waited for my family.

As we were all walking to the baggage claim, I was telling my Dad about the man and the car accident story. I wanted him to know that if a strange man came up to him and spoke of it, he needed to play along. I explained that I had made up a story about what had happened in response to his unwelcomed drunken curiosity. I also shared the story about breaking my feet when falling out of a tree. Although everyone, including myself, found them comical, I held shame in that I had not been truthful in who I am. As the family requested that they remain informed of character roles in my stories, I vowed to self to never allow it again.

I never did it again. From that moment forward, my rules of engagement were honesty or nothing at all. I was ashamed that the story took such an unexpected turn, all highly influenced by my own inability to process my trauma yet. The experience resonated over the years as the first of many that followed. The experience, and others similar to it, caused awareness of one's genuine concern and innocent compassion versus a superficial and insensitive curiosity. There is definitely a difference. Something I found myself assessing within every encounter when I had to choose not to care about a feeling within. Encounters that supplied materials for the shield unknowingly being constructed around my heart.

Once we retrieved our bags, we were one our way. The car ride from the airport to my Great Aunt and Uncle's house was full of fascination in the sights beyond the windows. I wondered how it would be to see family members, while everything was such a marvel to Quentin. I was reminded of my unencumbered youth while he saw everything as big and spacious, contrary to the tightly built communes of Europe that he was accustomed to experiencing. We arrived at Nanny and Rock's house, who were more like grandparents, and they welcomed all of us with open arms, including Quentin.

As we all settled in, it was quickly evident that it would be the same routine, just a different place. The grind was still very much the same. I woke up, ate, went through bandage changing, completed physical therapy, and then hung out until lunchtime. After lunch, physical therapy resumed and then ended with scar massages. There was time to relax and hang out before dinner, but then it was one more round of physical therapy before the day was over. When we were not sleeping, we were always either changing bandages, doing physical therapy, eating, or taking a break. Although the routine was in place before this trip, and would follow for many months to come, it was while on this trip that the daily grind found its authentic grove. The more I improved, the more natural things became. It felt like if I stayed committed and continued to work through the grind, life would again become easy.

23

My Own Version of Senior Year

It was our senior year. It was supposed to be the most amazing year of my time abroad. I was supposed to enjoy senior skip days, parties, and endless nights out with friends. It was all supposed to end with euro-railing across Europe, which included the infamous trip to the Pink Palace party hostel in Corfu, Greece. I had plans. Big plans.

It was nothing like I had envisioned it to be. It was not at all what I hoped and wanted it to be. I trusted that someone, something greater than me was showing me that Their plan was better, just as I did with the nurses when I took my first steps. I was still not convinced it was better, but I was following my unchosen path the best I was able. That was all I knew how to do as I surrendered to letting go of everything while embracing everything I could. Compelling forces continued to exist within me and around me as

I ventured through senior year. While my friends were embracing their senioritis, I was embracing me in my own new way.

It is interesting that even though I was on campus and at school every day, I only remember a few things from that year; the year that was supposed to be amazing and memorable. It was memorable, alright. I am sure it was great to be among friends in a familiar setting other than a hospital and at home, but that is not what I remember. The school campus had always been a place of joy, laughter, and friendships. Yet, short of the pillow I carried around to soften the hardwood chairs in class, I recall very little about my senior year on school campus among friends.

The memories of my surroundings were likely blurred by the thoughts that raced through my mind. As I traversed the parking lot and into the building for class, my awareness was only on my body and moving it to where it needed to go. With the acute attention and intent focus on each careful step that ensured my gait was held in balance, I was unable to be present in all the passing moments. I still had to think about how to walk.

My two classes were intentionally arranged on the first floor of the main building, so there were no stairs and little traffic, but it was just enough to incite thoughts and emotions. They were not pleasant, but they were healthy and needed as I continued to evolve back into life. It was the groundwork for existing beyond the walls of school when trying to live a healthy life.

With each passing face on campus, it was hard to escape the wonder of how much they knew about what happened. As passerby classmates scanned me from head to toe, I wondered if they realized I was walking beside them with bare bones exposed. I hoped that they knew nothing of it while simultaneously wondering if it was something they should know, needed to know, or would want to know. Since words were rarely spoken, I asked them in silence while in passing, that whichever it may be, simply look the other way. My walk was strange, but I was walking. My gait was lopsided, but I was walking. My feet pointed in with every step, but I was walking. I had to wear braces on both feet, but I was walking. Please, just look the other way. I was just trying to be.

I became acutely aware of people's reactions, and how everyone deals with circumstances differently, approaches things differently, expresses themselves differently. Including myself, and those I knew well. I was thankful that it was in small doses every day and within a supportive community. The school campus became a safe place to reacquaint myself with where my life left off while figuring out how to start growing into the changes before me.

Unexpectedly, one day at school, I was informed of my Homecoming Queen nomination. I do not recall who I voted for, but it surely was not myself. I never engaged in the hype around football and homecoming even though many of my friends were players and cheerleaders alike. I enjoyed the school dances, but that was about it. When I was nominated court Queen, I humbly accepted and pondered the motivation of my classmates to make such an election. There was the Homecoming Court and Queen appointment at the football game, the pre-dance party, and then the celebratory dance. All of which never made any sense to me. It was as if I was just going through the motions and accepting whatever was happening while trying to feel normal. Really, I did not do anything extraordinary. I lived. We were all living. I still did not understand the big deal.

As I continued to accept my senior year as it unfolded, I aspired to do the few things that I could keep doing. One of those was to participate in the school theatrical performance. Once the play *The King and I* was announced, I was cast as Buddha. It was an ideal role given the circumstances although at the time, it had more to do with the part requiring minimal mobility. Decades later after my life was influenced by eastern philosophies it serves as a poetic reflection. I find a tremendous sense of peace in the synchronicity of it all.

Outside of a few school events, I was engrossed in physical therapy and sorting through my reality. So much of me still wanted to have my old like back. I held many silent thoughts and emotions centered around not being who I wanted to become, and not doing what I dreamed I would do. I wanted life to be like it was. More importantly, I wanted my dreams of the future back intact.

As I continued to rebuild my life, piece by piece, the grind went on. During my waking hours, my thoughts were often consumed with physical therapy, and therefore Quentin. As my physical therapist, he was the most capable person to care for me. I know I trusted him the most, and so did my parents. They trusted me more with him than they did with themselves. They also knew that even though I was seventeen, the ballgame changed completely when I got sick. The normal struggles of a teenage girl were now compounded tremendously. They provided the space and freedom to allow me to navigate through every aspect as I needed to, with their love and support, I was free to be.

It was Quentin who showed me the world again. He showed me the world while I stood on my traumatized legs with bones exposed, protected in braces, now bearing my weight which felt like the weight of the world. He was the one that literally guided each physical step when the terrain was unstable; holding my foot secure as I shifted weight. He was the one that re-introduced me to seemingly normal things even though they were tremendously challenging. He helped me every step of the way. The range was endless - from helping my arms swing naturally when walking, to finding shoes that would support the braces, to relearning how to ride a bike, therapeutic horseback riding, physical therapy in a swimming pool, and visiting the beaches and snowcapped mountains. It was a privilege that the experiences took place in Europe, but that did not glamorize nor belittle the very real challenges of my experiences. It was just where I lived at the time. Although every experience may have seemed effortless from the outside, every experience held moments of pain and struggle in the acceptance of my new interaction with the world, and with myself.

All things I had done before were once again before me as I felt forced to embrace them in a new, unfamiliar, and scary way. Quentin helped me through every action, emotion, every thought, every barrier I thought I faced. Why wouldn't I love such a caring person? Why wouldn't I love someone who devoted so much of himself to me? What made me worth such an investment of oneself? I was very broken and damaged. I am forever grateful.

Many months of the grind had passed. It was the same thing every day even though more activities were filling the space. It was always about learning and re-integrating. I was always pushing to become a better version of myself. I just wanted to make the best out of an experience that would never make sense. To break up the monotony of our routine, Quentin requested permission from my parents to take me to the mountains over a weekend. Never sure of what to do, they agreed knowing that he would take care of me. They had almost a year of confidence and trust entangled into their decision of allowance.

I have always loved the mountains. Especially snow-covered mountains. I had never seen them where I came from in Louisiana, and it had only snowed one time by the time we moved overseas at age thirteen. There were definitely no snow-capped mountains in the swamplands of Louisiana, the bayou country of the South. The moment I saw snow-covered mountains for the first time, there was something about nature's beauty that captivated all of my being. There is an innocent beauty in the white covered landscape. I had seen their majestic beauty many times since we moved to Belgium. Before getting sick, I had explored and skied the alps of France and Switzerland. My family had gone on several vacations, and I went every year on the school ski trips. I loved to ski. It had become one of my favorite sports. But that was a different time. As many times as I had been before, it had always been for different reasons and with a different perspective.

This trip to the mountains was different. This time there was a different intended interaction which came with a different perspective. We stayed in a quaint cottage within a small village on the side of a mountain in Switzerland. It was isolated from popular lifts and crowds. It was difficult to walk in the snow and icy grounds, and it was extremely cold since my body struggled to regulate my body temperature. It was oddly perfect in the quiet, private escape.

During the day, Quentin skied for several hours while I rested at the cottage. Upon his return, we cooked, sat in quiet, read, and talked by the warm fire. Although we did the mandatory physical therapy, it was not the focus as it was during the daily grind. Instead, it was a pause to allow life to become the focus. It was still, quiet, and beautifully peaceful.

Most of the time during the day, I sat on the balcony, looked at the snow blanket that covered the undisturbed mountains, and thought about what life had done to me. I thought about what I still wanted to do to life. I thought about everything, and I thought about nothing. I let the thoughts come and go like the breeze on my face. The view was absolutely breathtaking. The air was crisp and cold, and the sounds of nature filled the space, even if with utter silence. While I was alone, feeling the rays of the sun reflect onto my face, and looking at the white snow that covered the world around me, I realized that the white mountains were representative of my life. It was a blank canvas, waiting for a new story to be painted. It was up to me to paint the scenes of my life - the scenes of my new reality.

I sectioned off areas in the landscape and began visualizing still images at the various stages of my life. The early years were easy. Those were memories that molded me. The current was fairly easy as well. My reality was so very blatant. It was the future images that required the most contemplation. The future version of me just wanted to be happy in this new life and new body. It was as if I could dream of an outcome, see it, and if I did not like the way it made me feel, and if it did not feel big enough, I cleared the painting away, and returned to my snow-white canvas to start anew. Dream, and then always dream bigger is what I told myself.

The images were not as important as the concept of being able to paint the images of my future. It was knowing I could change it. I knew this and demonstrated by my vision of walking, but it was during this trip that I gained a level of visual control. This helped me visualize how I wanted to see myself. My life. I would carry this landscape with me throughout my recovery. I referred to it often as I reflected, added, and changed the trajectory of my life through recovery and beyond.

As my friends prepared for their voyage through life, it felt like I was preparing for the voyage of my soul. It was during our senior year, at the young age of seventeen, that I unearthed my soul's internal blueprint of life. It was on the side of snow-covered mountains that on some level I knew that it would be a co-created masterpiece of art.

While I became a master artisan, I had no idea of what I had truly discovered within. I just trusted what I knew I held close in those moments. It was the gift of youthful awareness that I created my reality. Something I knew from the choices we make, but even at that moment, I knew it meant something grander than I could explain. I knew I needed to stay attuned to the blueprint and trusted that it would lead to happiness and love.

24

Mid-Year Exams

My senior year was taking on a life of its own, but it was really just more of the same. There were doctor visits, bandage changing, physical therapy, scar massages, and tests. Even though I was going to school, I probably took more medical tests than I took for school. There was one particular test that required a week-long hospital stay. Just before the Christmas holidays during my senior year, the arrangements were made for the test. It was time to revisit the adrenal insufficiency that caused my skin to tan six months prior.

Recall when I was in the medium care unit, and my doctor asked if I had been sunbathing because my skin looked tan? Well, this was the test to determine the cause of my darkened skin. We had put off the test for six months while other treatments stabilized and phased out. The tests would assess my adrenal gland function, with outcomes that determined the feasibility of future operations. There were two upcoming operations that held the potential to change my life. These were more than just tests of my adrenal glands. It felt like a cumulative exam in the course of life. I really wanted to pass this exam even though there was no such thing. Just living and being was passing.

We already knew that one of the previously diagnosed illnesses was Waterhouse-Fredrickson Syndrome. This is a malady of the adrenal glands. From the onset of my illness when first diagnosed, and for three months that followed, I was given glucocorticoids to support my adrenal glands. My fight or flight response mechanisms needed all the assistance available. Once I was in the Burn unit, awake from the coma in intensive care, and preparing for continued recovery in the medium care unit, the medication reduced over time and stopped. It was shortly after the transfer to the medium care unit that my doctor noticed the symptoms of adrenal insufficiency. They restarted the steroids, and I continued to take them up until the time of the test. The time had come.

The upcoming surgeries required operating on skin grafted tissue, which inherently increases the risk and has a prolonged healing process. Along with everything else to consider, it was critical to reduce or eliminate the steroids from my treatment regimen since they are also known to prolong or compromise healing. The operating surgeon required the tests before scheduling the surgeries.

Once the tests were scheduled, and the time came, I checked into yet another hospital on a Saturday morning. I was prepared to stay a week for testing with the hopes that the truth of my adrenal glands would be revealed. Medical experts say that you cannot live without this gland. It has been proven to produce vital hormones that serve as chemical messengers throughout the body. The unknown was in the extent of damage endured, and whether there was a more appropriate, more specific treatment regimen available. I knew I did not want to continue a medication that did not serve an intended purpose. I already had to promise my doctor that I would take it until the tests were performed.

The tests started and went on throughout the days and nights. I was woken up every four hours for urine samples, and blood draws, and a specific diet for six days and five nights. They stripped me from all medication albeit I was only on the one, hence the reason I had to stay at the hospital so that I could be monitored for any adverse reactions. They controlled everything that went into my body, analyzed every exam and test performed while I played cards in my hospital bed, read books, and watched movies. I did have a roommate for a couple of days, but for the most part, I was just passing the time. I felt fine.

I remember walking down the hall one day, rolling my IV pole in tote, and I was told that I should stay close to my bed and that I should get an aid if I wanted to walk the halls. I always smirked and wondered why they made those comments, however, towards the end of the week, their comments began to make more sense.

After the six days of testing, the doctors came back and yet again, confused while metaphorically scratching their heads. They could not understand the data before them. They went on to explain that I did not have any trace of the oral synthetic steroids in my system, nor was there any trace of organically produced glucocorticoids in my system, and I felt fine. They could not explain why I showed no sign of severe vomiting, dizziness, and fatigue. I showed no sign of withdrawal nor any symptoms of adrenal insufficiency, which was generalized as being violently ill. As the doctors reviewed the test results, everything I displayed was contradictory to what the data dictated should be expected. They had no explanation to provide amid their confusion.

The doctors concluded the week-long testing as unexplainable with a recommendation to continue taking the oral steroids as a precautionary measure. They could not explain anything that the test results revealed, nor willing to encourage me to stop the medication. They had nothing to support a recommendation that stopping the medicine would be beneficial. If anything, they felt it could be detrimental. In honor of their medical oaths of treatment, their recommendation was to continue adrenal gland support with glucocorticoids indefinitely.

The adrenal glands, and the numerous hormones it produces, are generally associated with the fight or flight response, but it is so much more than that. These hormones affect almost every organ and every chemical process in the body. It releases hormones that help the body respond to stress and respond to environmental changes. Both of which seemed pretty critical. Not just for me, but for every human being and for life.

At the time, I did not fully appreciate all that this gland does and how it contributes to the overall survival of the human body. Then, I knew I had survived, and I did not want to rely on medicine if I did not have to. Although I knew we would need a more acceptable long-term plan, I left the hospital accepting the recommendation to continue the steroid treatments. Along with the unsettling medical recommendation, I left with a self-awarded A on my mid-year exam, an A for Another unexplainable event.

I continued the medication through the Christmas holidays and into the new year. Ten months had passed since the medication was started, and a month had passed since the hospital test before I began to challenge the recommendation. Indefinitely did not settle well with me for the long-term. Likely because I knew that meant a life-term. After significant consideration, I decided that taking medicine as a precautionary measure was not an acceptable reason to continue the regimen.

I made an appointment with my doctor, the same one that made the continued diagnosis from my tanned skin. My Dad drove me to her office, and she and I discussed my request to stop the steroids. She was uncomfortable with the idea but remained open to the discussion. We discussed the concerns and the need for a gradual reduction. After an in-depth conversation, my doctor agreed, and we came up with a simple plan. The plan was to systematically reduce the dosage with an agreement to report all changes in sensation. I was naturally willing to agree since we had a plan. I understood and accepted that it would take as long as it took.

I called at the end of every dose reduction to check in and report the activity of the week. I would share the things I did throughout the week and how I felt, and my doctor asked a series of questions. Each call ended with the summation that there were no changes nor symptoms to report. Each time my doctor cleared me to continue weaning off the medication. Once the medication was stopped, I stopped calling. There was no change, nor symptoms, and no apparent continued need for the medication.

Beyond the medical expertise of the testing doctors, it was documented that my adrenal glands are insufficient on paper, while presenting to be functional in reality. Meanwhile, my operating surgeon was satisfied with the findings, and coupled with my decision to cease the medication, he agreed to schedule the surgeries. It was his preparation for these surgeries that grew into my recommendation with every future doctor to use steroids as assistive treatment during stressful medical situations.

My surgeon taught me to advise doctors to take precautionary measures during potentially stressful situations by administering steroids. He indicated that in doing so, doctors would inherently understand the reduction of unexpected events that could occur amid an already stressed state of being. The surgeon of the upcoming surgeries handled it in this manner and planned for sufficient adrenal support during the operations.

Once everything was planned out, my surgeon scheduled the first of two surgeries that would change my life forever. They were surgeries that would correct my walk. They were the surgeries that would allow me to walk on my own legs and feet. Without braces. As ready as I was ever going to be, I began preparing for the next phase of the journey. These would be the most mentally and physically intense surgeries to date. In the summer of 1994, two days after my High School Graduation, I would return to a hospital once again for the first foot repair surgery on my right foot. The second would follow six months later on my left foot. Until then, there was a lot of preparatory work to do.

25

Let Your Light Shine

Shortly after the week-long hospital test for adrenal function, the family packed my suitcase, and we all headed out of town for the holidays. It had been planned many weeks prior, but the time had come for the adventure. I saw it as a time to recalibrate after the extensive mid-term exams.

A short two months after the last trip, my family decided to go on vacation for the second time during my senior year. This time we traveled to Rome, Italy, during the Christmas holidays. With that decision, it meant that Quentin would also join the family. I don't recall being a part of the decision to go on vacation, and I tried not to think about the feasibility of my involvement. I trusted that it would be figured out along the way, similar to the last trip. I was much further along in my recovery and much more capable than the last time I had traveled, and with Quentin present, I felt confident that any physical barrier would be removed.

Although we generally did not travel or vacation with other families, my parents chose differently on this vacation and a close family from our school community would join us. Our family knew them well, and I was close friends with two of their three sons. It was an unexpected, and welcomed surprise. My older Sister, Dina, was also very close to the same two sons. Josh and Chad were like brothers to us, even to my little Sister, Diana. It always felt like brothers and sisters amongst us, so naturally, it would only make the trip more fun. Plus, I had always wanted to go to Rome and had not yet had the opportunity. It was something for me to look forward to in the very real continuance of my recovery that never took a break, no matter where I was.

This trip remains one of the most impressionable trips in my life. There is so much that I remember about this trip because it captivated my senses so intently. My senses got lost in the beauty and wonder in everything around me. Unlike ever before, nor within anywhere I had ever been.

Lights illuminated the winter gloom, Christmas markets buzzed in the streets, and the unbelievable architecture and art history were on display with such magnificence. Our days were filled with museums, shopping, sightseeing, and dining together for almost a week. I really enjoyed the carriage rides and shopping at the Christmas markets. A piece of memorabilia that I still possess is the menu from a restaurant where we celebrated life and broke bread together as one. My Mom later framed it as a memento from abroad, eventually passing it along to me. I hold a lot of memories from this trip.

The most impressionable experiences of this trip occurred within Vatican City. To my youthful self, it was the most sacred space to visit. As a born and raised Catholic, there was always this idea that the Pope was as close as one could physically get to God. As we entered the Vatican City, there remained a sacredness to the roads beneath my unstable feet. There was a veil of honor that filtered the experiences as I contemplated my own relationship with God and my sense of questionable faith. There was something very surreal about the experiences within the sacred space decorated to celebrate the birth of Christ. I, too, felt reborn into a new state of existence.

Although I questioned my own beliefs, I humbly admired and respected that of those around me, and of what was before me. As we ushered in for Christmas mass, my prayer remained the same in the infinite ethers within. I trusted that I would one day know the truths in God and my purpose to serve. I remained patient for understanding the purpose of my continued survival. I prayed I would one day understand why I was the chosen one to journey a path that I would have never chosen for myself nor another.

During the Midnight Mass in St. Peter's Basilica, I was captivated by the elegant voice of Pope John Paul II as he offered his blessings in Polish. Even though I could not understand a single word, it felt like I knew the message he was delivering. It was one that I knew from my upbringing and one that became intuitively molded into my own interpretation. It was my message within that resonated with the voice of the Pope even though language separated us in the moment.

Our families were also privileged to be included in a private papal audience. It was a tremendous honor to see and shake the gentle hands of the Pope as he spoke blessings upon us. Our families and the rest of the small audience huddled around to receive his sacred energy. As I witnessed all of us receiving his blessings, I felt oddly at peace in my spiritual confusion. I settled into the idea of my physical proximity with God, and I concurrently honored my truth that a connection to God did not have to go through another human. That moment molded my belief that if there were a God, then I would be in direct contact. With a guarded and confused spirituality, I embraced all that was around me and chose to be a part of the blessings. They were blessings that allowed my memories to remain pure and not tainted with the hardships I was enduring. Amid tragedy, it was a very special time. There was a deep sense of honor and gratitude.

One afternoon we were enjoying the sights from the streets in Rome. It was a cold and windy day, but what I remember most about the weather was that the sun was shining so brightly. While exploring cobblestone streets, there were many times when my legs became tired and either Josh, Chad, or Quentin would give me a piggy-back rides to give my legs a rest. I used a wheelchair when visiting museums and places as such, but on the streets, I either walked or was assisted by means of a piggy-back ride. It was during our walks on the streets when I noticed something occurred.

It was during the transitions between modes of transportation that something changed in my sight. It was a change so apparent that it caught my attention every time. The occurrences in Rome were not the first, but they happened so frequently on our short trip that it became the example of the collective. It must have been the golden rays of the sun that illuminated the sacred cities for me to see the experiences for what they truly were.

As my feet settled into walking, my view shifted. I saw with my eyes, but the view became one of me, looking down below and upon me. It was not a mental image that I could redirect elsewhere. It was through my eyes yet from above. I was seeing through the body that was walking, but I was me from above watching me walk below.

It was a view only known through my eyes as I floated higher than the rooftops. I looked down upon myself, watched myself walk, and interact with the world around me. I always saw myself from behind, and I was never drawn to look elsewhere. My eyes were on me, and because I was above, I could not see what was before me, yet somehow, I could always see what was coming.

This used to happen quite often after I got sick, especially when I was mobile. I always took note of the experience and then carried on my way. I never put much thought into it, and certainly never linked it to my own mortality and the truths behind the journey of my soul. Even when I unknowingly was taking flight after this trip, I acknowledged and dismissed it as if I had already reserved a memory slot for the experience. It was preserved without choice with an understanding that would reveal its purpose later.

It took years of life to acquire the understanding and language to unpack and filter my experiences with enough kindness, patience, and love for self to arrive at the space of acceptance. I unknowingly allowed my soul to take flight in full control to keep my body alive since it was clearly not my body's time to cease breath. It was how I navigated through the tremendous pain that was experienced on all levels of existence - physically, psychologically, emotionally, and spiritually. I left my body while my consciousness floated above.

It was a humbling truth to accept that in order to survive, my soul left my body, and allowed the physical being the space to do what was needed. On this trip, when my body needed to walk, my soul left my body. As the truths revealed themselves to me over the years that followed, I became intrigued as to what anchored my soul for safe return. I became curious about the level of choice I really held, for I did not choose my illness, nor for my soul to leave my body. Or did I?

It was in the unexplainable that I found I had to trust the most because if there was a purpose for all this, I had to trust that there was a Maestro conducting a masterpiece. I had to trust, that somehow, my brokenness of many pieces was a masterpiece itself. I wanted so deeply to feel and be a part of the universal masterpiece. In a shallow way, I knew I was, but I wanted to feel it. I wanted to know this truth deeply. Being a mystical part of the masterpiece in my brokenness was the only storyline that made sense. It felt like I needed it to be true. So, I believed without knowing, as I floated in and out - serving as my own guardian angel looking down upon myself as I walked my life in uncertainty.

The more I recovered, the less frequent the occurrences became, or at least in my awareness. For many years my lack of attention created experiences that would later require me to reconcile my truths. As days and years passed, I sensed deeply that the truths were working to set me free. Throughout life, these experiences remained some of the most prominent memories. They contributed to the uneasiness of what I later discovered was an untethered soul.
It took decades of devotion, patience and resolve as I waited for my time to voyage the journey that would anchor my soul within the physical realm of my existence where I belong. Where I am. Until then, I floated along.

26

A Graduation Gift for Life

Senior year had come to an end. I graduated with my senior class, received a standing ovation as I was assisted up the stairs and across the stage to accept my diploma, and Headmaster's award. With braces shoved in high-top basketball shoes, barely hidden under my wide-legged pants, Robin held my hand and provided the strength I needed when my name was called. He likely is still unaware of the magnitude and depths of the strength he offered in that moment. Not only to make it up the stairs without falling, but the strength to actually take action and do it.

There was a tremendous amount of strength and courage needed to accept the support and love being shown, and the expression of acknowledgment in what I had achieved. It still felt silly, and that I did not do anything extraordinary. I was simply doing my best to recover the best I knew how. That was likely when I began to learn that the allowance to be loved takes tremendous strength. To love deeply, in return, takes an equal amount of courage. It felt like I had neither yet walked my body along in overwhelming confusion while supported by both from others.

It had been a year that was nothing like I had envisioned it to be. And although I had accomplished so much, there was still a yearning for things to go back to the way they were. A sense of a life lost and experiences missed. While everyone was planning for senior parties and the senior celebratory adventures, I was preparing for the first of two surgeries to correct my feet. Parties and European excursions were part of my original plan, and it sounded much more exciting than the surgeries in my new life plan.

Two days after graduation, I was admitted to another hospital in preparation for the surgery the following morning. While friends were starting the next phase in their life, so was I. For most, it meant university studies, settling into a new phase in life and a new sense of freedom. I had always dreamed of the day that I would move out of the house and start university. I suppose I was doing the same, university of life, new phase of life with a sense of freedom from braces. The summer after graduation turned out to be the time and space for many things to change. It turned out to be a summer of separation, and not just from the braces that allowed me to walk.

It was this summer when the real separation began. Separation from the me I was before. Separation from the trauma endured. Separation from the only real community I ever knew. Separation from the only group of friends that I really had in my life and the only group of friends that I felt knew, accepted, and loved my authentic self. Separation from the old me and the community that supported me through the transformation into the new me and my new state of existence. And after the first surgery, separation from my family while confronting the new experiences alone. I had to take one thing at a time.

I had lost so much muscle in my legs and had been wearing braces for over a year. During that time, the curvature of my right foot was bending more and more inward. The muscles were contracting inward, but there were no muscles contracting in the opposing direction to straighten my foot back out, similar to the mobility limitations of my feet in the upward and downward motions. The surgery would serve a dual purpose and correct this issue in my right foot, whereas both feet would benefit from the elimination of the drop-foot.

Being that my right leg and foot were the most traumatized and the weakest of my lower limbs, it was the first to receive the surgery. Although also extremely traumatized, my left leg had less overall tissue and muscle loss and was better able to endure the first round of support. While the right leg and foot recovered, my left leg would become my primary leg for mobility with the use of crutches. My left foot would follow six months later, giving my right foot plenty of time to heal so it could support my left foot during a similar journey.

I had mentioned that we would find a unique way to resolve my falling foot, and anything, everything, was worth consideration. Collectively, we figured there was nothing to lose by exploring all possibilities. I would much prefer to try and have the worst possible outcome than not try and wonder about the best possible outcome. And this time, I was aware of what needed to be done. I was now a part of the discussions on how to achieve it. I had a say in what was happening. This experience inevitably would influence all future encounters with medical professionals throughout my life.

Dr. Vanderkelen, the head surgeon, the same one that fought to save my legs, was friends with a hand surgeon, Dr. Hoang. I was never sure of the scope of their friendship nor even how I came up in their conversations. Even so, they discussed my case. Together they reviewed possible solutions that could permanently fix the drop foot that prevented me from walking without braces. They also discussed the possibility of maximizing any muscles that remained intact.

The hand surgeon had been challenged with similar circumstances of the hand, and although slightly different, the concept was the same for the foot. He believed that if they could find one muscle that remained completely intact, that muscle could be used to lift and flex my foot. If one intact muscle existed, it could be rerouted to perform the needed function. It would require retraining the muscle in its new role, but it could be done. Dr. Hoang had performed many surgeries like this on the hand, and he had seen it work. He believed it could work on the foot as well.

Long before the surgery was scheduled, we began assessing my feet and legs to determine which muscle could serve that purpose, if any. In each leg, among the almost twenty muscles between the knee and ankle, I had only one fully intact muscle. The lone muscle was the tibialis posterior muscle, which is a relatively small and slender muscle that is nestled against the bone, under the many layers of the calf. It travels down the back of the leg, with a tendon that wraps under the ankle bone and secures to the arch of the foot. This particular muscle contributes to overall stability in the ankle, yet it is one that is rarely isolated and used independently. It was the only muscle I had to make the only movement I could make. I miraculously had the one muscle is each leg needed for the recommended surgery.

The hope was that these lone working muscles would give me a lifetime of walking without braces. It was proposed that rerouting the muscles would allow me to flex my feet, clear each step, and walk on my own without assistance. I had to decide that it was unnecessary to understand how each leg and foot could operate with one muscle and perform the lifework of many. I had to trust and believe that my muscle would endure, and it would be so. It felt easy to believe in the unbelievable.

Once my miracle muscles were isolated, physical therapy included specific exercises that would build their strength and endurance. They had a lifetime of work to do. While I was busy strength building, my medical team was busy securing a surgeon to perform the operation. Not only did a surgeon have to agree to the recommendation, but they also had to agree to operate on my severely fragile and traumatized skin grafted body. That was riskier than the surgery itself. Finding a competent, trustworthy, and willing surgeon was not an easy task.

When it comes to managing my health, there is a lot to consider, a lot to understand, and a lot to risk. Especially when it involves surgery on a skin grafted body, coupled with autoimmune deficiencies; both of which intrinsically elevate risk factors. Then, everything was still so new and in discovery. Everything about my medical state had to be considered even more. That was one of the challenges they knew they faced even then — the challenge of finding a doctor willing to perform the very risky surgeries. Dr. Hoang appeared unburdened by the risk and aided in reaching a solution. He became a team member committed to improving my quality of life.

Through the many discussions, Dr. Hoang, the hand surgeon, was approached to consider fulfilling the role himself. The request was that he perform the sophisticated surgery that he himself had recommended. My doctor expressed that he was the most qualified, and most capable, and reminded Dr. Hoang of his own validation that the foot and hand are similar in function. Dr. Vanderkelen may have even shared his own situation when confronted with taking the risk to save my legs. Perhaps it was the truth behind the risks already taken, which allowed for a new risk to be taken in continued faith.

All of us felt there was nothing to lose while holding tremendous faith that it would work. It was really the only option we had at that time. Somewhere and somehow along the way, Dr. Hoang made a life-changing decision. He agreed to perform the surgery himself. Although he had never performed surgery on a foot, he knew the concept was the same, and he felt confident that it would work. He became the hand surgeon that agreed to transform my feet.

Dr. Vanderkelen, the head surgeon of the Burn unit in a sense faced the same challenge and found within himself to take the risk. Dr. Hoang, the hand surgeon, made the same decision and agreed to do the surgeries on my feet. The only common factor I could see was me. They both chose to fight with me, and for me. Because Dr. Vanderkelen took the initial risk to save my legs, Dr. Hoang was able to take the next risk to transform my feet, and the infinite possibilities made it bound to work. Dr. Hoang was so confident in his ability, and the success of the surgery that it became the obvious choice.

In order for the procedure to be a success, the surgeon had several steps to follow. Although most familiar to the hand, he prepared for the operation on my right leg and foot. First, he had to detach the tendon from the arch of my foot. The plan was to then, from behind, pass the tendon through the opening between the tibia and fibula bones in the shin. There is a natural space between these two bones, but it was too narrow, so the medical team had to widen the window. It was critical to create a clear and smooth path for the tendon to pass, and to do so without creating friction. Once the opening was widened, and the tendon was passed through, the surgeon drilled a hole through one of the cuneiform tarsal bones in the center of my foot. The tendon was then passed through the hole to the bottom of my foot. The tendon was fed through the hole, extended out the bottom of my foot, and held in place in place with a button. A plastic button just like a button from a jacket. A big plastic button. I had just received a complex and sophisticated surgery, and it was all being held in place with a plastic button.

While the button held the tendon in place on the bottom of my foot, a metal horseshoe-shaped clamp was wedged around the cuneiform bones on the top of my foot. The clamps held the tendon in place from above and the button from below, while my bone closed in on the tendon. I crutched around as I waited for the hole to heal, and I could begin walking upon my foot. In the meantime, it was all about the exercises in preparation to do so.

The hole in my bone took about three months to heal closed and to completely secure the muscle into its new home. During that time, physical therapy consisted of the same scar massaging and modified physical exercises, but the main focus switched, once again. This time, it would take an interesting turn. One that I knew was coming, one that was part of the overall plan of how this would ultimately work, and one that would be the underlying element that would make the surgery either a success or failure. This is where my ultimate focus would be for the next year. First, with the right foot, then with the left.

Before the surgery, one of the many exercises in physical therapy revealed that when I contracted the muscles normally used to flex my foot, the remaining fragments would contract even though no movement would occur. I had lost the overlaying muscles, and the extensor digitorum longus muscle, the foot flexing muscle primarily used when walking and climbing stairs. The small section of this muscle that remained would oddly contract when trying to perform the movement. The muscle was not intact, and I witnessed the cell memory of a muscle movement that once used to flex my foot. Whenever I tried to flex my foot, the muscles, albeit not functioning, remembered the automatic contractions to flex my foot and would twitch in attempts to perform as before. This would play a critical part in the recovery of the surgery.

The next phase in the foot surgery recovery required the coordination of many functions. The exercise would make use of the muscle memory without function, the functioning muscle that had been rerouted, the memory of how to contract the muscle before rerouted, and the re-association of all of them into the task of walking. I basically had to retrain my brain as it related to these muscles, and what their new function would become in order to walk. It turned into a mastermind game. I was mastering the mind in every sense of the word. I had to retrain my brain and muscles on how to walk anew.

After figuring out how to do this, which took considerable time and focus, it was unbelievable. If I contracted the muscle which before moved my foot sideways, because of where it was now attached, when contracted, it pulled my foot upward in the flexing motion. So, if I thought to contract my foot sideways, my foot would actually flex and pull up. Over time, the foot flexing muscle fragments that would contract with cell memory began to automatically contract in sync with the new rerouted muscle with every practiced contraction.

In the end, if I think to flex my foot, the muscle fragments contract, perform no function, and my foot flexes from the new muscle. It was unbelievable. It actually worked. My foot was capable of flexing again. The real test would be if it was enough to clear a step. Of course, it would be. Everything had fallen into place since this all began a year prior. It was part of my intended journey to be able to walk again. It had to work.

Soon it was time to start bearing weight and exercising the muscle movements with the actual task of walking. I was nervous and hopeful. I was scared and proud. Everything was as perfect as it could be. It was everything that it needed to be. The new muscle lifting my foot was just enough for me to clear each step. My right foot was able to function and walk on its own. It was small, but it was enough. It was enough to clear a step.

When I threw my right brace in the garbage was when it truly felt like I celebrated my graduation. In a sense, I had graduated from one life and was entering into a new phase of my journey. Albeit considerably different than I had hoped for, it felt exhilarating just the same.

From the time of the surgery and for three months that followed, my foot could not bear weight while the bone was healing. I used crutches to get around, and although it was often against my will, I relied on many in my daily navigations. Once I was able to start walking on my foot, it was only able to do so during physical therapy sessions. For a couple of more months that followed, I used the crutches whenever outside of the home.

I was able to enjoy about three weeks of walking without crutches, and on my new foot, before it was time for the second operation. A lot transpired between the two surgeries. Not just with bone healing, muscle strengthening, and walking, but in healing, strengthening, and walking within my new existence. As life continued to unfold around me, I continued my journey to heal and grow into the new version of me.

27

Summer SOULstice

It was the summer right after my high school graduation, and I was recovering from the muscle transfer surgery to correct my right foot. In the midst of it all, my family was preparing for a big transition. During my senior year of recovery, my Dad received word from his employer that his overseas assignment had come to an end. It was time for the family to return to Louisiana. The five-year adventure abroad was over. We likely had a family pow-wow to receive the information, but there was no discussion to be had. It was a fact. There was no option other than to follow suit. Movers packed our home furnishings to begin the trek across the Atlantic, we moved out of our home, and into a furnished apartment.

It all unfolded so quickly around me, yet I felt I was moving in slow motion, enhanced by my slow pace with the crutches. Oddly, the rapid changes and adjustments that I had navigated throughout the year prior with trauma somehow made it easy to sway with the ebbs and flows of life. I did not feel a part of it, but I drifted along with it. It was this sensation that always gave a sense of being carried, in the most peaceful and graceful interpretations of meaning.

As I floated along in the gusts of everyone around me, I never felt committed to the actions of returning to Louisiana. I never entertained the notion that I was leaving. It was not in defiance. It was in clarity and certainty. It was the same factual truth that sourced the notion that I would walk again. I knew I would stay. I never thought of how it would be so, I only knew the truth that I would.

The time came and my Mom and little Sister headed back to the United States. I do not recall the details of all that transpired, but my Dad ended up flying my Mom and little Sister back to Louisiana to start life anew. All I knew at the time was that the immediate plan was for my Dad to return my Mom and Sister to Louisiana, and then come back to Belgium to close out final affairs. At some point, I said goodbye, not knowing when I would see them again. And that was it. They left, and my Mom and Sister never looked back.

My Dad was scheduled to return to settle affairs and to be present through my medical requirements. While he brought my Mom and Sister to their new home, I stayed behind. It was unrealistic for me to leave with them since I was still recovering from the surgery. It was also unrealistic for me to stay alone in the apartment. It had been eight weeks, and I was still unable to bear weight on my foot. I used crutches and needed assistance with most things, not to mention the continuous, albeit modified, priorities of physical therapy, bandage changing, and medical observation. Those requirements, and my medical team, the ones that saved all parts of me and my life throughout the past sixteen months, were the very reasons that made my continued stay the most logical option.

While preparing for my stay during the transition of my family, suddenly, seemingly out of nowhere, the most unexpected person entered my life. It was the presence of someone at precisely the right time that made most sense in the storyline of unexplainable events. It could have been anyone, yet it was Kelda. The fact that it was Kelda made the unexpected gift even more lovely.

I knew of Kelda. She was a student at the same international school. She was two years older, the same age and class of my Sister, and they were friends. I knew of her more through sports than I did through my Sister. Even so, I did not really know her. I had never spoken to her other than a cordial greeting. She had graduated two years prior with my Sister and remained in the Brussels area. We also held common friends within my graduating class that she was still in contact with over the summer before they departed on their ways. I do not know how she learned of my need for assistance, but there she was ready to serve in any way she could. She reached out and offered to stay with me at the apartment while my Dad traveled to Louisiana with my family. Surprised and mystified of how she knew of my need, I graciously accepted her extremely kind offer.

Kelda prepared for the arrangements, and we spent two weeks together. She spent every night in the apartment. She prepared meals for us, walked with me while I crutched around the block for physical therapy exercises, we watched movies, and played games in the evenings. She taught me how to make a delicious banana milkshake and spiced orange pomander balls, which are oranges with clovers pushed into the rind creating a natural air freshener. We made so many of these while she stayed with me.

I remained deeply touched that she mysteriously, yet perfectly became a part of my journey, especially when her journey ended too soon. A short year and a half later, while exercising on a treadmill, Kelda returned to her true home. I recall when I received the news and mourned the loss alone. I am fortunate to have known her and to have spent so much quality time with her precious and authentic spirit. She was so kind and selfless in her actions.

I was always intrigued by her unique beauty, her inner, peaceful, and genuine beauty, coupled perfectly with her unique facial features brought on by her mixed nationalities. She became an example of authentic beauty, inside and out. I always celebrate her as part of my life journey and how she touched my soul while she walked her life on this earth. She was a dear and close friend to so many others whom I do not know well, and yet I feel connected to them through having known her. Kelda's spirit dwells within each of us and connects our human hearts.

This encounter marked my awareness of my interpretation of a soul connection. I only understood it in the awareness of my youth, but it was enough for me to know that it was a connection within another plane of existence and brought into my experience for a purpose. The prior year of recovery, leading to those moments with Kelda were full of moments where this truth was blasted before me. Even so, my focus remained in the physical experience with my body but I remained aware and attuned.

After the appearance of Kelda, I was able to more clearly identify the other souls that appeared for me to serve, or to receive service from. Those mysteriously placed to save and heal me, the unexplainable encounters with encrypted-like messages all bearing clear evidence in the spiritual alignment of perfection. The most sacred were those sent to mold my heart and to grow me in love. Each known for the teachings, from past, present, and the duration of future breath.

There was a deep sense that the souls would teach me the lessons needed to gain an understanding of why it was me and what it was I was destined to uncover.

I had always believed that when it is my time, it shall be so. I wanted to understand what made it not my time, especially since within the space between, my physical body actually ceased breath, twice. I did not want to understand through physical, scientific, and medical explanations. I wanted spiritual explanations. I saw Kelda as an Angel gracing me with more than just her physical presence in a time of need. She was a gift from the ethers of my faith, inviting me to lean into my beliefs. Whatever they were. It was this connection that opened my eyes to the eyes of the souls that were sent to teach me. As long as I stayed honest and attuned, I trusted they would lead me to understanding.

28

Tested Faith

    The medical trauma challenged my physical experience down to every cell in my body. Literally and figuratively. I was unable to escape the truths of the trauma to my body, but the trauma was much deeper than I could even process during those times. I was also aware that it was changing me emotionally and psychologically, merely from their forced involvement. While my mind was clearly managing my emotions and acutely focused on my body, I was never quite clear on how my spirituality was transforming.

I was aware of its presence in the perimeter of every moment, floating in bubbles of seeming perfection. It oftentimes felt like I did not have the energy to do anything else but to acknowledge the perfection and have faith. It may have been disconnected and ridden in doubt, but it was faith. I just had to trust that it was enough, and I would get through everything and get back to life.

And then I did. I was living again. It was a modified life, but I was living. It was when I went back to living that my spirituality just lingered. Although it was experienced in the youthfulness of who I was, my spirituality lingered in the background of life while I remained attuned to the experiences and souls that would lead me to truth and understanding.

Within days of my Dad's return, and what turned out to be my final farewell to Kelda and her compassionate soul, I chose to lean into my beliefs. It always felt that it was Kelda's spirit that gave me the strength to find courage in my spiritual honesty. It was after she stayed with me that I leaned into my shattered faith while stripping myself naked within.

I had no clue where to source my beliefs, and at times, I had to balance the Atheist thoughts with the truths of my experiences, even those leading up to my illness. The storyline of my life was crystal clear - before, up to, and beyond my illness. Everything continued to fall into its place of precision once it was time to wake up. It took decades for me to discover the truths at the source of my evolving awareness.

During the passing hours of the days, I spent a lot of time in inward reflection, even when going about my day. There were so many unexplainable events, so many mysteries and miraculous findings. There were gaps in understanding, doubt when trusting blindly, fear that everyone was wrong, and there was nothing beyond us at all. It was very overwhelming and almost paralyzing to entertain for my youthful and unevolved being. There was a life of precision leading up to each continued breath that reflected a path that seemed intended. I just wanted to make sense of it all. I was confident that I did not intend for this to happen. Or did I? Did you? Did God? My life replayed over and over in the background, looking for clues while I crutched forward and discovered my seemingly intended life.

I was accomplishing so much, and I finally started to act human again, even though nothing about me felt human. Maybe subhuman, or superhuman, I was not quite sure, although I hoped for the latter. It felt like the clarity resided beyond what any human could explain, although they continued to try even without an inquiry from me. It felt like everyone sought similar answers that were beyond any of us yet could only be found within each of us, independently.

Within a four-year timespan, from age thirteen to seventeen, I transformed from a mindless believer to a cautious observer to an almost Atheist, to a nervous and guarded believer, in something. I have always been very aware of my spiritual space, no matter how accepting, inquisitive, humbled, abandoned, quieted, or guided it may have been. Honoring the truths in my spirituality was something that I struggled with immensely for a long time, even while being taught the Catholic doctrine in my childhood, but especially after my illness. It was a struggle that I never spoke about with anyone. I never knew how to talk about it in my youth, especially within the spaces of the deeply rooted faith of my parents and the generations before them. Then one day, it became too much, and somehow, I found the words. It was the mystical presence of Kelda that gave me the strength to lean into my broken beliefs.

My Dad had already returned my Mom and little Sister to Louisiana, and it was just my Dad and me in the apartment. One Sunday morning, I heard my Dad approaching as I was standing in the kitchen, balanced on one foot with crutches while trying to prepare something to eat. I had just placed my food on the other side of the counter and was leaving the kitchen when my Dad stopped me in the hallway. He said he wanted to ask me something. I could tell he was unsure of his delivery, yet it was somewhat masked by his directness. Standing face to face, inches apart, he asked me if I wanted to join him at morning mass. I will never forget the look on his face when he paused for me to answer. I informed him that I would not be joining.

In that moment, I decided that I was not going to pretend anymore. I was not going to pretend that I understood that my struggles were for a greater purpose. I was not going to pretend that I was not suffering spiritually. I was not going to pretend that I didn't feel betrayed. I felt very betrayed. Betrayed by the very Deity that he taught would forever protect me. I was not going to go sit somewhere and have someone else tell me how I should feel. This was between me and my God. No one else was invited, and I did not have to go anywhere to address it. We were addressing it within. It was alone and in the privacy of our sacred connection, even though it was one based on confusion and doubt. I prayed there was a God hearing my cries that echoed throughout the ethers within.

My Dad listened to me proclaim the reasons why my faith was challenged. It was incomprehensible to him as to how I could speak such words when we had all just witnessed the many miracles that proved the power of faith and prayer. I know. I lived it. I agreed in the power and truth of my reality, but that was not it. I never doubted that truth. In fact, I clearly saw the perfection in everything.

In truth, that was the most overwhelming aspect of my illness to process — the overwhelming sense of perfection from the spiritual planes of existence. I just wanted to know why. Not so much why me, but more so why did I live. I felt more honored that there was a sacred mission designed for me than concerned about the sorrows of my reality that I could not change. Why. I wanted to know the purpose of why I continued to live, and I wanted The One, The God, My God to communicate it to me.

Although every word I spoke was more and more foreign because of his own unwavering faith, he accepted my sentiments. Heartbroken and in tears, my Dad left me at the apartment while he went to mass alone. I am sure he prayed heavily about me that morning at mass. I am sure he prayed many days about my faith being restored. He would later influence my understanding and acceptance of a different, more fulfilling kind of faith and spirituality. One that would not have a voice for many years to come.

I knew it was healing in the background of my existence. The fact that it was not in the forefront of my experiences became the indicator that it was not time. At varying levels along the way, I must have known the very sacred, scary, and vulnerable process to overcome merely because it would require complete surrender to gain the fullest potential of what it could bring. I did not understand what that would mean, but I knew that it was a truth to be honored. I waited for my time. My time with my God. I waited in the ethers of my faith.

Although I did not perceive myself to believe in God, I trusted so deeply within the ethers of my faith that I truly believed that whatever powerful force continued to align my life would certainly not abandon nor betray me now, not after all that we had been through together. I became more and more accepting of the very evident truth that it had never been, nor would it ever be so. I always trusted, for whatever unexplainable reason, that I was always where I needed to be, doing what I needed to be doing. I never needed convincing of this truth. As long as I kept crutching forward, I would get where I needed to be and become whomever I needed to become, and it would somehow be my perfect contribution to the masterpiece of our collective experience.

I was no longer running around my lake, but it was the same sense of moving forward with intention. Only the intention had shifted, and I was on crutches. Still moving forward just at a slower pace and more focused. There was a desire to discover the journey that would make this worth my time here on earth. The journey would encapsulate the answers to the deep and dark questions of why my continued existence was so important. It felt sacred and overwhelming. I believed in time I would learn what was so unbelievable and amazing that would make my trauma make sense. I wanted to know what it was that I would bring to the world in this unbeknown, yet purposeful masterpiece. It felt like there was something powerful within that would need to get out. During my final year abroad, it felt like I was the powerful being that needed to get out, set free from the cage where I had become entrapped. The cage of my physically traumatized body.

It was a journey I knew would take place, and it was a journey that would heal my spiritual brokenness in whichever way it was intended. When the time and space were right, I would know. I continued my conversations within the ethers of my faith until the spiritual path was illuminated, and I could choose to walk it, or not. I desired enlightenment. I dreamed for enlightenment. I prayed for enlightenment. Even at the youthful age of seventeen, I knew enlightenment meant levels of understanding that I could not yet fathom. I believed that my mind would be sound if I could achieve enlightenment. Somehow in my naive unknowingness, I knew I was practicing patience for enlightenment. What I did not know of were the magnificent truths that awaited discovery. Not just by me, but by humanity as a collective.

Until that time, I quietly prayed, I begged, I pleaded into the ethers of my faith. My inner cries echoed throughout the infinite space within...

Is anyone, or anything, out there?

Is there a God behind the truths of who I am and my purpose here?

If so, please, please show me the way on this dark and baron road.

My light is not bright enough to find my own way.

I am trusting but please know this does not come easy.

I trust, but my doubt makes it feel empty, so I nervously continue to do my best.

Please do not betray me. I will be forever shattered if you do. I have already felt abandoned and betrayed in my humanness.

I am listening and following the best that I am able.

I vow to remain open and aware to the messages embedded within my life experiences.

I will love and be kind and forever go in peace, please just make this life easy since I am still here and must now live like this.

Please have mercy on my soul and be gentle with my mind, body, and heart.

I am fragile in my brokenness and weary at heart.

I pray that all I do and all that I become is good enough and deserving of the most glorious and magical life experiences, for I feel worthless and shameful in this body.

For that is why I am still here, is it not? To enjoy this life?

To shine my light and experience the magic in life? I love magic.

Please help me love this new life.

Please help me love me.

I will forever hold hope and faith in love.

29

Who Am I?

As the summer of 1994 came to an end, and my Dad and I finalized our arrangements, I held my silent questioning and patient desires close within. As everything unfolded, it was more and more clear that I would journey forward alone. My Dad would leave, and I would stay. There was never a doubt in my mind that I would stay in Belgium until everything was considered complete. We all knew it would never be complete, but the physical therapy and medical interventions as they related to the illness would eventually be complete. It was not that time. It was not complete.

I recall requesting my Dad to really think about what was being asked of me. With the truths before us, there was no way I could leave. Not if I was still recovering. I had been told that if I was in the United States, my legs would have been amputated at the waist; the very legs I was walking upon. It was a truth brought on by fear from a societal notion that if a risk was taken, and the outcomes were less than what was perceived as favorable, then the family would seek restitution. I had two surgeons that were hesitant to move past the fear in the face of that very real risk, but they had.

There was no way I was going to move back and build up trust and understanding with a new team that had no idea of what I had experienced while standing nervous in the uncertainty and risks and hope they would have the strength to choose me. There was no way I was going to risk all parts of my fragile being while others prodded and experimented in the newness before them. No way. What they were expecting of me was unconscionable in my mind. Although it seemed that my physical body could endure anything, I knew I did not have the psychological nor emotional strength to endure the wonderment beyond medical expertise again; they were both still recovering from the first round. I perceived moving as more trauma and I simply wanted the trauma to stop even though, on so many levels, it felt like it never would.

I am grateful that my Dad understood. He knew my Mom would understand, or at least he believed he could explain it in such a way that she might. My Mom always claimed that she thought I was returning home and that I somehow convinced my Dad to let me stay once she was gone. I can understand how that may have been the perception, but I never saw it that way. I knew I was staying long before the surgeries were scheduled, and when it was known that they would be six months apart. I knew then I would be in Brussels until the end of the recovery from both. I knew I was not leaving. I couldn't. I wouldn't.

Somehow, I guess that was not completely evident until it was time for me to actually leave to return to Louisiana, and I did not go. I stayed. The unknown was in the silent swells of emotion that crested with the truths that my Mom was not there and present with me, for me, beside me, in any way. We both felt it yet never spoke of it, nor labeled it. We never even told each other goodbye. She saw me as her fragile child, a sacred being birthed from her womb while I saw our tethered chord stretch across oceans. I was her vulnerable and broken child while I was focused to get on with life. I truly believed that I was not going to die therefore I knew I would be fine. I also knew I would see her in six months for the next surgery, if not sooner. The overwhelming emotions that had continued to swell for sixteen months, and over time had made me numb, somehow, shielded and protected my heart, emotionless without my own Mom. While I recovered oceans away from my Mom, I rested safely in the care of another. A gifted Mom at just the right time.

Everything aligned once again, and the details fell into place for my extra year without my family. Physical therapy schedules were set, I was enrolled in a post-graduate course as part of a thirteenth year in high school, room and board were arranged, and there was a means by which to pay for it, my employment.

In reflection, it is overwhelming how everything unfolded and worked out as it did. My entire life outlined in mystical perfection that could have only been orchestrated by a masterful maestro. How brave, angry, and scared my parents must have been to leave me while still recovering from such a traumatic experience. How brave, angry, and scared I must have been. Or should have been. Those are sentiments that seemed unfamiliar for many years but were expected along the way, even within me, given the circumstances.

I was confused how at times it seemed as if I felt nothing yet knowing that I felt everything and deeply; perhaps too deeply it numbed me. The capacity of strength, courage, and love needed on so many levels, by both of my parents, and of myself, to agree, support, and then follow through while being oceans apart. They almost lost me. I almost lost myself. I reflect on how they just left. I reflect on how I just stayed. I reflect on how that is what we did.

When framing the context of my experiences during this final year abroad, I oftentimes must remind myself of the trauma to my physical body from the nineteen months prior. At age eighteen, oceans apart from my family, all my friends had left the area, and while going to school and working I was learning to live with all the outcomes of the illness which still consisted of physical therapy, medical appointments, and pressure garments that covered my scarred body. All the while, I crutched through life actively retraining my foot and mind muscles to walk without braces. That was just the physical experience without consideration to the parts of my being beyond my physical body. I was clearly determined to live and get on with life. There was clearly a force that carried me.

It is difficult to recall the source that drove the determination needed to crutch along for days. For months. For almost the entire year. In the physical sense and metaphorical sense of the expression. It was not so much that I was on crutches; it was what I did throughout the days while on them that is overwhelming in my memories.

My daily routine required a strength beyond the physical strength of my body. My upper body was physically strong, but there was something deeper within. I may not have been able to decipher and feel my emotions clearly, but I could feel the deep-rooted strength that provided a recognizable source of energy. It existed from within the same space that made up the ethers of my faith. I was clearly drawing upon strength and courage from somewhere, which I always perceived as being carried by the Global Wave of Healing

Energy. The love of humanity carrying me until I was able to carry my own.

After graduation and while in the apartment, there was an awareness that my life was no longer being molded around physical therapy and my recovery. Due to my continued progression in the proceeding months, physical therapy became molded around my new living circumstances. There was a sense of freedom that accompanied the shift. It felt like I was standing before my mountain with a snow-white canvas awaiting the masterful next scene. I knew I was finally living the glimpse of the life I had experienced when Quentin took me to the same mountains where I discovered my blueprints.

I often wondered if it was the same sense of freedom my friends were experiencing as they began their life as a youthful adult, fresh out of high school. I believed that we were all experiencing a sense of freedom into life, albeit I was dissatisfied with how I was experiencing mine. I constantly looked past my circumstances in order to engage in what was around me and ahead and carried on my way the best I was able. It was a mechanism that propelled me through a very interesting journey. Step by step, I reentered the life experience, and it was during this last year that I was led back to the sense of wonderment and passion. Unbeknown to my youthful awareness, I was back at the source of who I am.

As my physical recovery continued to improve, the need for physical therapy continued to decrease. During the start of my final year of recovery, the only focus was on my foot surgery recovery, scar massages, and preparing the left foot for the next surgery. The frequency of visits was down to one visit a day for a couple of hours during which Quentin and I carried on as before. Among many things, this would be the final year for physical therapy before my official return to the United States the following summer. Everything as I knew it would come to an end. The life of my youth abroad, the onset, diagnosis, treatment and saving graces that encompassed the medical experience, life as I knew it even in my new state of existence would come to an end. My final year abroad was the end of an era and the start of another. As I was closing out one life, I was preparing for the next. In a sense, another death and rebirth and so soon from the last literal sequence. It seemed critical that this all stayed in the forefront as I journeyed through the experiences of my eighteenth year in life.

The year started off in the wonderment behind the generosity of a family from school. They invited me into their home and offered safety and protection while my parents were oceans away. In my mind, it was another perfect alignment. They invited me into their home, which became the sacred space for me to mend myself on my own time and at my own pace.

The father was my softball coach, the same coach that took us to Germany prior to becoming sick, and the one I sought out after school on the last day I walked the school grounds before heading home, hours before the trauma set in. He was also an elementary school teacher. The mother was the school nurse, and someone I had visited before throughout the prior years for nicks and bruises acquired on campus during school hours. Together, they had a son who was a student in the middle school, who I believe was five years younger than me. The Tomlinson's took me into their home and loved me as if I was their own. Mr. T., also referred to as Coach, Mrs. T., Sam, and I coexisted for eleven months. They became exposed to my world and me to theirs.

One of the most vulnerable experiences of this year was allowing

Mrs. T to know the truths of my trauma. Beyond the realms of my family and my medical team, no one knew the story that my body told behind the clothes and strength in character that disguised the trauma. I still see her sweet, gentle, and saddened face as it never shuttered while cleaning the wounds upon my traumatized legs. I know it was unlike anything she had ever seen, like many. Behind our soft-spoken words, her gentle and compassionate touch, and my bashful smiles of gratitude, I remained embarrassed by my trauma. I was ashamed of my body, yet proud for surviving. It was hard, complicated, and confusing, but I trusted in her love. Just as I had to do with all other hands that showed up to heal my being. She was the mother I needed when mine was so far away. Mrs. T. was the perfect Mom at the perfect time on what I believed was the perfect path. My gifted Mom.

Although there was no real way to repay the Tomlinson's for what they gave to me this year, there was monetary compensation arranged for my expenses. To pay for my boarding expenses, it was arranged for me to work part-time at the place of my father's employment. It seemed as with many things, I was not involved in the decision, yet recall when my Dad informed me of that caveat. As he explained the public transportation routes, I was surprised, yet knew that if my Dad thought I was capable, even with consideration to everything and the crutches, then I must be. I knew and believed I was capable as I accepted the circumstances in the awareness that self-imposed limitations would be critical to avoid. It all would be so if I wanted to stay. It would be so if I wanted to live.

I became the assistant to the administrative assistants of the CEO in the Belgian office of Albemarle Chemical Company. The position was comically made up just for me, yet I was humbled and thankful just the same. Inga, Marie, and I sat outside Mr. Betlem's office while we worked. I mainly processed resumes and response letters for the HR department, and in exchange, they paid my room and board.

Every morning, after maneuvering preparations which began on the second floor where I rested my head, the family and I headed out the door. Most days, I rode with the family since we were all headed to the same place, school. We all had to fulfill our independent obligations, whether it was as a student, nurse, teacher, or coach. While the family fulfilled theirs, I fulfilled mine.

I chose to remain a part-time student since I was not going to university as originally planned. Attending school gave me something to do outside of physical therapy. I had already graduated, so any class was considered extra credit so I ensured to review options that carried over to university studies for whenever that time would be. It was never clear to me of how the financial obligation associated with this choice was satisfied, all I knew was that I was advised to select any courses I desired. I picked one course, AP Biology. It was in-depth, of great interest as I learned the full scope of my body, and intense enough to engage my mind in between the rest of life as it returned to a sense of normalcy. School brought a familiar, consistent balance and focus especially since I continued to experience so much change and separation.

Each day I attended school for a couple of hours and then crutched down the long driveway on the backside of the school property to the public transportation bus stop. From there, I rode the public bus, switching lines once along the way to the downtown area where the departure was several blocks away from the Albemarle Office. I crutched to the building where I worked for several hours before reversing my path back to school. I made my way back in time for the end of the school day, when I met up with the Tomlinson's, and returned home together. As we settled into the evening, Quentin arrived for physical therapy, we ate upon his departure and then we closed out the day in our own ways. Sometimes collectively, and sometimes independently.

For the most part, this was the schedule of my eighteenth year in life. I knew it had to be better than the last. Anything and everything in life would always be better than the last. There was a deep knowing that this was the life event that I would spend my lifetime healing from, and it was the experience that would inevitably make everything else seem trivial.

There was an incredible amount of life experience from that prior year that still needed to integrate into my youthful, traumatized being. As I slowly re-entered the world, my layer of comfort and trust evolved beyond the hospitals, home with family and within the school community, and into the next realm of society. The path of the footprints widened, and at times I wondered if they were mine, or still those of another. The strength needed during these times is unfathomable to me; therefore, it must have belonged to another. I was clearly being carried while I floated along.

While working, I was invited into interesting, diverse experiences that left a wonderment in the wake of my social re-entry. It was interesting to see where I floated, especially when I drifted into social encounters beyond those known from school. Not only was holding a job a new introduction in life, but it also brought about new social interactions with Belgian citizens. I had never cultivated relationships beyond the perimeter of our neighbors, school, and church communities, which generally overlapped in some way. All my close ex-patriot friends had left the area, and I had made new friends within the city where I had lived for five years. It was all very strange in the moments that it was occurring, yet inspiring and motivating, especially as it unfolded primarily in the French and Deutsch languages.

Many times, I would equalize my experiences with the normalcy of what my life was becoming. The youthful freedom, school, work, friends, socializing, inner strength, courage, and love, it seemed pretty ordinary to me, even though my circumstances were extraordinary. I would normalize into the similarities amongst us until I caught a glimpse of my leg brace shoved awkwardly into the shoe of my "good" foot or my reflection as I crutched my way through the world and seeing my metaphorical baggage in tote.

As the physical part of my life continued to unfold, there was an allowance for the other parts of me to heal at their own pace. My body continued to get stronger, and medical interventions continued to decrease, except for what was needed for the surgery recovery and the preparations for the next. I was living and crutching along.

My mind was focused on my body and the world around me while my emotions tried to keep the pace while still numb from overstimulation. Most obvious to me was that my heart and soul still needed deep healing. I was by no means perfect, but I was all that I could be. It seemed as if the hardest work was done.

My new arrangements, my new sense of life, all felt like a clean slate — sort of. I was out of the hospital, I was covered in my own skin, I was crutching with only one brace, I was living with a family albeit not mine, and I was in a sense on my own in life. In a weird way, it was my version of continuing education. My university teachings arena was life. Yet it seemed different than how I had imagined merely because I was different from when I imagined it.

I knew I was the same me on the inside, but even though I knew it was the same me, I did not yet know who that was. Before I became ill, I was a social, athletic, energetic teenage girl working through self-identity. I was pubescent and experiencing the truth of intended and unintended consequences that come with choices while navigating the physical and hormonal changes that accompany growth. Then, suddenly I was ripped apart to start anew. Shattered into a million unrecognizable pieces. It occurred in the presence of the unavoidable irony that I grew up snuggling Dumpy pillows that my Mom crafted throughout my youth.

Uncertain of her chosen nod to the nursery rhyme, nor its intended meaning, in my brokenness I felt like Humpty Dumpty that had fallen off the wall, broken into pieces. I related to the very Dumpy that rested beside me in the hospital bed that my Mom created specifically for the experience. As my Dumpy remained whole beside me, it reminded me of how to rebuild. Unlike the broken Dumpy that I had been taught was unrepairable, I witnessed all the King's horses and all the King's men put my body back together again. While I rested beside my Dumpy and shared in our wholeness, I knew it was only the exterior shell of my being. I somehow knew that the sense of wholeness and independence I created, especially in my final year abroad, would be critical in my lifelong relationship with myself and with life. As my emotions tried to normalize, my mind and body led the way of my weary heart and soul.

I had no clue how I was going to interact with the world, nor with myself for that matter. At times it felt like I had no clue what I was supposed to do next. Even though I knew I could create my future, at the same time it no longer felt like my life path to follow, yet that of another, the masterful maestro's. Even though I knew I was making a choice to follow the journey, it seemed like I did not know what I was doing, nor where it was leading.

From the moment I opened my eyes from the coma, there was a sense of surrender that I had to consciously choose within each passing moment. It was blatantly apparent within those same passing moments that I was not, nor never would be in complete control of even my own life. I was always aware that by surrendering to the circumstances I was trusting in something greater. Despite holding the trust, it never seemed quite clear where that trust would lead me. In hindsight it was the deepest faith possible even though I never saw it as such. It took decades to expose that at varying levels of awareness throughout my life, I always knew where I was headed.

As my soul was carried in my foggy bubbles of faith, my heart continued to try to stay the pace with the rest of my being. Integrating the trauma into my heart proved to be the hardest yet the easiest space of self to receive my efforts. Hardest because it is the most sacred, authentic, and vulnerable space of me, and easiest because it was the most important space of me to heal, and for the same reasons. Not that my other parts were less important, but it had always been the matters of my heart that led me through life.

My heart had to heal if I was going to survive in this life like this. The relationships with my heart are the most authentic connections that expose the nakedness of my being if I allow it. It was important to create the time and space for my heart to heal, as the organ of breath and as the emotional compass of my love.

While in the hospital, I spent many hours in silence contemplating the matters of my heart. How would I exist in the space of love? Love for self, love for a different unknown life, and most terrifying, was the wonder of love with another. My life vision always held dreams of love and romance. A family with kids. That was what I was taught encapsulated love, and the children I wondered if I could still bear. If I was going to have a family, that meant I would have to let someone in. The idea of love for me seemed lost, yet there was hope that it would once again be found.

The scars from this experience would be something that would stay with me forever. And not just the physical scars. It felt like every skin graft that covered my body was a mortared stone around my heart. I wondered how my heart would learn to love through stone. I was definitely not loving towards anything about my circumstances. I was so young and thriving in my potential, and I could see infinite possibilities in my life ahead, and then everything had changed. I had to maintain the same outlook with a new, forced reframing into the unfortunate circumstances of my life. I could barely breathe through the rapid pace of transformation.

I have not spoken to the matters of my heart until now, solely because it is the most sacred space of me. The matters of my heart make me who I am. During this final year of many things, it was important for me to stay attuned with my heart so that I could remember who I am. It was my experience with Kelda several months prior, coupled with my spiritual awareness, that shined light upon the relationships with my heart. As young as four years old, I recall making construction paper bound books for my Mom about love and joy. It was the only space of me that I felt I could trust. It is the matters of the heart that matter most.

The love in my heart guided me through my childhood, my adolescence, through to when I awoke from the coma as a teenager and was depleted within every aspect of my existence. At the core of who I am, I knew that mending my heart would be a fundamental part of the me I would become. The love that I somehow managed to safeguard in my heart is what continues to ground me throughout my passing days, especially through days of weakness. If nothing else, there is always hope in love. I was not always clear on what it meant, where it came from, where it resided fully within, nor how to access it, but there was always hope in love.

As it relates to the intimate gift of love to experience with another while here on earth, Ahmad was the first matter of love within my heart at the tender age of fourteen. We shared sweet, young love for nine months until his family moved away for two years. Upon his return, we reconnected and shared a more mature, yet still young love. Ahmad and I had been dating seven months for the second time when I became ill.

There are no words to explain my relationship with Ahmad. As a matter of fact, no words can fully explain any relationship that make up the matters of my heart, nor many things I desire to express about my love. The relationship that we shared, its evolution, and the impacts that my trauma had on us both was unfathomable at times. Not just during those moments, but how knowing each other before, though, and after my illness has molded our hearts for the world to experience. There is a deep truth that our shared love became part of the foundation that built the best versions of our love to be brought forth throughout our life experiences. Ahmad and I were in love. It was young love, but it was real love. Our youthful and eager love knew of the possibility of choosing to share many more years, if not a life, together.

Ahmad was introduced as my boyfriend, alongside my friend Julie when they received special intensive care unit visiting privileges on my seventeenth birthday. He gifted the red velvet jewelry box and picture frame, and it was within his presence that I initially discovered my inability to feel, through touch, nor emotionally within. It was not until the second year of recovery and my final year abroad that I lived that loss in the full awareness of my days.

Early on in my recovery I learned to treat everything as it was and in the rawness of its truth. Part of my truth was that I was out of love. Not just out of love, but out of emotion. It seemed like I had no love within me. I seemed empty, like a vessel being kept alive by machines. I even knew that was sad, yet it did not seem like I felt that sadness. I just was. A mind blasted in focused awareness within a shattered vessel, trying to figure out how to move forward in this life. With a sense of abomination, my weary heart and its overstimulated emotional system existed in a newly mended vessel to navigate in the world without a compass.

While processing my trauma in the intensive care unit and trying to figure out how to survive each moment my body stayed alive, just like my family viewing from the glass windows, Ahmad was there. To me, he became another viewer from the sidelines, just like everyone else.

I had nothing to give. I felt like I was barely hanging on to life, especially the hope in love. Not just intimate love within a relationship with another, yet that seemed to be the path that love most often led me. I surely didn't understand the experience. I only knew the experience was sad, unfortunate, and lonely as I stood with only a mask of hope, especially in love. It felt like whoever was to share my love would have to love me deeply to see past my body and into my heart. I prayed that the love energy that I believed sourced the Global Wave of Healing Energy would heal my heart in the same manner that it was healing my body. I cried tears of hope that there was truth in what had only been a saying in that love and inner beauty always prevail.

When I transferred into Medium Care, and there were no visiting restrictions, along with many others, Ahmad visited as often as he could, knowing the days that he was unable were sometimes due to the psychological and emotional distance needed for his own sanity. I knew that truth more than anyone yet had no means by which to escape it. Through his own processing and navigation, he created videos of our friends, he made cards and letters, and he always brought anything he could put his hands on to uplift my spirits and to express his love.

When he was away from me, he spent many hours with my family, in particular my older Sister and Julie, as they processed the trauma together. When away from my family and me, he tried to fill his days with anything that replaced the reminder of my trauma. It was very difficult for our young hearts and young minds to process our young love in the space of such horrific trauma. In an instant, what we thought we knew in love was shattered into fear, doubt, anger, sadness, and every painful sentiment that is possible to experience. Love was blasted into its opposing forces. My love was numb to the world and to myself.

Due to the overwhelming need of every aspect of my being vying for healing potential, I was unable to nurture the relationship with my heart and my relationship with love, therefore I was unable to nurture my relationship with Ahmad. We both were molded deeply by my trauma, while our ideals of love were shattered at such a young age.

It turned out that Ahmad was one with whom I was unable to be vulnerable in my nakedness, on any level of my existence. I was unable to figure out how to connect knowing that he knew me before, and neither of us had any means of knowing the unexpected ways the trauma would change me. I never questioned the truth that our young love was not intended to journey through the trauma together, nor what was to come ahead. I knew that. I was still trying to accept myself in my broken nakedness. He knew that. While we both struggled with love in silence, we met each other where we could. We could only meet as friends, and sometimes not even that.

As we evolved into the organic transformation of our relationship, it became easy for us both to become who we needed to be. During our senior year, he molded one of the biggest impacts of my social recovery. It was Ahmad that grew me through one of the most awkward events of my senior year, the Homecoming Queen nomination, and all associated functions. He was my date, and as friends, he stood beside me as I navigated through the early stages of my re-entry back into the school community. He stood beside within our huge circle of friends, while I found my footing upon my mental legs and my tightly braced physical legs. I wish I could remember more from that night, but I like to imagine that I tried my best to dance the night away, with both braced legs in high-top sneakers covered by my bell-bottom pants. I know that I enjoyed the moments, no matter how early it likely ended.

As I sensed the shield around my heart strengthen and the more I woke up to the world, I knew the contract between our souls had ended. I certainly did not phrase it that way in my youth, but once I found the words, I knew that was what I sensed. My heart was ready to rest without obligation to anyone other than myself while

I learned how to recover. It was a time of utter physical world focus, and I shielded my heart and my love in preparation.

I knew that there would be another time when my heart would regain the reigns, but until then, my heart nestled into the silent transformation within that provided a shield from the gusty winds swirling around in life. Although the easiest way for me to navigate life was by falling in love, and I desperately prayed for love, I was not going to seek it. I did not have the interest, the concern, the desire, the energy, nor anything else I thought was needed to fuel a relationship with love. Not only did I lack the strength and courage to show up for love, but I also did not believe that it is ever anything to be sought. To me, love has always been the most sacred space of me to be honored completely. I have always believed that if I protect and follow my heart, then love will always find me.

At times I was surprised at my own ability and level of allowance considering my sheer vulnerability. I had closed off my heart from anyone entering, but what I did not expect was that it was already there, trapped within the confines around my heart. It was not that I fell in love; it was there waiting patiently for me. Once my heart found the love that was waiting for me, I simply chose to lean into it. My heart needed to lean into it. My life needed me to lean into it. My soul was grateful that I listened and chose to lean into it. More than anything, I always wanted to know that love still existed for me. During my senior year, after eight months into knowing Quentin, I leaned into his love.

After all the time spent together, a level of intimacy was bound to develop, especially given the intimate level of involvement in my recovery. As it continued to be unavoidably nurtured due to physical therapy, it was after Homecoming and the school's October Fall

Break when he traveled with us to Louisiana that the attraction led to more intimate and personal encounters. It was unexpected, yet it was easy to nurture the new version of love to be shared. During my senior year, when my friends were carrying on in their youthful eagerness, I was re-learning the world through youthful doubt and with a weary heart. Quentin was the soulful guide through this part of my journey, for the new physical body navigation, as well as the matters of my heart within my new body.

During my recovery, within and outside of the hospital, up to the time that my parents returned to Louisiana, Quentin and I were around each other on average of six to eight hours a day, every single day, for fourteen months. That does not include any encounters in the intensive care unit when he aided in the baths when identities were hidden behind face masks. At age seventeen, we spent the majority of my waking hours together doing physical therapy and engaging in experiences that re-integrated me back into the world. He believed in me when the odds were completely against me. He kept me focused on my goals by making them his goals and pushing me beyond comprehension. He comforted the uncomfortable uncertainty about everything.

I understood that I had to do the actual work. I understood that fairly quickly in my recovery. We were all very much parts of a bigger whole, the mysterious masterpiece, yet it was equally evident that I was at the core. Although the work was up to me, without Quentin, I am not sure of the level of successes I would have achieved. In every space of my being, and within every space of my life, he was a critical part of my continued survival. He became many things to me while growing and molding me into who I would forever become.

He became a caregiver changing bandages. A physical therapist building strength and mobility. A cheer-leader chanting inspiration. A friend who laughs and jokes. A confidant that listens and supports. And in time, a lover with whom I was able to express my timid version of a newly evolved love. It became one of the most special and unique relationships I have ever held. It seemed inevitable that my fragile and traumatized seventeen-year-old being would fall in love with the hands that were healing her.

On the surface, it appeared to be for all the wrong reasons, sometimes even within my own mind, and those around me, yet deep within my heart and soul, I was aware of what was transpiring. I trusted in the transformation of my heart more than the opinions echoed from the distance. Right before Christmas and the impending trip to Italy, it became known that I was dating my physical therapist. Not everyone understood it, yet they accepted it for what it was.

During the nine months that held space for our intimate love, Quentin gifted me with the most precious treasure in this life. For if it was not for his gift of love, all future versions of my love would have gone quite differently, and so far, the last is by far the most glorious. During our time together, in whichever way he managed to do so, he kept my heart alive. He shielded my inner spark from the extinguishing life forces while I learned how to follow my heart again.

Quentin tossed the embers within my heart by nurturing the sentiments of love and compassion, emotions that took time to remember how to grow and evolve. With every healing bandage he removed and reapplied, he cleansed the space around the fire in my heart. With every pulse of love that fueled the flame, the idea of being loved seemed more and more possible. It was his love and compassion that allowed me to gently evolve into a new love in my own time, in my own way, as my new me.

I was always curious about his attraction for me and in me. He met me in the depths of the most broken state in my existence – at all levels – physically, psychologically, emotionally, and spiritually. I was a patient, a severely scarred and debilitated patient. Over time I improved, but I still had the scars at all levels. He was the first person to teach me that the scars did not matter when it came to inner beauty and matters of the heart.

Everyone wants to feel loved and to be loved. And every woman wants to feel beautiful. For whatever reason, he incited both within me. They were feelings I definitely had not felt in a long time and was terrified that I would never feel them again, let alone with someone else feeling the same towards me. I did not believe that the scars did not matter, and I definitely did not understand how they could not, but I was not going to resist love. Nobody should ever resist love.

Once the new schedule of my final year was underway, and as I continued to heal, I made the personal decision to reduce physical therapy even more. It was easily validated by my recovery, plus, I eventually had to learn how to exist without therapy, so it was a natural progression. As everything continued to shift, so did my love. It had everything to do with me. Not that I wanted it to, but my heart was all I had to go by. I was humbled in my own truth as I accepted that my relationship with Quentin had served its purpose. I no longer depended on him in every way possible. It was possible that I no longer depended on him for anything. I had to ensure that love was not entangled in the trauma, nor my need to feel safe and protected. I needed to trust myself for those. As a result of my own growth, my own actions, and my own journey, our romance faded, while my heart continued to heal.

As a result of the organic decrease in physical therapy and our love, we naturally spent less and less time together. As winter months approached, I was beginning to bear a little weight on my right foot, yet still crutched everywhere, even within the home. The next surgery was a couple of months away, and I could modestly massage my scars in-between visits. I do not recall what the schedule turned out to be. I only recall what it turned out not to be. All I know is that I was not doing physical therapy every single day.

As the year continued to unfold with school and wok, I just wanted to be me in whichever way that meant. It seemed like a pretty isolated and lonely world when I removed the hustle and bustle of crutching through the city. Same world, new me, no close friends, no physical therapy nor its romance, and no family presence. It felt like I was more welcoming of it all versus defending a space. In time, with the new social work interactions which opened me up to connecting even more, I turned to the school campus. I hardly knew any of the students that remained and decided to change that. I wanted friends. I needed friends. Especially ones that spoke English.

While allowing my protected heart to assist me, I kept my eyes open for those I sensed would be kind to my vulnerability and shyness. Instead of physical therapy, I found myself trusting in the unknown and making new friends; one in particular that lived around the corner from where I was staying. It seemed convenient and hopeful.

I first spotted Alex on the school bus when I chose to ride the bus home from school one day instead of riding with the family. All I knew was that we attended the same school and rode the same bus. That was it. He always kept to himself, headphones on, and listening to his walkman radio. I liked that about him. He was doing exactly how I felt on the inside. It was his silent and private disposition that I noticed from a distance.

I had no idea how to be anything more than friends. I had no intention of connecting with anyone in the space of love. The love prior with Quentin existed because he was already there through my trauma. He was part of the healers that mended my million pieces back together as best they could and gave me extra thread for my journey alone. I still had no idea how to open my heart back up to love. I had no idea if I would ever be able to relate to anyone again in that way. I welcomed the clean slate. For everything. Even my heart and the love it yearned.

Both of us kept to ourselves, which was eventually the element that connected us. Soon enough, we exchanged small talk over lunch, and I became friends with the mysterious Brazilian with a British accent. The connection was one that felt like it had existed for many years by the time the first words were spoken. Although I knew then that Alex was another soul mated with mine to guide me along my journey, it was at such a young level that it was unframed and pure.

We spent a lot of time together and with his small circle of friends, but it was not until after my second surgery in January that we began spending every possible moment together. After my surgery and spending time with my Mom and Dad while they visited, I slipped right back into my routine. Physical therapy picked up a little while I recovered from the surgery, but somehow it didn't seem to interfere with anything. That included my time spent with Alex and my new circle of friends.

Alex and I took long walks, well, I crutched, or he carried me while we toured around the neighborhood streets and alley ways. Our talks were even longer. We talked about everything. We talked about nothing. We talked into the nights as we talked about what had happened to me. He was the first outsider, the only outsider that I had allowed into my heart.

As we grew to know each other, we learned that we were both struggling to overcome tragedy. Even within our brief connection, we had to make hard choices that I prayed would forever be in the name of love. Although our stories were very different, the psychological and emotional impacts were profoundly similar, again highlighting that although our experiences are different, we experience life the same. We allowed each other to be raw and vulnerable. We allowed each other to be who we needed to be and to help each other through whatever it was we needed to get through. It was this connection that formed the purest of friendships.

I held such deep love, respect, and appreciation for him. He was such a gentleman, and although we were both only eighteen, there was a maturity about our relationship that was indescribable. It always felt as though I was too young to be experiencing any of what I had faced, forcing me to grow up before I was ready. We journeyed through the rest of the year sharing time together, sharing time with his family and with our friends. What I remember most are the sincere smiles and the laughter that we shared.

During the many hours that we spent together, we used to play a lot of video games. We also spent a lot of time playing pool, but those times where usually centered around other events. It was the video games that always created a lot of laughter. I really liked to play Donkey Kong because I was good at it, but my true favorite was X-Men. There was something about the mystery, the superpowers, and the hidden identities of the X-Men characters that sent me soaring into wonderment. What if humans could nurture their senses to become superhuman like those in X-Men? I felt superhuman and wondered of my own powers.

> Wolverine has enhanced physical capabilities with bones and claws coated in adamantium, a fictional metal alloy with an attribute of indestructibility.
>
> Beast has super-human physical strength and agility.
>
> Cyclops is capable of projecting powerful, concussive force from his eyes which requires him to wear a specialized visor.
>
> Gambit holds the ability to manipulate kinetic energy and there-fore objects; and
>
> Psylocke, the character with the most techniques, has a primary ability of telepathy and is capable of forming a psychic knife from her fist.

When Rogue joined the crew, she quickly became my favorite character, likely more because of our similarities versus her superpower I desired to hold.

> Rogue is a female. As am I.

She is a mutant. I certainly felt like one.

Her power is that she absorbs the memories, superpowers, and sometimes the life of whoever comes in contact with her skin. It seemed pretty fitting, especially since she had to clothe her body and cover her skin to protect herself and those around her. I related it to my pressure garments that hid my scars from the world, shielding both from the truth of the trauma that exists in the world. I was hopeful that my new skin would have an awesome new purpose. More likely, I believed that if anyone got close enough to touch my skin that I may absorb the life out of them. I was likely more terrified that my unhealed inner trauma, buried deep within, would suck the life out of another. It felt like it was suffocating me. It felt like there was so much power entangled in my illness that if I did not heal, it might kill another, and use my body as the vessel. Like Rogue, I would need to harness my inner power of manifestation before exposing my skin to the world; heal my trauma before exposing my heart.

It was the deep intuitive connection between us, expressed through sincere love and appreciation, that at some level felt like it was grounding the superpowers within me. Unexpectedly, it was from within our deep authenticity that the passion eventually grew. Passion to live. Passion to love. Passion to be in the moment and embrace everything. Just be present in the moment and to let that be enough. Slowly, my inner flame that had been safeguarded by Quentin's gentleness was being fueled in an unfamiliar and exciting new way. From the lens of my soul, Alex was a sacred being with a purpose to fuel the flame within my heart with passion.

Through our interactions, over time, the passion and intensity continued to grow deeper and more powerful until neither of us could resist temptation. Love manifested into a kiss. There is a beautiful sweetness in a slow intended, simple kiss. Once we traversed the bridge, the flame in my heart grew and began shining through the mortar cracks framing my pulsing heart. I knew it was love in all my flaws. Not from any physical experience, although those were sending the same messages, but I knew purely from the intensity I felt within my heart. I had never felt that before, and I felt alive. My heart was truly awakening. This kind soul acted and loved exactly how my vulnerable heart needed, in a nervous yet calming way. No boundaries, no judgments, no expectations. Pure love.

I was aware that our bond was growing stronger and deeper the more time we spent together. I also knew that in a few short months, everything was going to come to an end when it was time for my return to the United States. Long-distance relationships have never been a desire of my heart, so if I was unable to stay, then I was unwilling to love. Therefore, I tried to change the path. I allowed my mind's idea of love to take the lead and attempt to prevent the inevitable.

When I reflect on the truths within, I knew, even then, in the depths of my heart that I had to return to Louisiana. I just did not want to leave the new passion burning so intensely within me, nor did I want to leave the safety in the temporary life I lived. I remember thinking that it felt like I was going through the motions just so I could say that I tried. It never felt like it would actually work out in my minds favor to stay. I tried to divert the path of where my soul was sending my heart next.

I could not imagine leaving my life and passion behind. It was so joyful and fun, with a mature intimacy that felt seductive and sensual. It made me forget about the trauma and gave a hopeful sense to life. It was completely unexpected given the journey I had traveled but welcomed every aspect as it awakened every cell within me. I was awake to sensual love.

Knowing that the end of the year was approaching, I did everything I could think of to secure arrangements to stay. I applied to the Université Libre du Bruxelles (ULB), the Free University of Brussels and was accepted to receive four years of instruction in French. It was attending ULB that would have given purpose to my continued stay in the place I called home. Not long after I received my acceptance letter, it turned out that it was not free for me as a non-Belgian resident.

At one point, I recall speaking to my Mom about financial options, and she indicated that they did not have any available funds to assist with college because they had used their savings on my medical expenses. This meant that no matter where I planned to attend, Europe or USA, I would need to figure out the finances on my own. It was good information to know since all my enrollment offers were at out of state universities which resulted in higher tuition. This financial constraint impacted every aspect of a life plan I was trying to build.

I started writing letters and seeing where or how I could possibly secure financing for tuition expenses. I wrote letters to my treating hospital to inquire of participant opportunities in studies as it related to my recent illness, especially since medical journaling was conducted throughout diagnosis and treatment. I inquired if there was anything I could do to offset the cost to attend ULB, their affiliated university. I wrote extensively back and forth to the ULB administration to determine credit transferability should I return to ULB in the second year, while securing the funds in the United States during the first.

I was hopeful, but piece by piece, the plan fell apart, or should I say fell into my heart. There were no opportunities with the hospital, there were no financial opportunities, and I never even considered getting a job. It soon became evident that it was not meant to be. In the depths of my heart, I knew it was never a part of my continued journey. It appeared as though Louisiana was where I was meant to be. I wondered why that was. I really did not want to go back there. What could possibly be there for me, especially after all this time. Six years had passed. I was thirteen when I left and was nineteen when the time came to return. Even so, I deeply knew that being in Louisiana was part of the masterplan. When my efforts did not work out, I surrendered again and held faith that there would be great purpose within whatever awaited my arrival.

Seemingly all a sudden, everything quickly came to an end. We had to say our goodbyes and go our separate ways. The hardest part was that it was purely by circumstance and not due to feelings, or lack thereof. Alex was the one who showed up at the airport to send me on my way. And although there had been celebrations with my Mom and Dad, the Tomlinson family, and Quentin, it was with Alex that my heart truly celebrated the freedom of throwing my second brace in the garbage. Right before my final departure to the United States, I was finally able to walk on my own two feet without assistance. After two years, I was walking free, without braces nor crutches. It was exhilarating and I walked in the fullness of those initial steps of freedom in the presence of Alex.

There was a deep sadness and equally deep gratitude as I waved goodbye while walking to the airport gate. It was almost surreal in the awareness of everything I was truly walking away from. Six years of the most mind-blowing years of existence contained within my vessel departing to fly off into the sky to never return. It felt like a dream.

I didn't know what would come next, nor where I was headed, except for that the path would be found in Louisiana. I had a tremendous amount of life experience that still needed to be integrated, yet life kept moving. It felt like I needed more time, but I did not want it to take more time, nor did I want to give it more time. I wanted to be finished healing and live life just like everybody else. As I tried to calm myself and start life anew, I entered a life that molded my body, mind, heart, and soul in ways I may never fully understand.

Most importantly, it was a life that molded the passionate and intimate matters of my heart. From Ahmad, who sparked the flame to Quentin, who kept it burning, to Alex, who fueled it with passion, my heart was forever molded. Deep within the depths of my heart, I knew that no matter what I do in life, there must be passion at the source of my love, and I must never lose sight of the wonderment in life's perfection.

30

Where Am I?

I made it back to Louisiana. I made it home. But was it really home? It was the place I was born, the place that grounded the roots of our family, but it was not home to me anymore. I had not lived in the area for over six years – from ages thirteen through nineteen. I had just left home, my home.

Teenage years are very influential years as it is, and further coupled with my experiences only caused my roots to be more firmly grounded in Belgium. Back in Louisiana, all the people I knew before had moved away for college, or we had lost contact over the years apart. So basically, I was transplanted again into another foreign place. At least this time they spoke English.

There were some family ties, and most of my immediate family was there, but it felt like it was me against the world. A very familiar feeling. Culture shock set in again but now coupled with a new dimension. My new physically, psychologically, emotionally, and spiritually changed being seeking a path, answers, and understanding about what those years abroad were supposed to teach me. There had to be something to gain from the experience. Something more profound other than my continued existence. I was desperately seeking affirmation that my suffering was not in vain.

In the never-fading presence of my soul's desire to find the true meaning in my experience, there was always an innate acceptance that never allowed me to question the situation. Believing and knowing that in time it would all make sense. I just had to remain patient. I knew I had to find joy in every moment before me and continue to move forward like my running, and to move forward with intention. In whatever situation, and whatever state of mind, I was always accepting and focused on how to keep moving forward.

There has always been an acknowledgment that all along, even before the moment that I entered the emergency room, that my life journey was as it needed to be. Everything seemed to be perfectly placed along the path, perfectly placed for the experience to occur. It was as if the religious background of my parents, the move overseas, the questioning of my Faith, and the fact that I began running to keep my body healthy only months before the trauma all seemed too perfect amongst the horrid chaos. More so, it was all seemingly in preparation for the journey it was now destined to take.

It was all so mysterious. Even how Aunt Max was in Brussels with an unexpected doctor's appointment that I joined, and by my own intuitive actions. There was the doctor that inevitably saved my life when on vacation and just happened to be passing through the hospital at just the right moment to intervene. There was the terrifying truth of being resuscitated back to life twice, the seemingly unexpected awakening from a five-week-long medically induced coma, and the surgeons that fought for me after debriding over sixty percent of my body. There was the artery in my leg that was switched at birth, and I watched my body grow skin to cover my bare bones. It was a series of otherwise unexplainable events, most seeming to be miracles, that harmoniously became a life-saving experience. Even the surreal connections with so many people along the way that profoundly resonated with the core of my being seemed mystically perfect. There had to be meaning in all it. I could sense it deeply but had no idea how to set it free. I knew that life would reveal the many meanings to me over time when it was time for me to learn them. I knew I had to remain patient and hold enough trust to continue onward.

I recognized early on in my youthful quest for self-enlightenment that these struggles of adjustment, whether it is physical, psychological, emotional, or spiritual, were not unique to me. This is part of humanity and every man's quest for purpose. But I was only able to truly experience what was happening within me. I knew I deeply wanted to experience every moment and appreciate the worldly beauty to the fullest, and yet felt so constrained by a new limited body. It was a constriction never experienced before and therefore lived a life believing I was alone in my experiences of such restriction. This eventually became my silent struggle. A struggle that would lead to the feeling of a disjointed self for many years to follow.

When I became ill, it was as though I became divided. And in a sense reborn. I had to change every perception, every dream, every idea of who and what I thought I would become in this world. I had sixteen years of exploring possibilities and growing to achieve those dreams. And then all a sudden, everything changed. Childhood dreams of being a professional dancer were over. My daily ritual of running would never happen again. Exploring every corner of the world faded into a memory. My physical body would never be the same.

Meanwhile, my soul and inner spirit were charged with infinite possibilities. There was electric energy that charged my own belief that I could do anything. I could do anything that I wanted to achieve. I knew that anything was possible. More and more, I became my own reminder of this truth as my body became the arena that represented both the constrained being and the infinitely free being. Integrating into balance from a space of opposition became a soulful desire.

Once I was able to identify that the sentiments were sourced in feeling split between two worlds, I understood why it felt as though I was split between journeys. The conflicting forces are what I eventually referred to within as my Inner Spirit and my Physical Spirit.

My Inner Spirit remained unchanged; perhaps even more energized. My Inner Spirit remembered the dreams, the hopes, and the possibilities. It remained free and light and full of love and gratitude. It could dance and run and hike and climb. It could travel the world in amazement and wonder. It could do all things in grace and peace.

And my Physical Spirit was changed completely. It became constricted, limited, and difficult. It became a fight, a focus, a constant awareness. The two were no longer in sync. The Inner Spirit still wanted to live life to the fullest in whatever way imaginable. I was always good at dreaming the impossible. That is what got me through everything thus far, making the most of every moment. But my Physical Spirit would confine my Inner Spirit in unimaginable ways.

It was two separate paths. Diverging before me with no wonder if they would ever reunite. It felt as though it was not up to me if they reunited on this earth walk. I used to imagine the bliss; what it would be like if they ever realigned again. I believed so deeply that it would be amazing and liberating. I used to believe that perhaps they would only realign when my physical body had been defeated and only my Inner Spirit lived on.

I carried this sense of split self throughout my life as my Physical Spirit took the lead, as it needed to. The time and space was for the physical earth walk experience. It was as though my Inner Spirit knew that it could continue to exist beyond space and time, being energized by the connections of past, present, and future. Independently, they somehow knew their intended paths. Even though they were very separate.

When I returned to Louisiana and began building a life was when my journey transformed into a spiritual existence within a physical experience. The intriguing part was that I never identified myself as being deeply spiritual. Therefore, I had no idea what such a life would yield, only dreams of the heart to know. All I knew to do was to trust my heart in love and kindness, be passionate about life, and continue to choose to grow and heal.

With as much strength, courage, and love I could muster up within, and upon each new day, I stepped into the start of a new life. It was broken, and messy, but it was a life full of unexpected beauty and endless possibilities, both of which held a dream of passionate love. Somehow, I knew that it would be discovered on the journey through Louisiana.

31

The Beautiful Life in Between

THE RAINBOW THAT LED TO LIFE'S POT OF GOLD

The chapters you just read were the memories sourced in the childhood sentiments of those times, the vulnerability in those moments, and the remembrance of the experiences. It is a story that had been held silently within for over twenty-five years, preserved in the voice of my inner child. During the journey to reach you, I found that each moment I stepped towards your light, the more light shined upon my darkness, and the depths of our collective experiences were exposed. I am humbled that you stood beside me on this journey and trusted that it was for a reason.

The level of detail that was found within the deep recesses of my mind was overwhelming even for me in the midst of the unfolding.

The more I uncovered, the more I understood why the journey took as long as it did. For throughout the journey of discovery, the greatest story there is to follow, is a story of love. Not an ordinary story of love, yet an extraordinary story of love. A love of the Highest Order.

The memories always felt like the preservation of a story to share, and never a burden within that needed to heal. There are likely just as many memories that have faded into the past, yet there is a deep acknowledgment that those that remained did so because they were instrumental steps in the walk of my life journey, leading me through a mystical life. It was clear that my life was leading me to the expressions meant to be shared, primarily between our hearts. I knew I was learning the deepest parts of me in order to bridge our experiences that seem so drastically different, and to do so in a meaningful way.

It took four failed attempts, over four-times as many years, and all those ventures were ceased when authentic expression felt forced and not fluid; even once the book was underway and undergoing its various renditions. It took the experiences that followed in the wake of deep expression that taught me who I really am; beyond the vessel within which I exist. This was when I had to remember my truths as a spiritual being since that was the only way I could remain firmly balanced as I stood before you.

From the moment I awoke from the coma, I knew that I had been broken yet I never used that word. My body did break, and the healers among us repaired and nurtured it back together. By the time I knew what was happening almost two months into the ordeal, my body was fixed, thereby, to me, I was no longer broken. The various parts of me were indeed wounded, fragile, tender, and scarred, but no longer broken. And although I never saw myself as broken, deep within I could feel the once broken parts held together ever so delicately. I was never quite sure what was holding those deep parts together. The inquiry generally was never able to exist beyond the more intriguing wonder of how it was so easy to journey through the experiences, especially when I kept my love for you in sight.

It took over twenty-five years of life experiences, and with an awareness that each moment was growing me into the time and space of complete authenticity of expression, for me to stand wholly in who I am, while embracing that I may very well be different in my next breath. It took several more years for me to translate my inner voice with fluidity, and in a meaningful way that could serve just one singular soul amongst us; to serve you. I deeply believe, within the depths of every breath that I take, that when I heal myself, in turn I heal the world. I found peace in knowing I may heal just one heart in this hard and messy life experience of lessons. For I too have journeyed to the depths of a perceived space of demise.

It felt like my experience was needed for something greater, especially when it felt so easy to navigate through it. All the while a sense of wholeness and purpose was needed now, in this life, for me. I knew there had to be purpose, and it felt like it was linked to you. If I wanted to arrive at both, I knew that I had to maintain sovereignty in my life walk and discover how to honor the autonomous nature of our collective purpose. I often wondered why my journey would entail such suffering of epic proportions yet concurrently knew that the walk would reveal its purpose in balanced magical bliss. I knew that I was healing my way to something. I prayed that I was healing my way to love.

It felt like the most honorable walk anyone could ever endure, so

I had to find a way to do it. I knew I had to find gratitude in the seemingly horrid experience knowing that it was uniquely mine by design. It felt like it was designed out of love, and it was easier to see myself as a work in progress, especially when I allowed my heart to lead the way. I was never quite sure where love was leading me, but I always knew I was following something deep within. It was how I had recovered and created opportunities to live and grow into the new me.

I lived a life watching the universe maintain energetic balance, and it felt deeply as though the worse had played out through me, and in the most horrific ways. It took a tremendous amount of trust in myself, in you, and in the human collective to stay the course in order for us to finally meet, soul to soul and heart to heart. I patiently waited for the scales to tip in our favor, bringing balance to our scales in the life experience. Up against the trauma endured, I was pretty bold in my request for it to be amazing beyond belief. I knew I needed it, thereby it was easy for me to trust that you needed it too since we are one and the same.

Generally, that was the only pleaful cry I ever made from the depths of my heart; that whatever was to come would be powerful enough to blast me into bliss for eternity. It was deemed impossible by my own mind. Especially after the attainment of all the pursuits I was led through by love; education and careers, marriage and growing a family, and within the connections at the core of my experiences that were designed to grow me into this world. My mind could not imagine anything that would have the power needed to move my needle a micro-blip, except perhaps the experience of you.

What started out as the seemingly simplistic project to document my medical experience quickly gained the momentum of much more. It was as if I had opened the gates leading to a magical field of flowers within the core of my being. People around me continuously expressed concerns and doubts in what was ultimately the expectancy of pain and sadness. All the while my field of flowers continued to blossom with beauty, bringing me inner joy and peace. It became a delicate balancing act between honoring my inner and outer worlds, while simultaneously deconstructing both to ensure they were aligned with the purity of self and the purity of my universal intentions sourced in love.

As I released the captive words, it was quickly revealed that...

>   my **Soul** wanted to sing;
>   >   my **Heart** wanted to feel...
>   >   >   my **Mind** wanted to rest...
>   >   >   >   and my **Body** wanted to heal and enjoy the life experience in the fullness of it's comfortable potential.

I wanted them all to feel at pace with each other so I could walk wholly into each new day; instead of fragmented across time and space. I deeply believed that the more I followed the journey within, the more peace, love, and joy I would bring into balance within me, and thereby throughout the world around me. I felt deeply connected to a calling that if I healed myself, I would in turn heal the world. I believed that if I did it correctly, my deep soulful love would light my path to you.

THE LIGHT AT THE SOURCE OF MY RAINBOW

I searched for you everywhere. I scanned the crowds as I sought out for you through every experience, knowing one day I would see you within a pair of eyes before me. I could feel you within every breath. I sensed you everywhere yet could not find you anywhere. I knew I had to find you. Reaching you has been at the source of my life intentions.

For many years it felt like the Global Wave of Healing Energy was healing the deepest parts of me as I surfed to your shoreline. Still, I wondered if I would need it to sustain the power of my truths for life, or just until I could stand in my truths alone, and before you. While the seemingly infinite flow of energy washed my soul clean, I lived a beautiful, hard, and messy life, full of growth, following love and seeking joy, while silently reconciling the space I hold as an infinite soul in an infinite universe living a brief and finite human experience.

Throughout life post illness, I could feel a power accumulating intensity within the depths of my being. I was never sure what it was, nor what it meant, until life gave me a set of words to describe it. Every sense of my being was growing into the capabilities to reach you across spacetime by defying every possible preconceived notion that kept us apart. I could feel it up against every unevolved sense and ability of my humanness; invoking pressure up against the laws that defined the world.

Although I knew very little about what it was that I was feeling deep within, I hoped, prayed, dreamed, and somehow inherently knew that it had something to do with the day I stood before you.

It always felt as though neither one of us was ready. I had not yet learned what I needed in order to stand in the power of my authenticity, and in the fullest expression needed to tip the scales, and you were not ready to hear my expression of truth knowing it was incomplete. I trusted I would know when the time and space was right. It was never a question of if I would reach you, only a question of when.

I trusted that whenever it was destined to be our time that it would be perfect for both of us. I envisioned I was walking towards our golden chess board where you awaited my arrival for the final masterful dance in the game of life. You had to be. It was the only thing that gave me hope. It was the only thing pulling me away from the dark and heavy suffering I knew was the alternative experience. It was a reality with you that I intentionally, masterfully, and consciously walked towards. It was clear that you had something to do with why I never struggled along the way, and in ways that even I would have expected. Keeping you in sight left me humbled by my own abilities.

THE PRISM WITHIN
The Angles that Diffracted My Light

    Throughout life, I was constantly observing the scattered parts of me, choosing whether to pick them back up, leave them behind, transform them into new meaning. I was constantly discerning who I was choosing to become within the mess of my parts. It was all I knew, and I analyzed my parts with every breath I took, primarily through the reflection of me that I saw in the world.

For many years, I interpreted one's reaction of me to be more telling of my flaws than theirs. Not in the sense that I felt I was personally attacked, but in the sense that I felt I could be doing better since I was often times triggered in response. The reflections exposed the spaces of me that needed healing. I needed the alarms to stop ringing after every encounter. I suppose in a sense I was silently attacking myself. I could not fathom how I could possibly be doing more in life yet simultaneously wanted so much more for myself. I wanted to feel life, be unencumbered and moved by the beauty in life, become captivated by the mysterious wonder that each day entails and very much a part of my reality. The very wonder within which I existed yet felt so distant from. I wanted to feel the truths I held within, and not just an intellectualized belief in them. It felt like my body was in the way.

Once I reconnected back to a time of complete vulnerability, a time when I was in essence wiped of all preconceived notions of self, my own and of those around me, I remembered that in those moments I was like a newborn child. My world was as new as a child entering the world. The difference was that I had the memories from sixteen years of life experiences, a level of knowledge and awareness, and all associated thoughts and emotions embodied in a sixteen-year-old body; a body that was once again anew to me and the world.

I realized that during those times and for many, many years to follow, my heightened level of awareness was deemed ordinary in my own mind. I noticed everything and remembered the details of everything; primarily how an experience made me feel. The deeper I felt it, the clearer the memory. It was my awareness that gave me the courage needed along the journey to find my way. It was love that reminded me that the purpose was you.

It took many moments over many years to understand the truths of what my physical body had endured. In truth, I still am as humanity evolves and gives me new words. Often the reality was too overwhelming to process considering all the details I held and the implications I understood, perhaps too well. There was never a doubt in my mind that I would be the only one to translate and tell my story, and the reality that I live. I was my only hope for explanation, and possibly survival. A reality I lived many times over when face to face with family, friends, and society alike; most vulnerable was with doctors when seeking assistance to stay alive, make sense of my world and my body, and survive each day comfortably. A reality no one ever seemed to understand at the level needed, nor that made me feel complete.

It seemed like the world did not have what I needed to be grown within the deepest parts of me. It felt like survival status quo was being maintained across all aspects of my existence, while the spectra of my inner rainbow casted a false reality for the world to observe and incorporate into their own. More often than not it felt like I was your only hope. I held onto my hope. I held on to you.

Early on it took concerted effort to embrace and be proud of my new state of existence. I worked tremendously hard to heal the mental, emotional, and spiritual wounds, while the physical scars left their everlasting impression. I tried my best to see my scars as badges of honor worn with pride although admittingly I felt they never made me as proud as the skin I once knew. I have always believed that through my illness and the suffering endured I had experienced the worst that life would offer. I knew it was up to me to make that my reality. I deeply believed that anything that followed would be minimal in comparison, and I have spent my life living that truth. I lived a happy, messy, hard, loving, joyful, tough, and interesting life. A beautiful life was created. A beautiful me was grown.

There was a lot to be thankful for and to celebrate. Deep within I chose to believe I was living the life I was meant to live. I knew I was the person I was meant to become, and I was where I was meant to live, and with the people designed to grow me through life. I was still believing and still nothing made sense, a cycle repeating until finally broken. I had to believe that for absolutely nothing made sense to my thinking, processing and perceiving mind creating perspectives that drove the emotions of my heart, within a foreign vessel that felt was controlled by your desire to meet me. Or was it just my desire to meet you? Nothing made sense so I trusted in love. I just wanted to hold and be held by you.

I knew I had to believe in something greater. The existence of a greater force was never the question, I was just never able to identify who or what it was that I was trusting in so much. It felt unnatural to have such trust without knowing where it was being directed.

It felt like it needed more committed intention. I felt sloppy and wavering, uncertain and unfocused. It felt as though I was missing something deep within yet could not figure out what; it was blocked behind something.

There was an unspoken and beautiful dichotomy within every experience I encountered that was teaching me about fluidity and balance; a dance that was unlocking and unblocking something within. I knew I was fulfilling a sacred role by showing up in my best effort at any given moment to grow those around me, yet the same sacred experience always reflected an incompleteness back to me; somehow, and in some way. I saw the wounded parts of me, often before I could see the wounded parts of you. I knew I could not see you clearly if I could not see past myself. I trusted that one day I would be healed enough so we could see each other clearly.

Without knowing where I was going, I used the world as a mirror reflecting back the spaces of me that needed to heal and grow. I saw my perspectives as opportunities for change where needed or desired. I viewed them as spaces of me that held potential for mending in order to catch up to the world while I still lagged behind. I believed the world was offering everything that was needed for me to heal within my growth so that I could find my way back to the collective. I was living amongst a collective; a beautiful network of love and support that walked beside me throughout the days. Even so, my lessons were growing me towards a deep soulful love which made the process natural and authentically easy. I set out to grow through what I saw reflected back to me in the silent vulnerability of my flaws.

No matter how awkward I felt in my body, uneasy I felt as a wounded being, and distorted by being shattered across time and space, I believed that encounters with others were an opportunity for you to reach me. If I was willing to listen and be present, then I would grow towards you. And keeping in balance, if another is what I needed, then I was what another needed, bringing balance into their lives through my expression of a humbled existence. I generally walked away witnessing the impact of my presence, drained, and reflecting upon whether there were opportunities for personal growth. I patiently waited for my turn, for something powerful enough to balance and energize me. It felt like I was waiting for an encounter with truth. It felt like I was waiting for you.

It seemed as if whenever I chose growth, I discovered love; and whenever I chose love, I experienced growth. I was pleased with how life was growing me albeit never the life I had envisioned. Those visions were left in the past when I saw my new body. I surely needed your love to help me find the same deep love for myself. A dance with the most complicated steps for the mind, yet the heart and soul glided with ease cascading their way to love through the planes of our realities. It felt like I was a feather defying gravity and floating upward, cascading side to side through the growth found in connections, drifting towards a unity in the graceful dance of love. A dance that would usher me to greet you as a feather descending from the skies, together forming angel wings to fly us off into eternity. A love song of my soul.

All the while I was grounded into my human reality. A reality that felt like you were a co-creator of, yet only illusions of you could be found. When I tried to find you through all the mirrors clouded by the smoke of the human experience and forming false realities before me, I knew that I had to stay focused to find my way out of the maze. I was here and alive, and I was determined. I was motivated. I was driven. I was persistent. I was committed. I was inspired. I was the best I was able to be within every moment that I lived. I was ready and actively walking towards the freeing release when I stood before you. I just hoped you would be there after so much time had passed.

Nothing was going to get in my way, especially not me, nor any aspect of my human body. At least that was always the intention. It did not necessarily always play out that way, but I was learning and growing. I wanted to do the best I could to minimize myself, and others, from forming a perception that held potential to derail me. If it did, which was more than admittingly desired, I would take a breath and find my way again. Love and joy were always the destinations, and I always ensured the trajectory was intact. I physically kept my head down when navigating throughout the days, while simultaneously holding my metaphysical head above into the skies collecting everything my senses could absorb. I could breathe when I checked the course, yet often lost my breath when submerged into the reality of my life.

Love fueled the creation of life into my experience while the various parts of me tried to stay the pace amidst the overwhelming truths that continued to unfold within me. I remained incredibly grateful for everything. My physical world experience was relentless. It felt like I lived within every expanding sense of my youthful imagination pushing for the next dream to be realized; albeit no dream felt grand enough to tip my scales except the dream of you. My aspirations were young, limited, and uncertain. They felt fresh, naïve, and stubborn, especially since it was as if they were built from scratch only years prior.

As life continued to grow me, the scattered parts of me excelled at their own pace and in their own space, with an ever-growing distance being felt between them. In time, it felt critical that I reassess my life and ensure it was a life that was able to support all my parts, collectively as one. It felt like the only choice I had was to surrender and allow life to grow me into whoever I needed to be. It felt like life was designed to find you, and I desperately wanted to be all that I needed to be for that encounter.

I believed that I was always, in some mystical way, the exact dose of whatever was needed from my brokenness in the story I bring, as whomever I was capable of being, that I would in some way serve the walk of another. When I found a wounded heart to heal, I knew I was on the path to you, because I was finding parts of me everywhere along the way. I knew I was heading in the right direction because when I found me, I sensed I was also finding parts of you. Just as it was up to another to allow me to grow them, it was up to me to allow another to grow me. I was willing to do so if it allowed me to grow towards you.

There was a sense of finding you when I served others, so I dedicated my efforts to better serve those I encountered. I looked for how to do so in every experience. By doing so, it felt like I created space for the evolution of self, and that I had the strength and courage in my own ability to grow and expand into the remainder of my life. Each heart you sent me to heal in turn healed mine, which ultimately brought our hearts closer into oneness.

Concurrently, it became more and more clear that whatever I was doing for those around me I also needed to learn how to do for myself. I could feel my inner cup being depleted by giving, yet never replenished by receiving. I could feel that receiving the love of others provided a different sense of fulfillment. There was something deeper still missing. Within the space of the beautiful life in between was where I sought out to find the missing pieces of me.

It was the four aspects of my being that diffracted my light within, and from which my rainbow of life was created. It was the prism within that was being polished by the walk towards you that I hoped in time would reflect your pure light. I prayed my prism would be clear enough to serve humanity; to serve you. The deepest inquiry was to know my true purpose, and it remained nestled within the depths of every cell that made up my thinking, breathing, and living being. I was overwhelmingly aware that each inquiry, response, and decision brought me closer to that truth. When compared to the perceived reality in the world around me, the reality within was the one that was expanding with clarity, and it was most certainly the one that I wanted to follow.

My Body – The Space of My Physical Reality
The Vessel that Carried Me Through a Journey of Growth

Following the path to Louisiana was baffling because my skin grafts and the humid and hot temperatures never have agreed with one another. It knew it was for a reason that I would end up in a place that made no sense, but then again nothing did anymore. While initially trying to adjust to my newly scarred body amongst a university springboard into real life, I tried a variety of versions of self yet none of them were sustainable, nor felt authentic and real. Everything felt like an extreme effort, or like I was trying so hard just to catch up to something. This continued throughout life as I grew into more comfortable ways to accept my scarred body. And although there were many physical body experiences, they were unintegrated and even spawned from the wounded parts of my heart and soul. The parts of me that my mind worked desperately to keep hidden.

Upon my return to Louisiana, I had remained tremendously focused and aware of my physical body experiences, primarily because medical trials continued after a five-year reprieve. It did not take long to realize that I would live a life walking beside the medical community. In a sense everyone does, but the need felt vulnerable and crucial; critical even.

Over time, I experienced normal happenstances viewed through my abnormal circumstances which repeatedly required me to trust myself when my physical body needed assistance. This never felt as easy, sufficient, and complete enough when standing before any given medical team that I was entrusting would be present enough to help me. I wanted to imagine a life that did not require them yet was unable to trust myself enough with my body to do so.

There are many stories to tell of my journey alongside western medicine, modern therapies and the constraints encountered when my body required more naturopathic and holistic treatments. I could write books covering the medical anomalies that have caused perceived baselines to vanish beyond the expertise of great practitioners. I continued to foster my mind and body duo that led me through life, as I autonomously defied my own boundaries, and the ideals of what had been projected for me, across every realm of my existence.

By the time I became ill at sixteen, I had already had half a dozen surgeries for tubes in my ears, a surgery to remove a cyst from my elbow, stitches for two major cuts, a broken ankle, corrective surgery to lengthen the ligaments in both knees, three organ removals all which were considered contributors to the lymphatic system, and numerous other bumps, bruises, and scars along the way. I was very athletic, active, and pushed my body's physical abilities to its potential. This also left me intrigued, mindful and routinely scanning my body as if there was something impending and I was awaiting its arrival. Until it arrived.

Although many organs failed during the onset and initial treatments of my illness, I made it through with the loss of skin, muscle mass, the small loss of two fingertips, and the limitations that those loses themselves imposed. I was considerably lucky that my internal organs restored themselves to a functioning level even if it was not considered normal optimum performance. It became my new optimum performance. I was my own baseline. No one knew what that really meant in terms of sustainability so learning how to appreciate the uniqueness of my body, and within each new day was somewhat of an unwelcomed gift. In the years that followed, my body went through life with even more experiences that would test its physiological, biological, and anatomical makeup while I concurrently held the other parts of me together with something much greater.

There was so much that had happened and continued to transpire within my body. There were the illnesses themselves, the experiences with death, and the myriad of medications, especially the barbiturates, opioid analgesics, and corticosteroids that all impacted my humanness. I knew they all had multi-dimensional impacts on my body in some way, if not in every way. One of the most vital treatments that sustained my life for over twenty-five years has been scientifically suggestive that it pushes the limits of the psyche. Not to mention the hundreds of surgeries using general anesthesia, x-rays, CT scans, MRIs, nuclear scans that use radioactive substances, the hyperbaric chambers, and many more therapies of modern medicine used to save, repair, and sustain life to my body. In addition to the five weeks when my consciousness lived in another plane of existence, my make-up was constantly morphing beneath the scarred skin that covered my being.

As life continued, it was more of the same as modern medicine was needed to sustain life while constantly changing the makeup of body, primarily my heart, my life experience translator. There was no doubt that the chemical, molecular, biological, and energetic makeup of every cell in my body was being morphed into something unexplainable, with a super psyche overseeing the whole production across dimensions and planes of existence. For many years I could not even wrap my humble and feeble human mind around the implications of those truths when I viewed myself with the scientific leans through which I viewed the world.

Along the way I opted for plastic surgeries for scar revisions, hardware removal, and slight reconstruction of my derriere, all which served its healing purpose to find more comfort for the days ahead. The unsolicited medical needs gently resurfaced after a five-year reprieve, and just as quickly transformed into a life-long chronic ailment within my body. During pre-op lab work for a reconstructive surgery, I was diagnosed with ITP which stood for Idiopathic Thrombocytopenic Purpura. The translation in layman terms is, that by means of deduction, the cause is unknown but known illnesses such as leukemia have been ruled out (idiopathic), where there is a deficiency in platelets which causes bleeding into tissues (thrombocytopenic), and causes rashes, or purple spots were the blood vessels have leaked blood into the skin (purpura). The name has since been changed to Immune Thrombocytopenia since it is now known to be an auto immune system malfunction that causes the body to destroy its own platelets. From the point of diagnosis, I was considered a chronic free bleeder. I remember thinking, what's one more thing? I will make it through this too. But at that point I had no idea what the journey would entail. In essence, at my core, I was my own worst enemy as my body fought against its own self destruction, a mere reflection of humanity.

Oral medications worked, but when it was time to wean off of them, counts would drop again. Long term treatment with corticosteroids is not in anyone's favor yet my blood responded to it, and well. In time, medical studies suggested that my spleen was the cause, and the recommendation for a splenectomy was presented to me. I had to make the decision to remove my spleen, or not. This time it was solely my decision. I prayed I would make the right one.

The spleen is a critical organ that filters the blood as part of the immune system function. It is the spleen that houses the platelets and white blood cells. It is even known to help fight certain bacteria that cause pneumonia and meningitis, the very illness that the Center for Disease Control was unable to confirm was linked to ITP because there was no data on survivors with similar conditions. Would it really be wise to remove my spleen given the journey I had just endured? Wouldn't I need my spleen to stay healthy? Yet, that same organ had the potential to kill me. It could cause free bleeding, massive internal hemorrhaging, which could be fatal at any given moment without warning. There was only one clear answer. Remove my spleen and keep on living and rely on modern medicine, Mother Earth, and Father Time to keep me alive. There were other ways to optimize health, but not in correcting the destructive function of my spleen. Living without a spleen became a part of my life story by the time I was twenty-five years old.

Embedded in this experience is another extraordinary event where science failed, all the while my existence led everyone through mysticism. The scheduled splenectomy was intended to last forty-five minutes, and instead took six hours. Once the surgery was underway, the surgeons found something unexpected; they discovered something they had never seen before. I had one full sized spleen, and twelve baby spleens that were not fully functional, but were possibly contributing to the platelet destruction process. Finding thirteen spleens was incomprehensible to the doctors, yet the astonishing peculiarities of the story were very familiar to me and my family. A silent part of me knew that the baby spleens began sprouting when I was placed in the hyperbaric chamber every day, twice a day, for five weeks to rejuvenate my tissue health; back in the burn unit seven years prior. There was no way to prove that, so I held space for the usual reaction while the doctors processed in amazing wonderment.

In the end, the splenectomy did not address the issue with my blood, even though science dictated it should, it did however, expand the minds of many which felt more familiar than anything. Over time, platelet crashes became an almost two-year cyclical experience. While trying to live, there was a silent experience of impending death that resided within every breath. A powerful experience that I never honored appropriately. What was unbeknown to most, yet most prevalent in my reality was that I lived with the possibility of death at any given moment. We all do, the minute we awake each morning and choose to enter the world from the safety of our home, and even that has proven not to protect us fully from the harms of life. Even so, I experienced it in a much different, and in a much more intimate way.

My platelets would drop dangerously low, covering my body in petechiae and bruises, followed by a fast-paced attempt to administer rescue medications in time to prevent mass internal bleeding, a fatality. Once stabilized and able to hold counts steady for at least a month, the medication weaning would begin and generally last nine months. Once off the medication and my body was allowed to sustain itself, my counts would hold for about six months, and then the cycle would start again. Eventually the rescue medications evolved into a minimum three day stay in the hospital while intravenous immunoglobulin therapy were administered. Over the course of twenty-five years, I danced intimately with death over a dozen times. There was a heaviness that came with the truth that I refined the intricate steps with each passing encounter. I wondered if I would ever know the dance of life as well as I knew the dance of death.

With the sensitivity in my blood as the backdrop, I was committed to make it the best life possible, and above all it would be meaningful. The stories that fill the beautiful life in between and the colors that make up the most radiant rainbow of life could fill many more books with portrayals of the mysticism encountered along my journey; perspectives of how and where I found gifts of joy and happiness to open. Be it so, the storyline to share in these expressions is what transpired in the silent space in between a beautiful life, and the storyline of my soul that was gracefully unfolding.

Amidst acquiring two undergraduate degrees, marrying a soul mate, creating, bearing, and rearing our three boys, nurturing a home, managing my ongoing medical, health and wellness needs, establishing a career, completing graduate school, and filling the numerous chosen roles within my reality, within the depths of my being something mystical was in the making. Within the space in between a beautiful life, I was exploring the universe within while up against the world around me.

I continued to experience normal life happenstances met by doctors that were reluctant and even refused to provide treatment out of fear of medical malpractice, mainly because there were no scientific baselines to support what was being presented; presented in me. I had to convince doctors of seemingly unrelated occurrences in my body and plea for trust and treatment, while they pondered the validity up against opposing scientific suggestions. I had heard several times from various fields of specialties during different diagnoses of discomfort and pain that there was little to recommend because assessing a baseline for discovery would be unnecessarily traumatic, more painful, and potentially unreliable when compared to the benefits of doing the analysis. Throughout medical experiences I was left feeling more like my own doctor than those who grew into their purpose to become one.

While moving through the medical matrix over the years which included several more surgeries, three semi-natural childbirths, and another organ removal making five in total, time and time again I was greeted with the eyes of wonderment when it felt like I needed much more. My mind contemplated and tried its best to adhere to the inherent knowledge of my body often driven by the sheer exhaustion of fighting so hard to stay alive in comfort. I often wondered if people of my past had advised my to not push my body and I had just not listened. I honestly do not recall anyone ever advising me to consider slowing down and closing differently. I really fell like I would have adhered to the advice since my body has forever felt tired. In fact, my first oncologist had one phrase of advice. I recall the visit when I was still nervous about my new blood diagnosis. "Make babies. Make lots of babies. We are alive to procreate" were his words of guidance. I did just that until I stifled my body to the point of uncertainty. I had always wished to find a doctor to help grow me to better understand the aftermath of my body. It is not broken that needs fixing, it is just different that needs understanding. The doctors of my past were not those doctors which only left me to navigate experiences with them, yet very much alone. Well, seemingly alone until I discovered my true self.

As doctors marveled in the mystery and tried to rely on science to treat me, science continued to fail me, and I wondered if my voice would ever be strong enough up against the medical community. Even so, I knew together we would figure something out that would leave me feeling better, whether it was with a tilted perspective, a treatment regimen, or an opportunity for growth. I always left feeling vulnerable and embarrassed in my exposure while knowing that there was a great likelihood that I had changed their world more than they had changed mine. I was always aware that modern medicine would never be able to heal the deepest parts within; especially the parts that felt like they were causing the physical ailments.

I prayed that any practitioner I encountered would be open to all possibilities for it was the only way I was able to journey before them; believing that all things are possible. Above all I could sense the healing powers when before me yet was unable to reconcile those truths with science. I have had experiences where my truths have aligned with science, and those that only come with a spiritual explanation; a miracle before us. I needed my healers to see both if I was going to be truly healed to a state of sustainability. I had to learn to stand in my wisdom of self while before medical professionals who merely looked at generalized science, and not the truths of my body, nor the story that comes with it.

I deeply believed that I would not survive another round of multi-dimensional trauma. I was so exhausted and actively healing from the first. And thus far those memories have proven to last this lifetime. It felt like one of my greatest desires was to walk a day without concern over the health of my body. It felt like I had lived a life on guard, prepared for any impending failure that would catch me when I was not paying attention. I could not fully relax and breathe into any moment because I remembered suffering, was suffering, was afraid of suffering, or knew that I would suffer in the aftermath. All of that existed before I grew into the world. The choices I made may have exacerbated the symptoms, but the root cause was much deeper and went beyond the physical body. I just wanted to feel comfortable in my body; feel comfort and not suffer. I wanted my body to feel good, and not afraid, embarrassed, or vulnerable in its truth. I wanted the peaceful and beautiful reality I held within to transcend into my reality setting me free from the cage of my body.

I was proud of everything I had been through. Even though, all the experiences with my body left me feeling more embarrassed and ashamed versus protective and nurturing of its truths and needs. Instead of being commanding of myself for the attention, time, and space to take care of me, I negated exposure, powered through, and even felt weak and fearful when I knew I had no other choice than to expose myself; the most vulnerable weakness being the condition of my breath sustaining body.

I knew I had to keep my body alive and figure out how to get the other parts of me working in unison so that I could live within this life comfortably and enjoy it; live my purpose. I so deeply wanted to experience life in joyful and freeing ways that I had not yet discovered. My mind had proven its ability to lead the way, and my tired body continuously was prepared to surrender and follow.

My Mind – The Space of My Mental Reality
The Mechanism that Propelled Me into My Fullest Potential

I continued to be led through experiences that created choice points for me to push the limits of my potential. Everything in the world that was growing me was telling me that this was what we were supposed to do in life. Especially the voice within. I agreed with that notion, and it was my choice whether or not to do so. It was important to me to know that I had done all I could do to achieve whatever it was that waited my discovery. Everything in the universe, the physical, metaphysical, scientific, spiritual, and all the likes, were reminding me I had purpose for being here. Trust me, I knew there was purpose. I too was eager to discover it in its entirety.

I knew I needed to fuel my mind if I were to ensure it would be sound after a journey through life. I recall finding it extremely difficult for me to decide a field of study while choosing a focus for university studies. I remember feeling defeated when I as unable to commit to just one field, or focus, as my lifelong interest. All fields were relevant to a greater unknown story within, and picking one felt like a disservice to the others. It felt preposterous to choose only one thing that I was to do for the remainder of my life when I enjoyed and was good at so many things. The process of deciding highlighted that the life experience is the real educational arena and I needed tools to ensure that I had what I needed to keep navigating life with strength, wisdom, and compassion. I viewed university as a hardware store with many skilled tools, and it was up to me to fill my magical toolbox. I decided then that my studies would somehow have to serve me no matter my profession and be transferable across any and all roles I may choose.

I started in microbiology, and after criticizing and judging myself and the limited ability of my mind to memorize data, I shifted and made a scientific trek to psychology. Throughout the mathematical, biological, physical, and social branches of science, it was the minds of the great psychologists, philosophers and physicists, and their myriad of perspectives and ideologies that added new levels of intriguing inquiry into my view of the human condition, the human body, spirituality and intended purpose.

The most resonating of all were the teachings of Socrates and his ideology that all truths are obtainable through asking the right questions. It was as though his teachings validated every question I had ever asked. And I have always asked a lot of questions. It was in my university days that I began intentionally using the Socratic method to ground every aspect of my life. About anything and everything. This gave a sense of tremendous confidence in my ability to solve any problem in life, especially coming to know the purpose of my life journey.

All the insightful and inspiring teachings acquired during my studies inevitably added tremendous color to the fabric of my being. The wisdom of those before us became the building blocks for the psychological strength needed to navigate myself and others; to understand what it means to be human in this world. Even through the studies of religion, science, philosophy, and many other fields, it was not until I encountered hypnosis many years later that I was given a language to my authentic and natural abilities. It was the first time that the voice within had words to relate to on the outside.

Hypnosis was presented to me as a conscious tool to cultivate the belief in something. Anything. A conscious tool that takes a thought, and over time, becomes a subconscious habit. The concept is that once it is embedded in the subconscious, then it is at a deeper level of knowing, and becomes a more integrated part of your overall being. Although it resonated at my core, it felt manipulative to know that our human brains could be programmed to achieve whichever outcome we desired. The idea and the truth that I could convince myself of anything I wanted and in time it would become truth was overwhelmingly accurate. I had lived that very truth.

I recall reconciling my past with the present, as it was within those moments that I realized what I had done to myself during the most physically painful moments of my life. A time when I was left alone, with my aware and visual mind, for endless heart and soul hours, unable to move; open in trauma on the outside, and peacefully relaxed within, with only the remains of my physical body that once separated the worlds.

I held a silent sense of pride in the younger versions of self for intrinsically knowing how to get through the experience. Concurrently I felt manipulative and overruling; I felt unauthentic and aggressive. I felt programmed and not natural. I knew it would become a delicate balance as I learned how to continue to be me in the awareness of such truth. I was humbled by my own false perceptions of self and with a new self-perceived sense of weakness I was able to look through my aged and murky lenses to find the trust needed to remember that I had been grown and morphed into exactly who I was meant to be.

I never practiced hypnosis in the way that it was presented, nor did it ever feel right to make a profession out of providing it to others as a means of self-healing. It felt like I was invading a sacred space that was not intended for me to visit even though an invitation was required before entry. It did however give me a language that included the collective consciousness, manifestation, law of attraction and laid the groundwork for understanding energy. I also incorporated the parts that worked for me and applied a practice to my inner spectrum of self.

At one end there was my human self, ridden with expectations and all its constructs, self-imposed and societal based, and full of unknown limiting beliefs. On the other end of the spectrum was my radiant, divine self, a source of abundant love and light, and full of infinite possibilities. Hypnosis became a self-propelling mechanism that I used to move, evolve, and expand my consciousness from the realm of my human ego and into a state of divinity. It was a tool that I hoped would serve its purpose. The more I walked through life, the more self-enlightenment seemed like the only attainment worth pursuing. My mind was up for the challenge.

All of the teachings, practices, and ideologies alike sourced in the psyche had taught me in a compilation of ways that my brain was more like a machine than anything else, acting as a sub-machine to the mega machine of the body. So, I treated it as such and allowed my mind to take in, process and compute the data. Good data in, good data out. Bad data in, bad data out. I programmed my operating system for only good data to be allowed in through natural selection along the walk through life.

The good data criteria were simple. In order for me to be fully engaged and take in an experience, it had to be happy, loving, and compassionate. If it was not, I most likely tuned it out even if my physical body was present. It was complicated, yet my mind was equipped to lead the way and did so honorably as if a crusader waving a peace flag in a final attempt for an eternal peace treaty. The mind was always much more willing and capable then my body was able. My body felt desperate to try and stay the pace and longed for the day that it was able to rest in peace while alive. I hoped it would be alongside you.

What I was never able to wrap my evolving awareness around was that if I was creating my reality, why was I creating a life centered around a walk to reach you, especially when it felt like you existed through a portal to another dimension. This further incited self-inquiry as to why I would remain dedicated to a journey that made me feel less human than I already felt knowing that living the human experience was why we are here and alive.

I enjoyed how I felt when I connected with my authentic self, and the beauty my expressions brought into the world. It felt like I had to choose you, or humanity. At least it felt like you knew I existed, whereas I wondered of my impact in the life that I had already lived. I wanted to just breathe in a sense of normalcy amidst the journey to reach you while knowing I was bringing extraordinary and unexplainable circumstances before you. I deeply wanted to believe that it would not cause you to turn your back on me. Even more painful to consider was if you were to turn your heart away. I trusted that neither would occur during the journey through the illusions of separate realities especially once I learned that we are one and the same.

I constantly tried to reconcile the teachings learned with my real-world experience and wondered which side was more accurate, theirs or mine. I could sense doubt forming over my reality and wondering if the reality of the teachings was more real than mine. My experiences were surely real to me, yet examples of similarities seldom could be found. It felt like I was on a never-ending path of change, adjustments, and acceptance yet everyone around me appeared to be grounded, knew who they were and steadfast in purpose. I wondered why I was unable to achieve the same.

We are constantly changing and evolving beings. I knew this truth about the world, and I could intimately feel this truth about myself. It had become one of the most honored parts of my human experience; the fluidity to navigate change. Even so it left me feeling tired and weary after so long. We are not the same people we were just moments prior. Every moment changes us. Change is the only constant in our experiences. After many years, the change within began pushing up against something as if pleading for escape. My mind was intrigued with what was occurring within, for it had been orderly and ruly over my body as a whole.

I had already lived through the truth of what my mind could do, which was anything. I knew it could get off track and I knew it could change how I functioned. I experienced the potential impact each floating thought held over my emotions. I was a machine of parts, and I was acutely aware how each breath fueled its interworking dynamics. My mind calculated every move to ensure I kept my pars together, and to know what to do next. I did not even realize how tiresome it had become because the world was full of people living, thriving, and growing. We were all doing the same thing, so I believed my mind was working like any other mind. Almost like you too could see all the perspectives yet knew which one was yours. I just wanted to know which one was purely mine because there were infinite perspectives in my sight, and I could relate to all of them, all were valid, all held truth, and all were honorable. I just wanted mine.

Within every step I took I believed I was doing the best that I could, yet it never felt like enough within the deepest parts of me; enough to know my truths. Or else I would have known, and the quest would have been complete. I celebrated every step that felt one step closer, while simultaneously saddened that I was not yet there. I hoped that knowing my purpose would coincide with an experience that was yet to be enjoyed.

Tapping into my potential felt like it was deeply linked to you. I deeply wanted to experience both. It felt like my mind was dragging my body in tote to get me to the next checkpoint to rest until my body could take on another round. My body knew it had to hang on for the great reveal yet wondered how much longer it would take. It felt like I was losing strength from the walk, and not only physical strength. I was losing mental, emotional, and most weary of all was the spiritual strength which I knew I never held securely. It felt like I was disintegrating into dust praying that you would rebuild me with your healing love, and before it was too late.

Early on in developing the portrayal of my life experiences, I was ever so kindly reminded, within everything and everywhere I went, that I would bring about what I think about. I was very aware of this notion. I always have been. I used this tactic during my recovery, my relationships, my education, my work, my medical trials, during every navigation of everything. It is at the source of who I am. It gave me even more of a reason to create space for my mind to rest. It felt like the intensity, power and momentum of this truth was going faster that I could manage.

I knew what was happening at every point that this was viewed through the lens of my younger versions of self, and the various layers of dirt, even after a gentle cleanse. I may not have even been able to express it to myself, but I could always see it in clarity within me. One of my core self-talk mantras used to be, "everything begins with a thought so make it a great one!" I may have labeled it differently, but the premise was always the same. Mind over matter was another popular slogan for many years. My truth was that the entirety of my life had become a product of thoughts; mine and yours alike.

All the while, it was my normal and no one was able to share an expression of any kind that truly grew me deeper and further into life; into love; into who I am. I carried on my way doing the best I was able by always asking myself four critical questions. I believed these questions would keep my thoughts sane and rational while navigating against the grain. I made sure that every thought and experience was factually true, that an experience was in my best interest, I was getting what I wanted, and that my life would be protected and prolonged as a result.

This is an inherent truth of being human, to create a reality from our thoughts. I am not alone in this ability, yet because of who I am, I honor my sensitivity to this truth, and I have had to learn how to flow with this powerful truth. Just as many have done before me, as will many in my wake, the remaining stories to be shared in this book walk you through the experiences of what it looked like for me to unleash the power within me; to connect to my purpose; to connect to you. It was a journey that quieted the mind so that I only manifest my heart's desires.

The expansion within was constant and fluid and clear and precise, yet my physical body could not translate the dialect into any meaningful expression. My mind rallied the fragmented parts of me and tried to mindfully manage what was integrated into one and was doing so in a seemingly masterful way. Until all my parts were ready, I was evolving within an ordinary life with ordinary human experiences and producing ordinary life outcomes. Life was beautiful and great yet deemed ordinary from the depths within me.

My soul yearned to feel normal in the extraordinary life within which I lived. I knew every aspect of me was growing to support the story unfolding within and before me. My mind performed as the rest of my parts sat patiently on the edge of their seats waiting for the moment to jump up cheering in celebration. It took the journey through the integration process to learn that I was the only one standing in my way. It was the precise outcome I intentionally tried to avoid. It was sobering to the perfectionist in me that I had worked so diligently to make the right choices only to find that I remained the fundamental flaw.

My mind was determined to do what was needed to stay engaged until its assignment was complete and all of my being knew you were out there. My mind was convinced that the world had evolved to the extent to contain the tools needed to find you. My mind felt like a warrior out on an adventure; somewhere in the world that left me behind. Even throughout a marriage and a journey through love my eyes were always on you. I sought out for my tools throughout experiences and encounters, which made the chaos make more sense and gave the struggles meaning. I felt peace when I looked into the world around me to find that life was providing all the tools needed to catch back up to the collective, and more importantly to find you.

I looked into the world and intellectualized my way through anything and everything, even the most heart burdened experiences. I reflected upon myself and life experiences through all the lenses that humanity prepared for exploration to find purpose. Yet time and time again, the minds of humanity alone could not explain me, nor what I was intended to do. All the while, the world within continued to evolve with clarity and precision, and albeit there was a voice, it came mostly without words that my mind could not decipher. They were messages for and from my heart which held every vibration needed to understand the unspoken words.

It was a compassionate voice that guided me through everything. The same voice was waiting for me to open my eyes from the coma to pose my first inquiry. The voice that answered every question ever asked about everything from that point forward. The same voice that guided me back to my soul, where I found you.

The voice within engaged in dialogue with my human mind, guiding me through every experience my being encountered. It was the voice within that walked my mind through the analytical, intellectual, and systematic process of holding my parts together. It was the voice within that battled with my ego to ensure purity of heart was maintained along the quest. It was the voice within that ensured I discovered every clue you left behind. It was the voice within that my mind had to surrender to if I wanted to follow my heart.

For all my life I believed the voice within was just my own. My own built-in protagonist and antagonist playing out scenarios to ensure I chose best for my whole being. I thought we all had the built-in mechanism. It was during the journey to balance into who I am that I discovered the voice within was much more. The only aspect I knew with certainty was that the voice was mine yet originated beyond me yet resided within me and it was guiding me to you. I questioned my own sanity during the pleas for a sound mind. I prayed you wanted to share your love with my heart so that my mind could finally rest from the quest.

The gentle voice kept my mind humble and ashamed of its unruly actions. It was the voice that held space for the truth, and all I knew to do was to follow the clear guidance. The voice assured the heart that, in time, my mind would experience what was needed to relax and let go. The voice held tremendous patience for my other parts to catch up to its wisdom. The voice was the conductor in the authentic convalescent orchestra healing my parts; a process that was never mentioned as an essential part of my youthful experience. In time, the voice took charge and commanded attention from all my parts and all my senses and made it clear that my heart would now lead the way into eternity.

My Heart – The Space of My Emotional Reality
The Compass That Led Me Through the Universe

My heart was all I had to go by in the nonsensical world around me. My heart held a sense of deep longing that I would one day feel whole again however never truly remembered the sensation as a gauge. It grew up believing that life was a walk towards a deep love until my perspectives tilted and I could see the love that brought me to life. Then I realized that life is a walk of choice in love - towards, away, with or without.

I was also acutely aware that I could draw upon all the emotions associated with all degrees of brokenness, and hardly any of the degrees of wholeness. I knew what it felt like recovering from a state of trauma, yet not what it felt like to exists in a state being healed. It felt like a lifelong journey of its own and that I would spend my life healing from the traumatic experience in some way or another. I lived through some pretty intense situations and always preferred to honor the healing achieved and continued to move forward.

Still, there remained a deep sadness that accompanied a belief that I would never fully recover, but I was determined to always move in that direction. Once I began living the details of my reality, I lived a forever unfolding story to be shared. I knew that it was a beginning of a journey to learn and grow through experiences that would in time tip the scales into balance; and I knew you would be involved in some way.

Although I had been mindfully convinced that I did not hold a lot of fear, my heart's truth was that it held a lot of deep rooted fear, beyond my own physical body and experiences in this life. My heart's deepest fear was that I would feel the way I felt for the remainder of my life, incomplete and fragmented across the universe. I was not accepting of that notion as a truth of mine and trusted that I was being led to the space I was intended to embody, wholly as uniquely me. I just had to hold trust, faith, and patience.

I so deeply wanted to believe that my heart had been leading me through the very experiences to learn the life lessons to later be practiced in the space of living a fully integrated and abundant life. It was the only thing that gave everything meaning. In a sense it was what was keeping me alive. I had to trust in you even when it felt like all I had to do was trust myself.

The very notion of my ever-evolving sense of self was the most prevalent and integral space of my existence when making life decisions. The most intentional were those regarding my education to broaden my intellect, career moves and associated notions to establish a sense of security and stability. The most sacred were the experiences that involved the matters of my heart. It felt like I was living experiences that I had to walk through, navigate the awareness of what they meant, what the experience was like, and even more so what that walk felt like. My heart is what drove every expression of self especially once I invited my soul and my love to calibrate into a sensual dance of spiritual love.

As my pre-trauma dreams were remolded from a youthful enthusiasm out to conquer the world, and into a critically aware importance on survival and safety, I adapted to the rapid, and unexpected adjustment. I had no choice. I was no longer dreaming of international travels and diverse life experiences brought on by work and globally positioned friendships. Instead, I was dreaming of how to remain healthy and functional in a life that made absolutely no sense and wondered how I would choose to find joy along the way. I hoped it would lead to love.

By the age of seventeen, my own life had become the very example that anything, everything, and even nothing is possible when viewed through the lens of belief. By the time I was living back in Louisiana, I believed that I could do anything, yet acknowledging now that I was still limited in what I believed that to truly mean. My body and mind dynamic duo conspired on how to bring the dreams of my heart into fruition even as I continued the ever-evolving expansion of who I thought I was and wanted to become. It was an expansion of self that grew as my timid fragility slowly transformed into strength of self; albeit never transforming quickly enough, nor feeling strong enough when out in the world around me.

The early years upon my return to Louisiana now feels like a lovely dream of youthful freedom yet it certainly never felt that way when experiencing them. I always felt nervous and timid; fragile and uncertain; strong and courageous yet bashfully shy while plowing through every feeling with an intellectualized rationale that kept the pace. I had to learn that I never really allowed myself the time and space to integrate life into who I was being grown into. I hastily found activities to fill my time, avenues to socialize and privy of engagements that would help grown me back into love with myself and my body so that it could be enjoyed, and with another. It seemed like experiencing a deep connection with someone remained a deeply rooted calling. It felt greater than a mindful desire, it felt more like a soulful mission. Even so, I was shamefully embarrassed of my body and struggled with exposures, explanations, and judgements. Amongst friends was easy, but on an intimate level it was a spiritual struggle with love.

Although it was the only sense worth trusting, my heart was shielded by trauma that remained vulnerable, timid, and uncertain. My mind fought with my heart repeatedly as it was the most current in life, storing data and computing outcomes. Although it was mostly in opposition to how I felt, my mind was adamant to know best. I survived within these boundaries while my body warded off the manifestations of the fearful, wounded, and doubtful mind masking my wounded heart. Even so, my body and mind took charge while my heart remained traumatized and childish in its dreams of life and in love, trapped behind the uncontrolled erection of its protective shield.

As I looked into the world, my heart felt the dichotomy between what it felt and my mind's narrative, yet my mindful justifications and perspectives were more powerful, and my heart was unable to bust through the cracks. I was very aware of my parts and the roles they held in an unintegrated state of existence. This was perhaps more painful than the physical experiences endured by my body itself. It was clear that my heart was the compass of my experience and I needed to regain control of my heart to guide the way to love.

Since there were infinite possibilities, I always tried to come from a place of kindness and understanding, especially with myself. It does not always mean that I did, but I tried my best and would attempt to correct my limited self in some way for growth. If I found myself unsure of how or what that meant, I reminded myself of love. I would think about love and the ideals around love. I reminded myself of experiences I had with love. I enjoyed the experiences that I was living out of love. I contemplated what I thought I knew of love and the teachings that molded my beliefs in love. I honored those with whom I shared my intimate experience of love, which from behind my lens of love never had anything to do with physical, sexual nor romantic love. I had to learn that it means intimate, intuitive, and sensual love.

From the moment I chose to marry and grow a family, I inherently chose to push the unknown infinite capacity of my love. I knew that if I held the privilege of creating life, I would undoubtably hold unconditional love for my child. The trust was that I would be able to continue to hold unconditional love for another human being that had also journeyed a life, separate yet now joined with mine. It was a choice of acceptance in the totality of another being that was a sacred decision to make. I knew deep within that I desired to be accepted in the totality of who I am, therefore, I desired to hold the same level of acceptance for another. I believed that as long as the purity of our commitment to each other was upheld, love would always prevail and grow us deeper and stronger into love.

Knowing that I always followed authentic love when I sensed it, eventually I chose to join lives with another to begin building a beautiful life together. We spent twenty-one years growing each other into the versions of ourselves we are today. We grew into the best and worst parts of ourselves, while simultaneously growing and expanding those parts of ourselves into our children. Even the expectations of what it would be like raising three sons dissipated into the messy, hard, and beautiful reality as they continue to evolve into who they are meant to become.

I cherished what I had created out of love, the most prideful being the miracles that are my children. And although the relationship with their father evolved into what it was designed to become, there is an inherent love that will forever remain regardless of how the physical experience of our knowing each other plays out. Love is very sacred to me and if you share in my love, it is eternal. I believed love to be so much more than an emotion, or an ideal that inherently reduces its infinite capacity merely by framing it into a label of any kind. I knew every version of my evolving love that I continued to experience and felt nervous in the awareness of that truth. Love has always been at the source of who I am.

I lived the brutal truth of awareness that every action and word serve as a strand of silk that in time is woven with life's many strands to form the fabric of who we become. I honored the truth in that the circumstances of my life, and the choices I make will inherently mold the circumstances of the lives of my children. My breath is a part of their existence. They are of me yet separate from me. They were created through and of me yet are not mine to own. There was a great sense of responsibility to grow them into grounded and fulfilled human beings, and for a lifetime. How to do that remained the mystery, so I continued to be me the best I knew how as I journeyed trying to find my way. A child of the universe now raising children of my own.

Once I created the space to bring my best self forward for my children, I was able to see them for who they really are. They were my sprouting indigo children with natural gifts of interpreting the meta-physical world around us. As I grew them into the world, they became my spiritual teacher. It was evident that I had to nurture their authentic gifts, yet while unconnected to mine I wondered how I would manage to do so. It felt like honoring myself was at the source of teaching them how to do the same and it felt as time was of the essence up against the world that continued to grow us into dissonance.

I had created humans that would have a physical experience in this world. Parts of me deeply wanted them to encounter the same amazing experiences I felt blessed to have had, while concurrently praying deeply that they were not brought on by experiences similar to mine. For I would never wish anyone to endure the life I have lived yet prayed the experiences would be comparable in mysticism. I felt torn because it was the life I had lived that led to the beautiful experiences, mainly those after my illness, but aware that it was because of my illness that the wonderment unfolded.

I wanted to ground my children in strength, courage, and love in all aspects of their beings, but felt that I lacked a solid foundation in the most important aspect of our existence, spirituality; our energetic being. I wanted to ensure they understood what they should stand for and how to hold their own space in the universe yet felt uncertain of my own.

I held a deep desire to understand what it was I was to teach them beyond the physical experiences brought on by education, professions, monetary and emotional stability, and to hold sacred the love held within their heart. I felt as though there was something much greater that I was to guide them towards. I just remained uncertain as to what that was but felt as though it was sourced in a spiritual love; a love that required an open heart, my open heart. I also felt deeply that the soulful growth underway would tilt those perspectives in ways that would provide clarity in the unique role I held within their lives, and theirs within mine.

Just as with many aspects of my being, I believed I was completely competent to handle whatever the journey would be. I was always on guard and ready to defend my life. In my broken humanness, in particularly in my seemingly distant emotions, I felt capable of raising children and allowing them to have the space to grow and become who they are meant to become. I knew I deeply wanted that for myself, and knew that it was not my place, nor would it ever be my place, to dictate their life to them. As the creator of their body, I knew their inner voice would be what would guide them through life, just as mine had done for me. It was up to me to ensure that the voice they heard was the voice of their heart and soul, and to teach them to discern the difference between that of the mindful ego.

Furthermore, I wanted to ensure their heart was the compass of their life experiences because I trusted that would lead them to peace and truths within. My own powerful teenage ego was example enough to know that the voice could be loud enough to sway one out of balance, while concurrently holding the potential to manifest related outcomes. I wanted to ensure that if their ego was indeed preventing the voice of their heart and soul from expression, I wanted to ensure the mind was positive, loving, supportive, inspiring, expansive, and enlightened enough for them to know that anything is possible, while remaining compassionate, understanding, empathetic, and accepting of everyone and their unique experiential humanness.

The more I grew, the more expansive my metaphysical inquiries became and the more my heart became intriguingly more captivated by the journey of the soul while living a human experience, especially my own. This became the space of my freedom. This became the space of my infinite potentiality. This was the space my heart longed to be when not engaged in the hectic life activities. With a family of three growing boys, a marriage and a career, there was little time for the space of my free and authentic self. Over time my own expansive beliefs left my heart feeling hindered for my heart to dream within my human experience.

The dreams others held for me always seemed less glorious than the ones I was able to imagine on my own. Even so, I knew that my imagination was inherently limited, which meant that the potentials were even more glorious than my mind could imagine. The more dreams in life I crafted, the more dreams were realized and the less they felt like dreams to dream. As physical world dreams came and were realized, and in a sense losing their luster, I knew I would have to dig deeper into my heart to receive the dream that truly held a sense of fulfillment. It was a beautiful yet sad state of awareness when I realized the difference between physical world accomplishments and what real dreams of the heart feel like. When I viewed my dreams through the new lens, the only dream I ever knew for my heart has been to share a deep soulful love with another in the fullness of my vulnerable and intimate authenticity. I was humbled, excited, and nervous by the acknowledgement that dreams are always realized. Mine and yours alike.

While continuously up against them, it took many years for me to see that it was the beliefs of those around me, primarily during my illness and recovery, that formed the baseline of expectations that my heart always aspired to grow beyond. Even more impactful was the awareness that the sub-par expectations were sourced in a fear that I inherently lacked while aspiring to be more. The most noticeable messages were through unspoken languages which revealed that incomplete and inaccurate realties were being created about me. These were the messages that often set the backdrop for my life script; a script that surprisingly everyone seemed to have memorized in their hearts, yet I was unable to integrate the expressions into the role I held in the screenplay. The scripts seemed so vastly different while remaining desperate to reveal that they were indeed the same; just seemingly different. The most common oxymoronic expression of my youth; different but the same; similar but different.

Although encouraging and optimistic in their own way, the levels and standards of achievement were set very low. Even for my own state of happiness. It seemed as if through the eyes of the world, it was enough to have survived. Perhaps it was but I never saw it that way. Through my eyes, it was time to get the show on the road and discover why I was still alive. I clearly had multiple opportunities for my time on Earth to cease. It felt blatantly clear that the Mighty Maestro had other plans. The expectations of me, created by those around me, were not acceptable to me. I certainly doubted that if I stood alone in the realm of everyone else's expectations, that it would not be acceptable, nor would I be able to explain myself when I held my moment before you.

I was patiently waiting for my mystical explanation. It felt as if the same patience was being held for me to discover it; for the day I could speak from my heart in honor about my earthly actions. I promised within the ethers of my faith that I would continue to do the best I felt I could do in life and push the boundaries of my potential the best I was able. I sensed that there was something powerful and sacred within my heart that begged for my commitment. It felt like a deep soulful love was yearning to be set free. In time it was this very feeling of potential love energy that became the transformative catalyst in discovering my truths.

I had to fulfill my part and be willing to trust, receive and believe that there would always be joy in whatever was delivered. It was up to my response and impending choices to find the nuggets of joy; it was the same tactic that pulled me through every moment of trauma endured. Sometimes it was through fun, beautiful, and bright experiences where joy was easily found. Other times it was through hard, messy, and dark experiences when the joy could only be found in the love that guided me through. Combined, a beautiful life of infinite possibilities colored my world with love.

I hoped all that I was using to mold my perception of love was leading me to you. I was terrified to even consider that everything I built my life upon was false, while simultaneously trusting that every experience and every soul encountered was leading the way to you. More often than not, I did not even realize I was making a choice as long as I kept you in sight. The gift of the unknown was that by having the desire to fulfill my purpose more fully, and walking more wholly towards you, I was organically fulfilling my purpose. Years and experiences later when I understood how to tap into my self-perpetuating cycle was when the magic entered my experience and illuminated the final steps to reach you. Love was polishing my prism heart.

Until then, it was the belief that among the infinite possibilities, there was always one outcome that was perfectly designed for my heart, solely for me, at precisely the right time and would deliver exactly what I needed. I just had to trust, be open to receive and know there would always be joy in whatever was delivered. Belief was at the source of my faith that propelled me through life. At least until I met knowing, then belief felt lacking.

My heart has encountered many life experiences, plenty that I did not agree with, and even some that I could not comprehend as being on any path of love and joy. Even so, everything always felt peaceful and right when I believed in the unbeknown. My internal world was much more peaceful and graceful to navigate than my external world. I held on to the hope that there would be a day that I would feel the fullness of who I am, and I would know that I had unequivocally arrived in the space of love and joy throughout the remaining days of my life. I also believed that I would have to stand alone in that moment, physically and metaphysically yet unsure of what either truly meant. I deeply believed that joy with another can only be shared purely once one is able to stand in joy alone. I deeply felt this to be my truth. A truth that eventually ended a twenty-two year partnership with my heart.

It was overwhelming to experience others seeing my mystical truths before I could embody them myself. I needed a safe space to be human, be vulnerable, be tender in my experience. Not to be glorified as an example of a miracle, nor to be fixed with advice on how to do better, but to sit quietly, or through expressions, and simply allow me to fall knowing that I will pull myself up in the very next breath. I found it was hard being human more often than not and longed for my external world to reflect the quiet and still space I felt so deeply on the inside.

All the while, until it was time, and for some reason or another, my unintegrated parts continued to do the best they were able, acting out in their own accord while my heart busted free to reach you. Often times I was left with a sense that there was much to be done in the wake of my wobble. I knew everything was converging into one while wondering if I would experience it while still alive to fully enjoy it.

I decided that if I could control the input and output of my mind, I would be able to decipher all the truths that my physical world experienced and transmute the information in such a way that I would no longer get lost in the matrix of the human mind. In its place would be the transcendence into my heart to experience the sweetest and warmest love. After a life of collecting data, my mind and body duo longed to rest and allow my heart to feel truth like it was able to feel everything else. My peace came from setting out with forward-thinking optimism, self-growth, and to do the best I could to return to a sense of wholeness. Truthfully it was something I did not remember ever feeling in this life. Perhaps because I had never lived without fear and doubt.

I found that the true dreams of my heart were in exact alignment with the potential I held yet stood in my way from achieving. For me it was growing into my spiritual senses and flowing with Divine Love energy. It felt like the more I grew into the core of my being, the more nervous I became in meeting you. Each step closer was exposing my truths and my love for you; I was exposing them to me.

My Soul – The Space of My Spiritual Reality
The Song that Led My Dance with Love

I was born and raised Catholic in the strong Christian community in Southern Louisiana. Both of my parents served in Catholic Orders in their youth. My Dad was a brother within the Brothers of the Sacred Heart Order in New Orleans, and my Mom was a nun within the Dominican Order in Rosaryville, both in Louisiana and less than an hour apart by vehicle. They were known as Brother Lawrence, Sacre Coeur, and Sister Joan of Arc, respectively. This naturally led to a deeply rooted faith that was taught throughout my childhood. There was a sense of poetic irony given the plight I would endure, and the incomprehensible amount of strength, courage, and faith they would need on the journey. They were clearly being carried in faith early on in their lives.

They met when they were both still heavily involved in their religious Orders, and during their encounters and conversations, it was identified that perhaps they were both on their paths with the church for reasons other than their devotion to God. Due to his educational upbringing, My Dad believed he could only become a teacher if he was a Brother of the Church, and my Mom joined the convent to escape a troubled home life.

As part of the mass exudes in the 1960's, inspired and excited that their faith was leading them away from organized religion, they both left the church to start a life together and to form more liberal connections to their faith. My Mom left the convent first, and since my Dad had already taken his celibacy vows, he followed six months later after receiving the release of his religious obligations from Pope Paul VI in Vatican City.

Once they dissolved their commitment to the church, they made a commitment to each other. They wed and started to build a home they could share. They both became teachers, and they remained dedicated to the Catholic religion and the church community. Together they grew a family within a community of love and Christian faith.

During their lives together, they remained very committed to the Catholic church. Our family went to mass every Sunday, and the kids participated in Sunday school while my parents participated in the liturgical meeting and preparations. My brother was an altar boy, my Dad played the organ, both of my parents were eucharistic ministers, and we even baked the unleavened bread in our family kitchen at home, sometimes right after baking our family meals. As children we were also inundated with religious dogma all day, every day at the Catholic school we attended, with mass every Wednesday. We were friends with families from church and school, and our family was very active in the religious community. Therefore, it was part of who we were. Never discussed. Never Challenged. It just was.

Even so, the older I grew the more questions arose. I kept them quietly within while surrounded by what appeared to be questionless believers. I thought to myself I must be broken, especially given the background of my family, and the generations of service in the Catholic church. I was surprised to uncover decades later that the story I created in my youth laid the foundation of what I grew to believe. I grew myself to believe I was spiritually broken. Once I discovered the storyline, everything shifted more into its rightful space, albeit that did not occur for decades to come.

From birth to age thirteen, I was an innocent child wondering what would happen if I questioned the existence of God. Not that I did, I just wondered about what was being taught. The idea of an all-knowing and all-powerful Being, existing outside of ourselves, as a Heavenly Father that loved us and would deliver us from evil. All the while, it remained at the source of disharmony while humanity worked to prove or disprove Its existence while holding faith in their One. More fascinated by my childish mind was that there were communities everywhere that did the same. I used to chuckle on the pew when I heard the sermons that reference the flock of sheep, for we were the sheep being led by the shepherds.

I was taught for thirteen years to believe in only one God, and Jesus Christ is the only example of that truth while encouraged to ignore the truth that we all have the power to be an example too. Although I played my youthful part, I challenged my beliefs and God quietly within. I did not know anything about other religions, other than that they existed, and that I found it difficult to accept that all other beliefs were blasphemy, and the believers of those shall perish.

From an early age, I wondered if I myself would perish if I did not fully believe in the God of teachings. It felt like I was being asked to believe out of fear, and that never felt right. I thought that it should be a choice out of love. I never feared the truth of who I may be and the impending outcome of my spiritual choice. It was a choice to believe or not, and my framework was the Catholic religion. I believed yet I was being told I would perish for even questioning.

Then, at the age of thirteen, we moved overseas and began attending the international school. School became the singular setting that contained individuals from over sixty countries. I was exposed to diversity in everything. Diversity in nationalities. Diversity in cultures. Diversity in language. Diversity in cuisine. Diversity in fashion. And most prominent was the diversity in religion. I was profoundly aware of the diversity that existed within the belief systems that coexisted around me and lived harmoniously with me. I could silently hear them all proclaiming to have their own God. Meanwhile, my spiritual beliefs went from an innocently growing, youthful strength in one God, to a curiously confused adolescent exposed to the possibility of sixty more. It did not seem possible for there to be more than one God, especially when everyone believed they were right in their One. I quietly observed the spiritual space of my experiences transform while the inquiry of how there could be sixty-one Gods floated throughout my being. Everything I was taught seemed contradictory to what my reality was presenting. Everything that I thought I knew and believed about God was shattered into doubt.

While overseas, we still attended mass on Sundays, and I even received the sacrament of Confirmation. I chose to honor Santa Rosa de Lima, Saint Rose of Lima, Peru, and would hold her name as a reminder of love. I recall that the deciding factor in those times was that the Saint was canonized on April 12, 1671; April 12th is my birthdate.

In selecting St. Rosa, my evolving heart was awakened to the metaphysical inquiry of what someone is willing to do in the name of love. It was unbeknown that I would later connect deeper with the outcomes of her journey, which was a distorted physical being. Hers was self-induced in reverence of an unwavering love of God; mine delivered unto me, followed by a journey back home to the same unwavering love energy.

I also love the sweet sights and smells of a beautiful budding flower. They are a beautiful gift I give my senses whenever I have the chance. Coupled with my romantic Shakespearian heart, I always believed that to know me is to love me and to be loved by me. I believed that a rose by any other name would not smell as sweet and that I was the sweetest smelling rose, attracting the most beautiful butterflies—my princess fairytale of self.

However, none of the teachings of my youth provided the same sense of rooted faith that grew me for thirteen years, now with a blanket of diversity upon me. Over time, our attendance at the English-speaking masses started to decrease, and we started attending the church around the corner from our home. The biggest change was that they were either in French or Dutch. It was difficult to connect to a message delivered in an unknown language. It was this practice of personal interpretations of my faith that bridged me to the messages from the Pope and his elegant Polish voice during my sacred visit before him. The distance between me and the Catholic religion continued to widen with my own disjointed faith now patchwork pieces of many. The more I experienced and learned in life, the more I grew within the depths of my label-less faith.

I felt confused, intrigued, and curious to understand how it could be so. I wondered about the taught notions of coexistence, acceptance, and unconditional love within international belief systems and the misconception that it is impossible to achieve. It had been the source of wars between nations and religions alike. I did not understand how any religion could put limitations on who, where, and how one is to love. For me, it was through the teachings of Christianity, yet it was evident that others were doing the same, and before me in harmony.

The more people I met, and the vastness of beliefs encountered, the more I began to mold my own ideals of Christian love. The Christian love that I felt was represented in the stories of the Bible yet were never fully delivered, nor received, in such a way that I could embrace the purity of their intention. I remember navigating my youthful interpretations of the Bible and how the words resonated deeper than I ever understood while sounding silly to my unevolved ears.

My silent confusion, in essence, was fueling a passion to discover what spirituality truly meant to me, and not just the dogma that was taught, nor expected meanings. It was a part of me to know completely, and I did not. I never had. As a young teenager, I do not recall reflecting on spirituality as much as I was cautiously shielding myself from external influences. I was very spiritually confused, which left me spiritually shielded, for I knew no one would be able to clarify my confusion but me and my God if there was one.

It was as if I was constantly preventing the absorption of opinions, ideologies, and belief systems while I tried to understand my own. I felt spiritually on guard, not knowing if I was dealing with One, or Many. Instead of inviting more Gods of protection, I became defensive to all. As if I had been lied to and no one offered to provide the clarity it warranted. I slowly became a cautious spiritual observer. I had transitioned from a mindless believer in my youth to a cautious observer that was tested time and time again. It felt like I was testing my faith, more than my faith was testing me. Testing by questioning, and doubting, and at times almost commanding a presence so I could know with my being. My youthful being was processing the best I was able.

I was already timid in my faith and guarded in my youthful sense of disconnect when asked to seek God outside of myself. Then I became ill, and everything about my spirituality changed even more. When I awoke from the coma and learned of my reality, initially, I felt spiritually abandoned. I knew of my life experiences up to that point, life choices and resulting consequences, and inquiries of the afterlife if there was one.

I questioned if I was being punished by God, and the collective of sixty, for any of my actions, thoughts, or for my stubborn inquisitions. I wondered if my illness was the powerful message from beyond that was intended for me to receive, powerful enough to be received by every cell of my being, and to see it with my own eyes.

I felt ashamed to bear a burden that could have possibly been brought on by self. I contemplated whether I held such power. I felt spiritually shunned by what I thought was pure and protective, as if we could not look each other in the face exposing we knew the truth. I could not find one single God before me as I fought for life, abandoned and afraid. Even so, everywhere I looked I saw evidence of a mystical presence yet gone before our moment of reconciliation.

I wanted nothing more than to know the truth in the words of my reassuring poem. I desperately wanted to believe that the footprints in the sand were not mine, but those of whomever carried me. I wanted to feel it deep within. I cried myself to sleep many nights in the hospital, praying that my doubt-ridden faith would be enough. I prayed I would be carried because, at times, it felt like I did not have the spiritual strength to go on. At times my spiritual doubt felt more painful than the physical trauma. I had to trust in the awareness that my faith would be the only gauge of truth. I was willing to take the risk, since I was still here, and bashful since my illness somehow amplified the instability of my youthful faith.

Once I agreed to accept the truth that I was never spiritually alone, there was a sense of betrayal that surfaced. If I had not been abandoned, then that meant that God, or Many, knew of my trauma and suffering, and furthermore allowed it. Shattering my being was permitted in the presence of whatever powerful source existed. Surely a God would not allow the pain I was experiencing. The feeling that a God would allow such suffering felt like a deep betrayal. I could not comprehend how an all-loving Deity could allow such pain and suffering, and it be in the name of love. Betrayal felt worse than abandonment.

I felt spiritually betrayed, not by one God, but by sixty-one Gods. I felt betrayed by a belief that I was taught would protect me, along with the collective of sixty others that represented the same commitment. It felt like a huge misunderstanding that needed to be clarified. A teacher, somewhere along the way in life, potentially has misleading information. It could be anyone I have ever encountered. It was this misunderstanding that gained momentum over time that ultimately contributed to many years of living with the sense of a disjointed existence, with an existential trauma of sorts.

For decades I lived patiently disjointed until I discovered that I was betraying myself by doubting my faith and therefore denying the magic of a God. Until then, I didn't not know what I did not know. Throughout my recovery while in the hospital and during my senior year, I questioned my brokenness and how it fit into my beliefs. I still believed that there was a greater source to the mystical wonderment in life. I was less concerned about how it was labeled and remained curious as to how my brokenness was a part of the maestro's masterpiece. I sometimes even doubted there was a masterpiece at all because if there were, how could my experience be a part of that beauty. I wondered how I could be a part of that beauty because I surely did not feel beautiful. Nothing about my experience was physically beautiful. I felt tremendously broken and rejected, vulnerable and exposed, traumatized, and afraid, scarred, and damaged. I had to believe that if everything was true about God, and the master plan, then I would be ok. I would be better than ok. I would be amazing.

With that focus, throughout the sentiments of my humanness there remained a very clear infinite space where everything rested in peace. I could see it so clearly, along with my self-imposed separation between the label of God and what I knew as the ethers of my faith. Seemingly contradictory, while I repaired my relationship with the God I desired to know, alongside my uncertainty and doubt, I placed all my trust within the ethers of my faith and believed that my voice would be heard. Somehow, I believed they were unrelated to each other, and I could separate them and live within one without the other. I could see them side by side and my unwillingness to tilt my head to reconcile the truth in their oneness.

In truth, there was nothing to dispute; without question, there is a greater force. It felt more like the truth in spiritual perfection was more overwhelming to process than the truths of my physical body's trauma. It seemed like the physical changes progressed as seamlessly as possible, which in and of themselves were threaded with mysticism. I felt the energy behind the Global Wave of Healing Energy more than I was ever able to explain the truth of its impact yet carried it and felt it deep within for decades until balanced back into perfection. It was the ungrounded, uncertain, and doubtful spiritual navigation that seemed to throw me off balance more than my traumatized legs and my compromised physical experience.

When the notions of spiritual abandonment and betrayal had been acknowledged, I requested patience and understanding, and for personal allowance to grow through my trauma and into love. I knew deep within that I had to learn how to love myself in my new body and within a newly framed life experience. While I journeyed towards that love, there was a sense of spiritual acceptance in my need to establish rules of engagement and the boundaries needed by the humbling truth of my humanity.

There was a need for flexibility to mend my soul, a flexibility to use various labels that corresponded with my healing. The ethers of my faith, the universe, the mystical force, I was even embarrassed when I tried to use the label of God many times throughout my life. It took decades of life experiences and healing for the label to comfortably enter into my spoken truths. My bashful stubbornness felt accepted with the understanding smirk upon the face of my God as grace and mercy swept over me, time and time again. It felt like a gesture of tolerance in my childish ways until I was able to bridge the differences and accept the truths.

I found my circumstances were easiest to navigate when I honored the truth of my experience, and the perfection threaded throughout my life. Indeed, the illness itself was unfortunate, but that has always felt like it came from a different source, perhaps the same source behind the Global Wave of Healing Energy, balancing the power of its collective manifestation of fear and doubt. It felt as though I was a light to balance the darkness of my illness which reflected the darkness within humanity. It felt like the trauma of my illness needed the balance of mystical wonders and unexplainable circumstances that allowed for continued breath, furthermore, with legs to walk this Earth as an example.

I have always been attuned to the spirituality of those encountered, likely because I was always seeking to define my own. If you listen, you can tell just from the words that are spoken. I admired them all, especially since I felt lost within my curiosity. Although I did not know what to believe in at the source of the mysticism, I did know that religions, congregations, individuals, and collectives were joining together, because of the same shared vision. I wondered what they were seeing.

They all held a Faith in something greater. Everyone was set out on a journey of experiences, seeking their own path, answers, and understanding of their purpose; believing in something greater than ourselves; holding faith that someone, something, was leading and protecting us. It didn't matter which religion it was, nor the name that it was given, I held tremendous respect for the unwavering faith that everyone around me appeared to hold. It seemed as if everyone held a strong faith in something. I wanted to experience the same. I thought I should experience it at a deep level that I knew I was not experiencing.

My youthful mind did not realize that we were all one and the same. I did not realize that my version of blind faith was the same as everyone else. I did not know that it was the blindness that makes it faith. When you remove the labels, faith is faith. Yet even in the presence of my faith, it felt like a mindful act of choice to believe in God. I believed it should be experienced differently. I knew I felt deep emotions, but I wanted to feel truth. I wanted to know truth, my soul's truth.

I believed something powerful was indeed governing our existence. I also believed that I had already held the privilege of experiencing and knowing as a recipient of that direct connection. Even so, I was saddened that I did not feel it in my heart. I felt deserving of the direct connection and wondered if my spiritual perception was the same and enough. It must have been different since I did not feel the connection the way I thought it should be felt. I knew that every aspect of my survival came from beyond our physical realm, yet there was a brokenness, and an incompleteness that engulfed every experience. My inability to integrate the truths into my heart seemed like a huge misunderstanding that needed to be clarified, and it felt adamant that it would not occur through someone else, nor anywhere other than within me. I believed that feeling truth was possible which made it easy to hold patience as I evolved and grew into being. In doing so, I trusted that I would arrive and never question my faith, love, and God again. I would know the truths of my soul because I would feel it deeply in my heart. When the time and space was right the day would come.

Until then, my spiritual space remained unnamed, unlabeled, and as pure as I could maintain. It was the angelic space that held my heart and my love; my prayers, hopes and dreams; intentions, desires and all that is for my highest good while walking through life. It was the space where I knew you and I would one day meet and dance. It used to be the sacred space that patiently kept record of every breath I heard in the silence, every whisper you sent along the way, every clue you left behind, every nugget of joy unearthed, and every intentional choice I made trusting that it was leading me to our unity. All the while it was my heart that cried in prayer, with an ever-weary faith that one day I would spend my days with you and rest within your heart, and you within mine. I would rest in the truths of my soul.

A KALEIDOSCOPE OF COLOR
Turning the Wheels of Perspectives

I always recognized my perspectives as the easiest and greatest gifts to open every day. It was my perspectives that created the unbelievable storyline of my life. Without them my life would have been considerably different. I lived the truth that my experience would be a result of my perspectives, and I had a choice over every single one of them. It always seemed as though everyone held a saddened and broken expectation for my reality. Meanwhile I stood cheering silently in my stubborn determination to be proud of all that was achieved; all that I had done to be anything, and everything but broken.

Within every perspective created from the ever-changing angles of my prism, a reality was created. Within each reality rested infinite opportunities. For many years it was too overwhelming to live in alignment with the truths of my soul because I could see the infinite potential and not my unique gifts in this life; a sensation that exacerbated the fragmentation across time and space. When I became aware of the choices that would allow myself to connect more fully to my uniqueness, it made me wonder if we are designed to dream and aspire to hold and achieve that which we are destined to unleash within? I know this to be true for me.

I held a sense of pride in what now seems like a constant analysis of my own perception of everything, mostly in that balance was maintained within and throughout the world around me. Doing so was an attempt to understand the world so that I could do my best to never cast judgment, unknowingly being most critical of self. If a situation needed stillness and silence, I tried to hold space for that. If a voice was needed, I provided whatever voice I had. Admittingly, it provided a sense of control within the chaos of my reality, and what seemed life was all about. I was able to do so for others which is what added color and order, yet I was unable to do so for myself, which then only caused my colorful art to shift into chaotic messes, yet still beautiful in their own way. I could see that I was the same as those around me, yet so very different.

I took tremendous pride in the joy I was able to create in life, and honored, respected, and celebrated when others did the same. It is what drove the desire to want to understand the mystical screenplay so I could master my role in the live performance of each and every day. All the roles I had chosen to take on throughout life felt like sacred costumes in unrehearsed auditions. When the unexpected curtain opened and I was exposed to the world, generally one of my four parts was on display. As the unintegrated parts of me vied for center stage, I stood blubbering over words and stumbling over me existence.

Which would it be? Would my heart have the courage to love myself enough and trust in what would authentically flow in action and allow others to love what is seen? Would my mind show up and try to dominate the experience in calculated predictions of the next best step while simultaneously processing past, present, and future data inputs and the validity of any outcome? Would my soul show up as a reminder of infinite potential and the perfection in spiritual truth no matter what unfolds in any given moment? Or would my body show up tired and indifferent going through the motions until graced with intermission so that it may rest and regain strength while the others boast for attention?

After being organically grown into these roles, in time the incongruency of my parts became amplified by my inability to keep up with the unpredictable presence, and the rapid pace of entrance and exit off stage, leaving heart and soul baggage in the way of the next scene. I knew that in time they would funnel into the performance when they all showed up together as one and in sync for the most masterful and captivating experience. I trusted that staying true to my heart was the most impactful mechanism to calibrate my mind and body to hear the song of my soul while in preparation for the next curtain call; uncertain if the next would be the one I danced before you.

Every impending scene had the opportunity to be the live show yet in the unfolding I instantly knew it was not. I believed that all I had to do in order for them to sync was remain authentic and true to self and remain present in the world around me. I believed that eventually it would no longer matter when the curtain was pulled open, the storyline of my life would always be playing whether a curtain veiled the scene or not. It took thirty years of stubborn commitment and a steady emergence of self to play my authentic role wholly and proudly.

It was always clear that I was returning to wholeness, yet just not fast enough. I knew the parts of me would come together in time, but I had to take the journey to achieve it. It was a journey that I knew I had to take, especially if it helped you reach me. I used the four parts of me as the prism to reflect the white light I saw in others, while concurrently breaking it up into its constituent spectral colors within my being: my rainbow of life. The colors of my rainbow are what guided my heart into life's final act, a heart of golden love.

It was troubling that as humans we are only capable of expressing ourselves through a mask. A mask of the human body. I had struggled with the very division of inner and outer worlds with only my body as a veil of separation. No wonder I saw it all around me. It was this very awareness of my masked self that allowed me to find serenity in the intensive care unit when my body was torn apart. All the while, I felt like the veil of my body was a tuning fork within every space I entered, balancing what existed within and beyond my body, and yours.

Since the awareness of my inherent limitations is a part of who I am, my perception felt like it was a gifted tool to be tuned, yet I never seemed to find the uniquely specialized tuner. It seemed like life was a joyous walk collecting the materials to build one myself; collecting everything my senses could absorb without knowing precisely what was needed. Hope wondered if the right pieces were collected, while trust knew there was no other outcome than to be precise and perfect. Patience and Love threaded the fragments through life while crafting what awaited my discovery.

It felt as though I was walking aimlessly through life waiting on purpose. I was intentional in my pursuits, joyful and happy, and enjoying every experience and the encounters with those I met along the way. Even so, deep within I was wandering and wondering through life with a deep presence as if purpose was impending. A purpose that would only be delivered in the form of messages found beyond the ethers of my faith; my meta-physical reality; my spirituality before it held such a label. The sense of uncertainty was not in a lack of awareness in the choices being made, I was very much aware of those if nothing else. It was more in the sense that I did not know with all certainty where those intentional choices were leading me and afraid of choosing poorly. I just wanted to know what I was supposed to do. I had to trust that in time I would know with certainty.

I had my ideals. I had predictions, and my hopes. I had educated guesses, and calculated outcomes. I formulated plans and timelines of desires and goals. I felt as though I always did the very best I could to methodically do, while being the best me I was able to be. I surely had my flaws, but I was very proud of the unbelievable truths of my life. I was very proud even if it was only when I rested within, alone, and in the comfort of my own silence. Many seemed not to understand what it was that I was so proud of, nor joyful for in life, especially when snippets from my reality were exposed. My light-hearted spirit was misinterpreted for something much different; something that needed a much greater force than mine to sway.

Beyond the space of me, a disconnect remained with the world. No matter who it was. It always felt like me, and the world. As I lived life, I always knew there would be a cascading ripple effect of my choices and engagements in some way. There was always a sense of pressure to fulfill the role as it was supposed to be. It was all part of the master plan. There was always concern that the choice I was making was the free will choice that impacted the greater universal story, and while my story always felt like it played out upon the scale of the masses. It was important that my ripple was a positive one because like everything, it held infinite potentiality and capacity. Although beautiful beyond words in so many ways, the life experience had not yet balanced the trauma within the abundant joy that I believed was in order, so every flutter of my being felt more traumatic for the world versus healing.

While intentionally closing out the external world in order to ensure that the experience was uniquely mine, I had to settle into a more grounded state of existence that allowed my senses to guide my navigation. I had to create the time and space to experience through feeling before being concerned with any label, and only use labels if it served a purpose. I learned it was the very allowance and fluidity of experiencing my emotions without labels during my trauma that later was a barrier in my adult life. I discovered that I never knew how to appropriate label my emotions which thereby made it challenging to identify which ones where not serving my highest good, and thereby would not serve you.

I was not sure if I should follow love or follow God. I did believe that if there is a God, God is love and love is God, so I realized that if I followed either, they would lead to each other. I found it was easy to follow both. Along the way, I was no longer able to discern if you were God, or if you were love, yet I knew that if you were either or both it would be a glorious experience. I knew all my being would perceive both as an experience of Heaven on Earth. Either, or both would be a lovely sensation to experience, so I remained devoted to the journey to solve the mighty mystery.

I lived a beautiful life and all that my physical reality was fulfilling. Even so, it was within the metaphysical contemplations of universal laws, the human experience, and the deep and peaceful walk towards love that held my attention. It was in this space in between life where I felt at home and at ease. It was where time stood still. It was where the stillness of serenity still sweeps me off my human feet. I felt humbled while standing in my strongest and most courageous attempts to be as graceful as possible while simultaneously allowing each authentic moment to move me to the fullest. When I discovered my truths had led me to you was the moment all was indeed well with my soul.

Throughout my life, it felt like the most important job I held was to follow the calling towards love. As an adult, my path of attaining physical world accolades was a delicate balance of intention to demonstrate defiance of any preconceived limiting notion of my abilities, all the while honoring a deep love in my heart. With the delicacy of each carefully weighed option within every experience of my existence, I had to choose to follow my heart. When I let my mind lead the way, the physical world experience felt underwhelming when compared to discovering the playground of infinite potentiality within.

I believed in the infinite possibilities left impending with every breath, and in time I became inspired to see what would be discovered at the core of my soul, versus dreaming in and of the physical experience. I sensed that I would be moved much more deeply by the discovery of my soul versus a physical world pursuit. I believed I should be living the experience of my soul. If done right, my soul would manifest the deepest dreams of the heart into the world around me. This would mean that I would be living my dreams and the joy of discovering them in material form. It was evident that this very script had brought me through life. I believed it would continue to do so the more I aligned with the voice of my soul. But I was still missing something. As if I was missing the magical thread that would weave everything together into perfection and illuminate the masterpiece of the Magical Maestro.

I carried on my way while exploring ways on how to defy the limited expectations of the intellect. I envisioned creative ways on how I could heal my body. I imagined the infinite potential we have as humans. I metaphorically stitched upon the universal fabric of life with the intentions of strength, courage, and love for all, every stitch representing the beautiful souls in the world. I held tremendous gratitude for how everything has purpose and meaning if we choose to see it. I had acquired all possible fragments from my life experiences and teachings alike and dreamed about my space in the world as I continued through life repairing and mending from experiences. I wondered if it was your sonar signals that I felt insinuating it was time to rest in peace and that the day had come for everything to merge together in harmony.

I surely was not prepared to reconcile all aspects of my existence in the manner at which it unfolded although I must acknowledge that I prayed deeply for everything to be compiled into one explosive experience for I did not have the human capacity to continue dispersed across many. I trusted in the purity of my intentions, the love I was capable of holding, my presence in the experiences of life, all within the best of my ability as a singular soul on a journey through a human life experience. I felt reminded along the way to stay true to the tune of my soul the best I was able, and the rest will fall into place. This notion held my deepest trust.

I believe that we receive what we give away. Therefore, I remained committed to sharing the best parts of me, in whichever means I was capable of doing so. I did so while believing that as long as I acted in kindness and out of love, all would come back to me, somehow and in some way, and in the most magnificent ways. Living a life of love and understanding was a fundamental and deeply personal intention, for I wanted nothing more than love and understanding in return. As I accepted others, the more radiant my rainbow in life became and my perspectives were tilted towards you.

A Reflection of Love

Soon enough, while I tried to live life to the fullest, time floated me further from the past and into a life where those around me knew nothing about my yesteryears. Seemingly acceptable yet my past was very much a part of my present which caused a great sense of dissonance within the world around me. I am unable to leave my physical scars, limitations, medical ailments, and life adjustments in the past. I sometimes felt conflicted on how to let go and carry forward at the same time, but eventually would find my way and carry on.

If we were to encounter each other on the street, you would have no idea of the journey I have travelled; nor I of yours. I held close friendships, worked alongside many, and for numerous years, knowing they had no idea of the story that came with my actions, words, sentiments; my character of being. I acknowledged and honored the same of them and their journey.

I deeply cherished and protected the vulnerable truths that many felt comfortable sharing, often unprovoked. Those connections ultimately made me love them more for being brave enough to share, and I honored that they trusted me with their vulnerability. Those moments gave me the opportunity to love them enough to see and hear them, and not judge them. I offered unto others that which I was longing for within, and when I did, I found the yearning ceased.

Most were unaware to the truth that I barely had enough energy to make it through a day. Those encountered in the workplace undoubtably received the best, most energized, and enthusiastic version of me. That was my predominant worldly facing mask. Inwardly, during those same times, I was mentally assessing breath, stamina and energy reserves, muscle strength, mental clarity, and tasks lists to determine where I had the strength to exert myself. There was strength and courage that I was proud to present to the world, yet within there was sadness, shame, and embarrassment.

While my mind's focus was on infinite possibilities, the dichotomous opposite that is my finite body was out of focus.

My own actions highlighted that this was happening amongst us all; across humanity, as individuals living a life experience. It didn't take long to recognize the false realities being created by everyone, and that we do not truly know anyone. There has always been an unexplainable and uncontrollable desire to reach for a heart through the illusions of our existence. I didn't always understand those experiences, yet intrinsically I knew that each heart was leading me somewhere. Deep within I prayed it would lead me to you. I reached for every heart that felt guided by you, hoping that you would soon be reaching out for mine.

As I looked into the world, I felt deeply that I could relate to any and all emotions that any possible scenario could incite. I had walked through all of them at some point or another. I spent twenty-five years trying to balance the physical, emotional, medical, biological, physiological, psychological, sociological, and meta-physical aspects of every moment of our existence while inquisitively seeking the pieces to the masterful puzzle that gave it all meaning. I felt confident that finding you would be entangled into discovering the purpose of my experiences. I truly believed that if I found you, I would be able to relate to you. I just wasn't sure if you would feel that you could relate to me. Even I held doubt that anyone would be able to relate to my experiences since they appear so drastically different. That was until you removed doubt from my reality.

It pained me when I witnessed and experienced the mislabeled and misunderstood parts of others; and more so their silent suffering observed from afar. For some reason, when I experienced it for myself, I was always able to justify the actions as if my unbeknown circumstances made all the difference. The flaw in application was that I was accepting of when the hidden parts of me where dishonored, yet I was unaccepting of it upon another. I was much more available to others than I was to myself likely because it felt like I could innately relate to everyone. I could sense one's sadness for not being seen just as I had felt sadness for not feeling seen.

In time, life constructed the widest and longest bridge between our hearts with the rubble from my circumstances, creating distance between our similarities. Somehow, I could feel the energy shift during every inaccurate and incomplete reflection when I looked to find you within; a broken kaleidoscope blocking the light. I knew I had to clear the way for my light to shine into the world. My heart and soul welcomed the healing steps while my mind fought to keep my body alive.

Aligning with the Light

One of my truths is that my heart and spirituality have become so interconnected and aligned that it has become unnecessary to discern between the two. I consider that alignment a sacred gift and hold tremendous gratitude for the gift of wholeness and the peace such an awareness brings to my mind. It is, however, important to honor my previous space which was not viewed as troubling, saddening, nor intense. It was just there, in the abyss of time and space. There was a silent grace that protected that space which I honored with tremendous faith and patience. I believed deeply that the source of my essence and the scope of my love would surface in time from within that space.

I have always believed. I am unable to recap expressions of how I used to frame my beliefs, but I do know that it has always felt the same within the depths of me and within the ethers of the universe. Especially after my illness, I believed I was always exactly where, what, and who I was supposed to be. Holding onto that truth was the only thing that got me through many dark hours. In those hours of silence, I simply casted every cell of my being into the energetic vortex of time and space, and into the vastness of endless possibilities.

There are those that may call that prayer, others may refer to the notion as meditation and others as releasing the mind to God. My language continued to evolve throughout my life experience, but the action was always the same; to deliver my silent experiential reflections into infinite space with vulnerability for growth, return to gratitude, believe in my life walk, have faith in the deliverance of the most glorious gifts unto me, and to continue on my path. It always felt like I would continue to be mystified beyond my own imagination. This would in turn bring about joy and excitement because I knew of my own ability to imagine pretty amazing things. Thereby the reality would be even more glorious.

Through the space of my existence, I had become extremely aware of when I held the connection to my perfect experiential existence and the mysteries that surfaced with my beliefs, and when I did not. My mind was always scanning, capturing, processing, and storing data, yet was unable to construct and compute the algorithm to produce the magic. I was always overjoyed whet it presented itself in my experiences yet tried to mimic it when it was no longer present. It took a graduated walk into the levels of awareness that I had to experience in order to understand it in such a way that resonated within the depths of my heart and soul.

Over time, the journey of my ever-evolving heart began to feel trapped by my own mind and the space it was evolving out of, through, and into. It was the journey through the passion of my heart that fueled the most glorious of spaces within which ultimately set my mind free. For my soul was no longer willing to allow my mind to temper my heart.

In the complexity of my being, I simultaneously lived, saw, and experienced each unexplainable and mystic experience. It was my reality. The truth was extremely overwhelming because it was so unexplainable. Even so, I felt disconnected from what was causing it and it felt like it should be more sustainable than the fragmented and sporadic experiences I was living. The most overwhelming sensation was when others would speak to me of the truths that I lived; the miracle of my life walk; the Angel that I am. It was humbling and almost shameful as I stood bashful and untamed when some could see and feel that truth, yet I could not. I could see it clearer than the world around me yet felt disconnected from being able to embody that truth to feel throughout my being.

Every aspect of my being believed in the purity of my soul and how that belief left me feeling like an Angel soaring above humanity watching the world unfold beneath me. Concurrently, I felt that an Angel would be doing much better in the human experience whereas mine was messy, seemed very non-Angelic, and never feeling enough. I was left feeling the scale between ego and soul ensure the strength of my soul did not inflate my human ego, or even more so, the strength of my soul could withstand the mind's attempt to deflate my heart. My mind was always ready to deconstruct a situation and to walk my heart through any feelings before I could feel them. Over time my heart yearned to feel. It felt like the greatest contradiction to overcome. My mind remained perplexed and tried to find the ways to become connected to truth and feel it, instead of intellectualizing and shaming it every step of the way. The inability for me to feel truth caused an even greater yearning to seek out the path to you. It was a lesson of self-love that did not come for many years.

When it was just me within, everything was at peace and calm with grace, albeit shameful in my messy humanness that held patience for explanation, simplicity, and comfort. I always managed to fluff my sparse angel wings and float into another day on the journey to meet you. Yet when I opened my eyes, and even more troublesome my mouth, it felt like there was a wrecking ball within set loose to destroy what was trying to float to the surface. It was a wrecking ball controlled by my mind, destroying the bubbles that the chemistry of my heart and soul were brewing deep within. My mind was tearing down my strength and my hope for balance, and doing so in slow motion, one destructive swing at a time. The saddest experience was when I felt my pillars of love tremble from the wreckage.

My mind tried to maintain tactful control over my heart and soul within a never-ending evolving world within and around me. The clarity I saw in both my minds reality and the reality of soul caused considerable pause with discernment over which reality was indeed most real to me. Everything seemed like an illusion. Since everything was a matter of perspective and would thereby create a reality, and that reality would solely be mine no matter what, it was clear that I could choose the reality I was willing to follow. If my reality was based on mere perception alone, I examined which one made me feel best since I surely wanted to feel the best I possibly could. Following and creating a reality was a role that my mind filled naturally and honestly as it needed to. It had clearly served its purpose yet proved to be unable to relinquish its powerful control without assistance.

This is where I knew I would find the missing parts of me. This is where all the chemicals of my periodic table ingested along the beautiful life would alchemize into a mystical concoction with an explosion so bright it would eradicate the darkness within. I trusted that the data that supported my hypothesis would transform into a theoretical golden conduit straight to your heart; a pathway that extended into space beyond our physical experience and into a world we tend to forget exists and generally becomes overrun with a material presence or a cognitive rationale. The space where all parts of me would harmonize into one so that I could stand before you wholly and completely in all that I am.

I sensed I was fine tuning my senses that would reunite my Physical and Inner Spirits. Over time it felt like I became Physical Spirit, and you were Inner Spirit slowly rotating as the double helix strands of our realities joined to form the DNA of our existence, transposing worlds before us. With constantly changing and rotating perspectives, I always saw that there was purpose in what I was seeing and somewhere on the other side you stood there waiting to be seen. I hoped your trust was as strong as mine because it felt like lifetimes for me to make the journey. I hoped you wanted me to see you just as much as I wanted to see you; a union I dreamed of in the passing of days.

I was open to anything and everything. I felt I was prepared yet knew I would have no idea of what it would be like until it was before me. The part that I was not expecting was it would be a journey away from the physical world and into the metaphysical world while exploring the universe through the lens of my human experience. I had to trust deeply in the journey I was choosing to take and that it would lead to a return where I achieved the sense of wholeness and stood whole before you. There was a deep prayer in each passing day that it had purpose at the depths I had given it meaning.

I had to ignore the possibilities of anything contrary to the majestic, while knowing the slightest vibration of my thoughts would impact the outcome. I would not have the courage to stand in my truths until I had the strength to honor who I am, and to do so with love. I knew I would learn what was needed to become the master of me, so all I had to do was pay attention. Pay close attention. This was critical because my juvenile human body was growing forward in our perceived concept of time; yet my infinite soul had to wait for my humanness to catch up in order to integrate my soul and the wisdom from beyond. My mind led my body through as much as it could, but an incongruency came when my mind could no longer reach the depths of my soul.

My soul patiently watched my humanness grow through experiences to catch up for full embodiment. It was a slow integration that had been underway for most of my remembered adult life. An experience that held a deeper and more lasting since of pain than the one I journeyed you through thus far. It felt like every attempt to embody my soul was the very experience that caused my body to lose balance resulting in low platelets. Instead of healing my platelets through modern medicine, I believed that there was something deeper within that needed to heal. I believed that if I healed deep enough within, I would heal my body to the extent needed for balanced sustainability.

As I lived life and all that the physical reality was fulfilling, it was within the metaphysical contemplations of universal laws, the human experience, and a deep and peaceful patience for love that kept me alive. It was where I felt at home and at ease. It was where time stood still. It was where the stillness of serenity continuously swept me off my human feet causing my body to crash to the ground. It took many years to correlate my physical experience of platelets explained by science with the spiritual journey under way. Once I did, I was not longer able to live in wonder. I had to switch gears into actionable choices. I had to create opportunities to choose differently.

It felt like a game of tug of war between the truths within my soul and the truth my mind was programmed to believe. As one side pulled me, the other side pulled even harder. It was clear that there was only a meta-physical explanation to my physical reality. My inability to integrate the truths of my experience was at the source of my blood instabilities; they fueled each other with every broken breath of life.

My inability to look wholly at myself prevented me from seeing that both my spiritual instabilities and the resulting physical manifestations were fogging my clarity to navigate either realm well. Deep within I knew it was all linked together and that healing one would heal the other. The order of operation in the masterful algorithm made all the difference and for a long time was under analysis.

I felt humbled while standing in my strongest and most courageous attempts to be as graceful as possible while simultaneously allowing each authentic moment to knock me off my feet. It was easy to get caught up in the mystical bubble that housed my physical world reality that continued to drift me to you. I just was not sure how long I would be able to float around. It felt like I was not ever able to equalize, balance, and calibrate my core. While living a beautiful life with no real mechanism to do so, I gave each day everything I could. I would find within myself, whatever I could find, to stand on my delicate legs and feet of meta-physical steel to walk me through another day. If it happened to be the last, it was going to be the last best day I could put forth.

The experiences that added beautiful color to life concurrently creating tremendous noise around the voice within. What follows are the stories of how my scales were brought into balance when the voice within became louder than the noise in the world. It represents what we as humans have the capacity to do, as a singular being and as a collective. There is untapped potentiality within the focused collective intentions of the human collective heart. It had already proven to be powerful and real throughout my story. The balance came from reigning in the power as a singular soul that holds the same potential of the collective.

Since I saw me in the collective, and wanted the collective to be seen in me, I started at what felt like the most obvious place to begin. I began with me. I had lived, experienced, and learned enough to know all what I was experiencing, and feeling was sourced from within. I knew that whatever it was I was seeking could not be found outside of me. I knew early on in life as a child that I was the only thing I would ever have and want complete power and control over. Something I tried to honor the best I could during the younger versions of self. By default, I knew I needed to look inward. By doing so I was once again choosing to know all me no matter the consequences.

I motivated myself with a gift to be received when I was able to hold you autonomously in my heart. The gift would be to experience your healed vulnerability, in the purity of my healed vulnerability, and together experience a magical love while remaining true to our uniquely powerful selves. Like ships passing in the night, only sailboats floating in sync for a life. I knew I had not experienced the magic of real love because it cannot flow in its purity from a broken spirit, and I knew mine was broken even if I tried to mend the cracks along the way. I was always aware that the surface mending never penetrated deep enough to be felt at the core, where life had shattered it many moons ago.

I had certainly experienced the ever-evolving versions of beautiful love and experienced how love was growing me closer to its inherent purity, especially when I was led and called to share intimate love with another and joining together through marriage. It was the magic of love that motivated me to heal my soul so that I may be able to experience that flow of love energy with my partner and within our growing family. Many times, it felt like we were on the cusp of allowance, but then our wounded love shielded our hearts. My broken love, which blended perfectly with another's broken love synced beautifully together with laughter and joy. Hope in love remains the only thing that keeps me going, and it continues to show up before me.

It all sounds lovely and magical and blissfully surreal. And it was, primarily within the ethers of my silence. In my physical reality, everything was ridden with a lot of noise, limited beliefs, and what felt like an imposition on my ability to expand and evolve. What at first felt like lifetimes away, began to feel closer and more powerful. It felt like the core of my soul trying to burst upward through my body and escape the cage around it. It was a very familiar feeling as it seemed to have existed for eternity, yet small enough to not sense the confines around it from this life. Over a life of living, it slowly grew in intensity until the power felt like a magnet beginning to move objects through space, magnetically pulling me by the chest into the universal abyss.

It never felt like I had any idea of how to do any inner healing, yet my heart forever knew how to heal its way to you. All I had to go on were the things I held to be truths in what I wanted to experience, and I definitely invited thoughts and opportunities towards those.

I wanted my heart to feel free to love at the depths it desired instead of feeling captive and trying to break free. I wanted my heart to swell with love and joy. I knew what that felt like and knew that it was lacking. The sound and feeling of a jovial laugh full of love always bring a tearful smile to my heart. We are meant to be happy.

I wanted my face, my eyes, my entire being to emulate the love and joy sourced in my heart. There is nothing more beautiful than an authentic expression of joy. It creates a glisten in the eye, and the facial muscles contract in such a way that cannot be mimicked otherwise. There is something captivating about genuine joy.

I wanted my mind to relinquish control and learn to relax. I wanted to trust in myself and the wisdom of my soul and use my mind to intellectualize those truths into expression.

I wanted to become more fluid with the ebbs and flows of life so that my body could navigate more gracefully.

I wanted to arrive at a sense of meaning and purpose in all that my physical life had experienced. I believed in all the unexplainable gifts the universe had to offer and remained humbled by my own life walk of extraordinary circumstances and experiences.

I wanted to feel whole, really whole, although uncertain of how the parts of me would integrate into one. I knew that it was all a matter of my perspective so I could tilt my perspectives to change the way I feel.

I wanted to experience the purest, sweetest, most sensual unconditional love for, with and from another yet knew it must first be achieved within for self; first, and foremost. If I was going to fight for the love in my heart, then I was going to have to know me wholly and completely first. I knew the soulful love I felt deep within must be known by me first before sharing it with another.

I wanted my soul song to be emitted into the universal abyss, transmitted across galaxies and dimensions so that you would hear it, feel it, sense it in some way. It felt like you were the only one who would recognize the calling of my deep soulful love.

I wanted to attract that which was of the essence of me for I knew of the purity and authenticity of my intentions, compassion, and love. It felt like there was a part of my energetic essence out in the universal abyss. I felt a magnetic pull within my body to somewhere, out there. I wanted to attract that which was attracting me. It felt like the missing parts of me. It felt like love. It felt like you.

I wanted to be fully open to receive what the universe had to offer knowing I had to clear the path for deliverance. I trusted that whatever was on its way to my heart was in my highest good and was designed to return balance to my scales of life. I was ready and open to receive in all the abundant glory.

A sacred desire that I held close and dear was that I wanted to meet the Angels that had carried me through life. I had always felt a presence of being supported along the way from the realms beyond my physical experience. I wanted to expand my senses so that I could sense and feel spiritual presence. It felt like there was untapped love awaiting my discovery. It felt like my Angels were carrying me until I could integrate the truths of my soul; helping and guiding me along the way to understanding; leading me to the light.

It all was beginning to feel very much connected in ways that I wanted to explore. My body was awakening to a magnetic pull in my heart. I knew I was finally approaching the threshold to meet you. I could feel it within every cell of my being.

32

Deconstruct the Ego to Reconstruct the Heart

The morning that my Mom took her last breath was the moment that I knew I had to gain spiritual strength. I was not willing to believe in a construct that ceased her presence. I knew that her existence would extend beyond the physical reality even though my beliefs had become jaded by uncertainty. I could see how the worldly constructs prevented exploring what that meant to me. Yet, I knew and felt the truth was that it had to be what mattered to me. Unraveling the spiritual reality behind the physical loss of my Mom would, in time, reach the depths required for my soulful healing—another blessing she graciously bestowed upon me during her graceful transition.

I could see her. As clear as she was before me when living. She was radiant and beautifully wrapped in the hand-woven Balinese silk fabric we had adorned around her space during her transition.

She called me, as she always did, "Hey, you," for me to turn inward. Once we engaged, she explained that she had to go but would still be present. I acknowledged that truth and that I understood. Off to the side, there was a door ajar with brightness on the other side, and we embraced with a farewell hug and words of love. The experience ended with a slow fade of her essence and a profound resonance of her everlasting presence. This experience started the quest for a soulful strength and clarity that would allow unlimited connectedness to her infinite spirit.

I knew that I had to develop a new relationship with her, and I lovingly wanted it to be closer than ever. It felt like we could finally connect in the same space of love and light. For once, we didn't have worldly barriers jading our soulful connection. I truly felt the purity in our exchange of unconditional love for the first time. I celebrated that I could see her in everything, whereas before, I only understood how to see her in Los Angeles. I was honored that she wanted to reveal her presence to me, and the only deterrents to seeing her resided within me. If that were true, I knew I would see her for eternity.

This experience left me determined to connect with my spirituality because I wanted to remain forever connected to my Mom. To maintain our bond, I was committed to defining what constituted my spirituality. I wanted to know the space where she would now rest and where I would join her one day. I yearned to achieve unwavering peace in the moments of my physical life and that of my spiritual afterlife. For almost two years after her transition, my spiritual and physical beings were alchemizing into the most magical concoction and prepping the foundation of one of the most transformative journeys of my life. An explosion of self that sent me into the Universe to discover my truths and then back to live Heaven on Earth. All guided by the infinite love of my Mom.

Until then, my mindful ego kept a glaring watch over everything that transpired within my parts. Everything. Like a stern dictatorship commanding pristine management of all parts, orderly conduct zipped up high and tight. Exhausting. For many years I thought I wanted a construct. I thought that it was within a construct that I would find spiritual refuge. I was taught to believe that it could only be found within these constructs, but my heart knew it felt restrictive, which defied everything taught about infinite love.

I wanted to have unwavering faith in something greater than my physical body and beyond what my egoic mind could comprehend. I wanted to feel the unconditional love and compassion guaranteed in this sacred space. I wanted to feel my connection to Spirit and know the Source that created and carried me. I wanted to know the Source that saved me. I wanted to feel and experience the very Source of my miracles and the magic that comes from a space of oneness. My own operational constructs were unable to fulfill those desires. I wanted more. My heart yearned for more. My soul guided every aspect of my humanness as it sought for truth.

There were a lot of uncertainties. I had no idea what any of it meant except that I had to remain grounded and focused on authentic self-expression. When I did, I felt at peace. I felt at ease until I re-engaged my external world ridden with misalignment. I wasn't sure what that meant either, but I did know that my body would not be able to endure the impacts of rushing the soulful process. There was a resounding acknowledgment that it was somehow related to the physical trials I endured with my crashing platelets.

By this point, I had identified that the stress of my soul's misalignment was the trigger. However, it took several more years to learn how delicate it had become and easily tipped by external interference. I could feel that if I did not slow down, I would only further disrupt the imbalance within, and I most certainly wanted to get to the destination. It always felt as though the joy was in the destination, and I found stability and strength trusting the destination would be soulful, energetic love awaiting my arrival. I focused on the destination despite not knowing what that would look like either. Even so, It felt like the only choice was to trust that the path to get there would be equally beautiful and enjoyable, and that taking the journey of discovery would only amplify the magnificence of the destination.

To make it there, I had to adjust away from fear and only invite strength, courage, and love. I found that I had to cultivate the same power within and trust in self, albeit the strength of soul came much differently than in my youth within the hospital. This time it was by choice. This time, I was choosing to balance within so that I could balance without. It was my choice to reboot my life and figure out how to integrate every aspect of my being into who I am for the sake of feeling love. This time I could choose with love instead of fear.

The writing process unfolded as a walk through the depths of my humanness, through which I set the intentions to assess my life in terms of living or existing, discern if I was in alignment with whatever it was within and if I needed to make actionable choices to do so. There was a deep desire to align my whole being and remain open to receive the abundant glory from the universe that my heart and soul felt, and my mind and body hoped were impending.

The choice was very clear and before me. All I had to do was choose to take the journey or not. Once the self-analysis was underway, just the awareness of the "or not" option made me commit to my soul's "must" requirement. I felt a deep sense of betrayal when I considered the "or not" option, betrayal of my own soul. For that reason alone, I had to hold my intentions closer than ever, believe in infinite possibilities, and remain open to receiving whatever was on its way to me. And to take action.

I was prepared for the process to be easier said than done. This also proved to be true. When I started writing, the intention was to document my medical journey. Yet, the more I wrote, the more I found I had to say. And the more I uncovered, the more my essence expanded. The more I evolved, the more I wanted to continue on the journey. As I allowed the memories to flood my mind and I documented them with emotion, I noticed that light was shining upon other intertwined journeys on the path to oneness. It was the journey of my soul, and the reconnection to my heart. Yet, before I could get there, I had to deconstruct everything blocking the way, and my mind was blocking my love. I had to deconstruct my ego if I wanted to reconstruct my heart.

Throughout the spaces in between, I sought clarity within myself to discern what that all meant to me, what labels, what words, expressions and actions, fears, concerns, and doubts was I going to allow to limit me. It made me consider the design of the human body, the human experience and the programs inherently built into our operating systems that we then use to grow and learn from experiences. It felt like I had followed the path of my heart and soul yet all the while the exterior world was trying to program me into something I am not.

I found that I was inherently more likely to be positive, optimistic, and inspired by life likely due to my prior dances with death. I have had over a dozen experiences that felt like invitations to dance with death, and each invitation felt harder to decline. I love to dance. It left me needing to find meaning in the dance. I could tell each experience brought me closer to you while simultaneously I was losing the strength to get there. I had to tilt my perspectives if I wanted to reach the destination.

Over the years of my walk, I felt like I was warding off decisions made in fear, by me and those around me, all the while my heart desired something completely different. I wanted love to be my upgraded operating system, and every command to align with that intention. I wanted to evolve into the song of my soul which was only a song of love. I wanted to live in love and not in fear. I wanted to live as a being of love. I wanted to shift away from my mental reality of overcrowded, over controlled, over paced, over thought, over analyzed, over calculated and overestimated aspects of everything, and into a quiet and peaceful place of existence that I knew every cell of my being yearned to experience. Within that vision is where I reconnected with the truths of who I am, as a singular soul within this infinite universe.

It felt like I understood what the world was claiming as truths, about humanity, the human condition, spirituality, and a God. I understood it and I certainly believed it, but I did not feel those truths. I believed I should feel truth. About everything, especially the biggest mystery, at the core of all truths, the truth in God. Humanity's greatest inquiry indeed, yet my pursuit was very personal. Sacred.

Everything I deemed healthy and useful in life as a gauge of joy, success and love had been fulfilled, so I was left exploring complex topics and scientific theories that defy the limited expectations of the intellect. I envisioned creative ways on how I could heal my body. I imagined the infinite potential we have as humans when looking at all dimensions of our existence; primarily how they are funneled into this reality. I metaphorically stitched upon the universal fabric of life with the intentions of strength, courage, and love for all, every stitch representing the beautiful souls in the world of past, present, and future. I held tremendous gratitude for how everything has purpose within out interconnectedness.

Even with all of the fragments from my life experiences and teachings alike, I was unable to thread it in a way that made sense and gave it the deep soulful meaning it felt like I needed to sustain breath. I dreamed about my space in the world as I continued through life repairing and mending from the trauma. In the presence of it all, there was something that remained unfulfilled, my spiritual purpose

I kept the pace for as long as I could. It was a weariness from holding everything together to maintain order that became the impetus to start the book. I knew I had to reconnect to the story of my youth to embody the truths of spiritual mysticism that I desperately prayed would restore balance to my weary heart. It felt like my mind was evolving into eternity, my soul was unable to stay in my body, my body felt like it was going to die, and my heart yearned to be held in the arms of love. It was a do-or-die moment for me. It felt like my parts were ripping me apart to my death.

I found it hard to discern what would satisfy my life experience to bring about joy albeit knowing it would be found within. I believed that if I found joy, I would find love and when I found love I knew I would find you. I felt joyful in my life, yet with a lacking deep within I continued to explore and experiment in life to see what force would pull me into expression. I hoped you were still waiting for me, especially once the journey began. I wondered if it was your sonar signals that I felt prompting me that it was time to rest in peace and that the day had come for everything to merge together in harmony. It felt like you were waiting for me to start my walk so that you would know when to begin yours to meet me halfway.

The more time passed, the spiritual sound bites became louder within, merely because I was becoming more misaligned in my physical experience. As if the enhanced volume within was the indicator that I needed to realign my life by listening more clearly, but uncertain of what I needed to hear, nor what was truly transpiring.

All of the messages that had repeatedly replayed throughout the years fertilized the soil within which the seeds of my spirituality began to bloom. It was humbling to admit that my life choices were creating dissonance within. Choices that, at one time, were the perfect choices for my heart were now out of sync. It was clear that a soulful evolution was underway. I had no idea what that meant either other than I was willing to discover where it would lead me. I held faith and hoped that it would lead me to a sense of wholeness and love in my heart.

It would be the most critical, in depth, comprehensive human analysis I had endeavored since my trauma. I suppose the prior experience made it easier but there was nothing easy about the journey I was committed to undertake. It was necessary in order to know how I wanted to grow into the remainder of my life experiences. The only roadmap was to trust in love as I deprogrammed over twenty-five years of accumulated programming and automatic upgrades for every aspect of my being. It was a myriad of contradicting, over-complicated, strategically coded programs designed by everyone but me. I wanted to remove everything in the way preventing the authentic love song of my soul to run in the background of my being. I was slightly surprised by the depths of emotions and the tsunami waves that followed in the wake of this seemingly simplistic intention, for it was the beautiful life in between that had programmed my humanness that I ultimately had to deconstruct.

33

Trust in the Process

Once underway, it became evident that writing was the catalyst for the growth I always knew I would endure. I was never concerned about what the growth would entail because I knew I would translate all the experiences into beautiful growth of self in some way or another. That is just a part of who I am. My writing ultimately offered a gift to my soul with an invitation for deep healing and abundant love. I was honored to receive my invitation and considered it a privilege to accept and show up.

I was curious though as to why if I was creating my reality, why was I being called to create a life centered around a walk to reach you, especially when it felt like you existed through a portal into another dimension. This further incited self-inquiry as to why I would remain dedicated to a journey that made me feel less human than I already felt knowing that living the human experience was why we are here and alive. I was intrigued and trusted in the journey since it felt easier than many other things. Timidly, I knew it was the true and authentic storyline of my Soul. I tried not to wonder why since it felt like that truth was also buried deep within.

I was already a believer. My life was one big, mystifying reason to believe. I was just never sure what I believed in, how to navigate the unexplainable space of my mystical reality, and how to connect to and set free the power within that I felt I was constantly walking towards unleashing. There were so many conceptualized frameworks, ideals, and beliefs and none of them resonated within. I realized that I had to choose whether I was willing to accept the beliefs of others as my own or if I was willing and capable of identifying them myself. I believed I could and should do both. It felt like my soul was begging me to hear what it was trying to say. It felt like I needed to build my own framework uniquely designed to listen to the song of my soul. I believed that if I was indeed unique, I must have a unique framework, path, and purpose. I trusted that if I had a sound framework, I would be able to let my experiences guide the rest. I just had to honor myself enough to discovery my own truths and to trust in the process to get there.

Some may likely summarize healing my soul as a spiritual awakening, except it felt like I had been awake. I was awake within a world that I did not understand. I was awake within a fragmented and nonsensical world, a world that never skipped a beat while caught up in an ever-evolving culture that perpetuated the dissonance. I felt distant and separate in a world that left me behind as it hurried into the future.

I felt awake and stuck in a physical world experience versus asleep, now awakened to truth in a greater force. I already knew a greater force was present. I wanted to feel connected so I would forever know that I was connected and dancing with truth and love instead of wondering, hoping, and praying while feeling powerless in creating my experience caused by the pull to follow a voice within. I knew truths. Yet, I did not feel them. I believed and wanted to feel my truths and know through that feeling.

I was generally aware of when I became stuck in my navigation. I always walked while self-assessing, reviewing, and adjusting, in my thoughts and actions alike, for the path to become illuminated so I could organically and authentically continue on my way. The path I had traveled was long, with no end in sight, and deep within, it felt like I could not walk through life much longer. Even knowing it was by design, I was conflicted by the energy of my partner that had grounded my physical being for almost twenty-five years.

The grounding force allowed my Inner Spirit to traverse the world in amazing wonder while my Physical Spirit was living out all that life needed to teach me. The force grounded my ever-evolving heart to the fullest capacity until it felt as if my heart could no longer grow and evolve. I deeply sensed something more powerful was on its way into my experience, yet only if I was willing to allow my heart the space to evolve towards it. I intentionally connected to this notion and the feeling it incited. When I did, I felt a deep peace and sense of serenity, much deeper and more expansive than words express.

Accepting the invitation to heal my deepest parts felt more like a journey to consciously remove limiting beliefs and reconnect to the purity of who I am. I could sense that doing so would allow me to hold love for and from another between our hearts. I wanted to experience pure love and not conditionally ridden as it had become in the relationship with my heart and within my reality. Returning home to my pure love and sharing your sacred love were the silent intentions behind my seemingly simplistic book project. I knew nothing more of you other than feeling a magnetic pull within the universal abyss attracting us to unity, yet it was all I needed for my heart to follow.

The beautiful life in between secured the platform upon which I could finally begin mending and healing my body and mind, mind and soul, soul and body, mind, body, and soul together while allowing my heart to rest in love. It was now time to reconcile everything collected throughout the life walk and to form the masterful fabric of who I am, not just in this life but for eternity.

34

Finding My Soul's Light

Fainting spells were more frequent than desired throughout the years of crashing platelets. So much so that "it's happening" became the label used for the sequence of events underway. It was a label intended to expedite response time because it would be a matter of seconds before I would black out. If I could get through my mind and into the quiet, I could avoid a blackout. When I chose to honor who I am and to discover my truths, I was eventually led to the truths behind those moments, but until then all I knew were the experiences I had lived through. During each episode, once I was able to lie down, I always arrived in the same space of the most beautiful, serene expanse of white light. My mind followed in observance since it always appears conscious and aware, especially throughout the abyss of the averted blackout.

The visions in my mind always had me positioned as I was and the view of self was the same as if my eyes were open. I was the center of my vision, seeing all around me. As my body rested, a stream of white light would flow through me, enter into me, move within, and then exit. Sometimes there were defined entry and exit pathways, and sometimes it was all-encompassing, yet the white light was always flowing into, within, and then leaving my energetic body. The accompanying message was also always the same, clear, and precise.

Let the healing light flow through me and heal my body.

It was easy to follow since it was a natural script despite not being sure of what it meant. I would soothe my breath to calmness, see the white light flowing and feel my body balance back. These moments were always fascinating because there would be a quick onset of sweating, my senses would change, primarily hearing and my mind's eye, and my body would have an overwhelming sense of weariness. Then, I would lie down, instantly find myself in the visualization, experience the sensation of the white light, and within moments the sweats would stop, my heart rate would stabilize, and I would feel better than before. I always stood up cautiously, yet it felt similar to a power nap rather than what I would expect from an intermittently labeled fainting episode linked to an issue with my blood.

When the episodes first started, they were terrifying. Without warning, the experience would come and just as quickly go, leaving wonder as to what happened, assessing where I was left, and each time cautiously aware that the next could be the one that was too much for me to endure; my body would fail. I could feel my soul begging my humanness to figure it out. It felt like my most significant responsibility. The only real job I held was to stay alive. I knew I could not be afraid yet was unsure how to journey through the experiences with love. I did know I would have to figure it out.

I seldom shared my fainting episodes with my medical team because medical recommendations always seemed to contradict a deep knowingness that it was all due to the soulful imbalance within me, thereby causing the misalignments within the environment around me, and within my body. Doctors would want to label and medicate based on scientific data, and I wanted to restore holistic, organic, and authentic balance with my soul so that my body could heal on its own. The biggest struggle was that I was unsure of how to get there, and it felt like our humanness was the only thing in the way.

Limiting thoughts were prevalent during the onset of my soulful journey before I could align with the truth at the source of the episodes. I believed my broken spirituality and blood ailments were related, yet I could not find my spiritual medicine to heal. It took the process of writing the book to unleash the fear that my trauma embedded deep within the core of my being. It was a fear so deep that it became necessary to be deconstructed and eradicated along the way. It was only then that I discovered I was looking in the wrong place. I was looking within my physical reality when I needed to look within my spiritual reality.

As I started writing, I used the healing white light and trusted that it would heal me through the process, just as it had healed me through many platelet crashes. As I would close my day in meditation while nestled in bed, among the gratitude and blessings offered, I intentionally went to the space of white light and poured my heart and soul into writing. The experiences that surfaced while in the white light became the space of my inner focus, a space of healing. It was within this space where the white light exposed the dots within the matrix of my mind and illuminated the infinite fluidity of the universe. There were no points of connectivity between me and the universe. Within, we existed as one. I could see the micro-universe

I am, floating throughout the macro-universe from which we have come and within which we now exist. A multiverse within me.

The more I wrote and cleared my heart, the complexity of my egoic matrix was exposed. There was a lot of work to do: clearing, recycling, and creating. The space of infinite capacity was the space that I wanted to embody all the time, not only when I closed my eyes or wrote words on paper that tried to capture a momentary experience. I wanted to live in it. It was the space to reconnect with the purity of self and authentic love. It was the space where I knew I would find you.

The white light meditations that healed my blood were transformed into intentions to heal all parts of me. Two weeks into writing with heartfelt intention, I began having very unexpected experiences, yet also very expected. I expected to experience something while writing, yet it was so mind-blowing that it was difficult to remain aware of anything else, including life around me. The culmination of experiences highlighted that I merely held belief and lacked knowing truth. It was as if my writing was creating experiences that transformed every cell in my body into truth and love. More specifically, the truth in my love.

Once I committed, I was in for the long haul, and I had to experience the unfolding of all that was before me. First, it started with physical body changes. About two weeks into writing a powerful heat accumulated in my chest. It was felt throughout the day but demonstrated its strength at nighttime. I began to sweat. Profuse night sweats left me in a platinum chill throughout the days. Although I never sweat during the day, the heat was constantly emitted from my body, mainly my chest. It felt like there was a swirling ball of fire in my chest and that I was hugging a fireball while asleep.

Every night, regardless of the room temperature, I woke up several times with only my chest area drenched in sweat. I quickly began sleeping with three extra shirts under my pillow and a towel by my side. Multiple times amid the night, I blindly wiped the sweat from my body and changed tops while trying to return to comfort.

Once awake for a daily journey, it was as if my body was acclimating from the previous night and preparing for the next nightly purge. I ultimately saw it as the ebb and flow of energetic calibration. When I sat in meditation which had become a natural practice throughout the day, my breath slowed, and my body would organically fall into relaxation. The more my body relaxed, the more vivid the world within became and the easier it was to follow. It also felt like energy was accumulating within me during each quiet moment that pulled me into the abyss.

It did not matter how hot or cold the temperature was inside or out. I was constantly sweating at night and chilled during the day. I knew that my heart held the love energy it wanted to share with another. I later learned that the energy held captive was also for a greater, more deeply felt love for self and everything along the way. Until then, all I knew was that my heart had some energy to release in those moments. That much was clear.

The night sweats went on for almost seventy months, only ceasing once the transformation was over, and remains an indicator of when my humanness is unable to let something go. Initially though, the experience with the sweats led me to an internet search of "fireball heat in chest when sleeping," and to the delight of my inquiring mind, the results resonated deeper than I expected.

My search led me to the body's energy chakras. I had already discovered the chakras, the concept of universal energy, and being in alignment with the flow of energy. Those were part of the beliefs that anchored me on this unknown path. I had even read and studied the chakras and energy flow years prior when trying to sync my energy. Even so, there was a new connection to universal energy, which clearly linked to my heart chakra.

I had learned that various religious and mythological narratives source the chakras within the spiritual hearts of the Hindu and Buddhist traditions. The historical and spiritual backgrounds are fascinating and span a presence as far back as 1,500 B.C. in India's oldest written traditions. The most resonating statement encountered in the reacquaintance was a reference to the chakras as being the centers of spiritual power. Depending on the teaching, these energy wheels vary in quantity, attributes, and meanings. I was not concerned about what specifics someone else had labeled them to be; it felt like noise and unauthentic relatability. The history of the tradition and cultural meanings were certainly interesting for the mind, but my body felt it.

In a sense, I was seeking a level of validation that what I felt was even possible. I suppose that, yet again, I questioned whether what I was experiencing was real or could be real. It indeed felt real. And it felt as if my soul, my spiritual energy, was experiencing such a shift that it could cause an energetic purge so deep that heat radiated from my chest. I felt the energy living within me. The heat was unavoidable in the dance that was underway.

I recognized that I could choose whether it was true or not. It felt like the most engaging and exciting journey of my life. I wanted to believe it to be true, and it was clearly a part of my reality. If our realities are merely personal perceptions, I was excited to make this a part of mine. I found myself forgiving the younger version of self that just did not know the first time around when I had the choice. Now, I was intrigued that my choices led my spiritual energy to start the clean-up work. It was clean-up work apparently needed in order for my spiritual wheels to become the self-sustaining, balanced mechanism that provides the pathway to, and maintains the connection to my light within.

Once I had a framework and could feel my chakras, I integrated them into my meditations of the white light. The meditative visions held my energetic being with glowing chakras waiting for me to unlock their spiritual powers. This was the only past-time activity I engaged once responsibilities were fulfilled. I have always been very selective in my reading and listening to gain perspectives. There is a lot of noise, static and hidden agendas. I prefer to create the space and opportunity to experience what it is like for me and within me. I treated this exploration the same.

I knew deep down that it was cell history and stored energy purging from my body with every expanded thought. I could feel deep within that the white light of universal energy was clearing the energy of the collective consciousness I had absorbed along the way. I could feel the transition within my core after every typed word, soulful awareness, and soaked night. It was real and happening, and I could feel my humanness begin to struggle.

My mind could not process and accept that my soul was regaining control of my heart. It felt like my mind was under a surprise attack by means of its own stored data from life. It felt like my egoic mind was awakening out of fear to prevent the return of its sovereign ruler, my soul.

After nine months of intense inward reflection, I received my first reprieve after patiently removing one limiting belief after another. The first phase of healing turned out to be 264 days of sweating with a twenty-pound loss of un-useful energy. It only lasted a week or so and then the lessons resumed, and my body became the voice of my soul to ensure I listened.

As I continued to write, meditate, and sweat, my soul and heart continued on their separate yet intertwined journeys. Just as the heat from my chest led me to the spiritual energy wheels within, the light of my soul was guiding my heart back to love. I was willing to follow the light within and surrender to the passionate love burning to be set free.

35

Replacing My Heart's Fear with Love

    With a new sense of authentic connection to spirituality through my burning heart chakra, I was led through a myriad of ideologies and pedagogical experiences. One by one, they continued to unearth themselves before me at just the precise time. I navigated through other Christian-based organized religions, Ayurvedic medicine and practices, and yoga and meditation techniques of the Hindus and Buddhists. I was then energetically drawn to chakra energy alignment, the healing strength in crystals, and how to achieve spiritual alchemy. Unexpectedly I was then swooped away into meta and quantum physics, sacred geometry, astrology, astronomy, and the collective consciousness. All concepts of great interest at some point through life along the way. I felt them collectively looping in endless cycles within my being until they started to come together and form the cohesive spiritual fabric my soul was yearning; unbeknown, the foundation was always there. It was a foundation that sourced the truths in my beliefs. The truths my heart was beginning to feel.

I once again found comfort in reconnecting back to the Catholic religion of my youth. It was the only idea of religion or connection to spirituality. The new energy shifts within my body called for me to reconnect with the teachings of my youth, my experiences abroad, where life had grown me, and how it had done so now on display in the moments before me. I reflected on my admiration for those deeply rooted in their religious and spiritual faith. It was the greatest dream I held in life. I had not yet learned I had already arrived. Even so, I recognized that I felt there were errors in my ways for not being able to connect in such a similar way as others. It did not make sense in my mind, yet I knew that tightening my spiritual fabric was part of this journey's purpose; to break free from my own perceived errors and admire my own sense of connection.

Then the day arrived, and out of nowhere I knew everything was beginning to unravel. I was beginning to unravel. I was engaging in a mid-day meditation when I felt a suffocating fear. And I mean, really felt it. I was already experiencing so many physiological changes and the deep energetic sensations of those experiences. So, when I felt suffocated, it was literally taking my breath away, but not in a good way, in a very new, real, unnerving, and frightening way. I sat with the situation in silence as I regained my breath, waiting for a response to why it happened. There it was. As clear as I could read on paper. The word fear. It was flashing, bold, bright, and unrelenting in my mind's eye. I knew this was my starting point. Fear was where I needed to start the deconstruction of my mind.

The intention was to deconstruct the mind, remove the garbage from the psyche and make way for purity. I knew it was my starting point because in my experience fear had been the opposite of love, not indifference. Love and fear are incapable of existing within the same time and space within me. I knew I would be unable to love purely if fear was present. I wanted to know that I would always choose love. I knew I had unconsciously chosen out of fear during prior breaths. I wanted to create opportunities to choose differently. With love. For love.

I could not figure out why I had experienced fear in my space of white light. I was perplexed as to why there was such fear associated with achieving the brightest, most joyful state of existence my mind's eye had ever envisioned and where my soul was longing to return. I was surprised to find fear arose when I thought about the beautiful possibilities of strong spiritual faith. Then I realized where the fear was rooted. The fear was rooted in the constructs of God and death. The fear was rooted not in the act of dying yet knowing the truth that I would live on for eternity.

I do not fear death. I have been face-to-face with death too many times to be scared. Conversely, I felt more like I was patiently awaiting that glorious day. I sincerely felt I knew that space well, perhaps too well. I felt more fear from the idea of not succeeding at bringing the Heavens to Earth than I did about leaving Earth to go to Heaven.

I feared I would not succeed at decoding my light language, thereby not fulfill my soul's purpose. I was curious as to what awaited on the other side of the spiritual veil while blinded by the truths of humanity. There was an unknown of the afterlife with a simultaneous knowingness that it was not as taught albeit magical in every freeing way, and could and should be enjoyed while alive.

I discovered that my fear was rooted in what I had seen happen to loved ones due to an experience with death, while mine with my Mom was beautiful and peaceful; I felt her freeing release. I prayed deeply that I could navigate my own unavoidable and organic life processes with strength, leaving grace upon the hearts I leave behind. My fear was rooted in the idea that the beautiful space of white light and infinite love that I had been envisioning could only be attainable after my physical life walk was over.

I knew that the space of bright love and compassion was the reflection of God's love, taught as a child. I had my naming convention, but that is what it was in truth. I knew it was the same space we have all heard about when someone experiences a near-death experience. It was the same space the dying walk towards in their final breaths. It was the same space I journeyed to and from during my illness and saw clearly with each dance with death thereafter.

For me, it was a glorious and radiant space of all positive and amazing wonders yet to enjoy while in the human physical experience. It was the majestic space of the purest attainable vibration of creation, the vibration of love, bringing the Heavens to the Earth. It was a space completely contrasted to what I knew my reality was holding. The fear was a genuine and scary notion, purely mind-driven, and required extinction from my being if I were to make it to my sacred space to find love.

I realized that it was only a construct and that the fear was irrational. The fear was my limited mind trying to make sense of a dimension beyond comprehension. It became clear that I wanted to experience the glory of that space during my physical life. I did not want to wait until my afterlife to experience the magnitude of authentic and genuine beauty. Instead, I wanted to experience the limitless possibilities of infinite love while living a physical life. Once I deconstructed the fear erected around my heart, all of my mindful shadows were exposed.

One by one, I began deconstructing the myriad of constructs and limiting beliefs that remained. As I met each dark shadow within, I concurrently discovered the truth in its entirety as to what had caused its presence. As I tore each shielding wall down, it felt like I exposed the lifelong building blueprint of integral and meticulous design. As I deconstructed every aspect of my mind, I instantly knew where the building materials had come from along my walk and how to choose differently. Slowly light was able to break through the shadows and shine upon my heart.

For the first time it felt like I was affirming what I wanted spiritually, and my body felt healing as it followed. The journey had been so unexplainable in so many ways up to this point. The more it continued, the more I wanted to follow and journey on my soulful path. It did not make sense in my limited mind, and it likely did not make sense to those around me, even as I tried to explain the inner exploration and realignment. I felt misunderstood most of the time as I reconciled that those around me only knew that of which I had been able to extend into my reality, vocalized or portrayed in action. All the while it continued to be nothing more than a personal journey about my past from the exterior; my deeply inward, very soulful, personal journey. I myself sometimes struggled to accept the exciting uncomfortableness and had very few words to express the new dimensions I was expanding into and becoming. It was hard to explain to the exterior world, especially when the journey continued to unfold just as quickly as I held intentions, intentional and unintentional alike.

It felt like my Inner Spirit had led me thus far, so I trusted that the guidance would continue. I believed that my level of conscious awareness would expand into knowingness. I believed my heart would become full and swell with love and joy. I believed I would connect to the energy source of all creation, the same energy that healed me. I believed in the powerful energy within me, you, the collective, and the universe. I believed it had the power to heal; heal the body, mind, heart, and soul; mine and yours alike. I believed this so deeply that the choice to continue onward was clear and straightforward. I was not surprised to find that love remains the easiest to follow.

Over time, I found that the more I surrendered to letting every aspect of my being to be soulfully guided, down to the cellular level of my physical body, the more I discovered the truths in my beliefs. I was continually presented with the perfect experiences to embrace and integrate all that I believed in, and what my heart desired within each moment I was evolving. It made every moment a beautiful moment. It made every moment meaningful. It made every moment count. It made me realize that the combination of soulful bliss and the physical experience needed to come together to have the spiritual sense that every moment is *truly* beautiful. To make every moment *truly* meaningful. To make every moment *truly* count. At times I found I had to remind myself of my own intentions to reunite my Inner and Physical Spirits.

There is something surreal and peaceful when you allow your mind to surrender to the heart, release the oars, and drift upon the waters of serenity. That is the space of soulful love. That is the love that is unconditional. That is unwavering love. While knowing that the experience with another would be sublime, I knew that before I could exchange such a soulful, energetic love, I would first have to hold that same soulful, unconditional love for myself. Something I knew I did not hold, merely from the sense of misalignment itself. I knew I trusted the purity of my love for self within, but it was the lack of trust to love myself within the world around me. I also knew I had a slight fear of not being able to wholly hold my love for myself in the presence of such soulful love from another. My love felt powerful, so I knew I would have to stand strong to receive something similar in kind.

My challenge was navigating myself within the realms of those around me. It felt difficult to remain quiet enough on the inside to know what to do next on the outside. The noise of the external world always seemed loud up against the quieted mind needed to hear the whispers of my path. It was incredibly challenging when up against the hurried, buzzing energy often coupled with expectations of being incapable, medically fragile, weak, and thereby sad. I have always felt the complete opposite. I became weary from constantly warding off expectations and somehow would unknowingly and organically defy them by staying true to myself when given the space to be me. It felt like a space I rarely was able to visit. The last time I recalled living from that space was in the hospital in my youth and the year of recovery abroad. Once I returned to Louisiana and life took over, I forgot it even existed until I commanded its rediscovery

I knew I loved myself. I believe I am pretty remarkable. Fascinating to my own human mind. It used to be a challenge to own my life story because it is so unbelievably amazing, mystical, and magical. There are so many unexplainable and unbelievable experiences that it used to be overwhelming to contain the truths within my being. I have always been an optimistic and kind person. That is just who I am; sometimes, even the over-zealous optimist that is easily and quickly tempered by the so-called realist. I love to love. I love learning, growing, expanding, and continuing to be the next best version of myself. I love to laugh and smile. I love to create and spread joy. There is so much sadness in this world. I would much rather be happy than sad.

I have never needed nor relied on anyone to incite this within me. My existence was quite the contrary. Those who knew my life experiences held greater expectations that my life was limited, hard, and sad. It was at times. I was also determined not to allow limitations, hardships, and sadness to overpower the love and joy held deep within. There is so much to be grateful for in this life.

While married, raising our children, and working full time, I was left reconciling all this within my being for several years as I navigated the many chosen roles with my heart. Before starting to write, a marking experience within our family dynamic left me in a state of clear intention. It was an upsetting and troubling experience that left me feeling uncertain about the future of our family unit. Over the years that followed, although challenging at times, I remained devoted to the shared commitment we had begun out of love. Although this time was different in so many ways, it was no different in how I navigated it. I knew deeply that there was meaning in the experience, yet many times over, I had to dig deep to remember the silent purpose. I trusted that one day I would know that purpose. I never doubted that within my being, yet the uptick in occurrences often made me forget. Something within kept me grounded in the experiences while my mind questioned our connection many times over. I always trusted that I would know and feel what we both needed. I always trusted that within myself.

I meditated and prayed alike, for I did not know what would unfold in the coming moments. I leaned heavily into my intentions and trusted that I would receive the answers clearly before me and I would be able to navigate with peace and grace. I also stood fragile in the truth that where there is love, there is understanding. I loved my partner. I believed in the healing power of love and knew we were healing each other in our lives together. But after this one experience, it no longer felt healing. It brought my awareness to the actions and choices we were both making, thereby creating an experience that no longer held love; our connection to each other was no longer healing.

In time, my heart began carving its path when I felt the disconnect between my partner's heart and mine. I had to discern what I felt was lacking in the relationship. To my mindful surprise, my soul revealed that our soulful resonance was not magnetizing our essence, the swirling of energetic love that alchemizes the hearts was still, the chemistry of the souls that defies time and space was inactive, and the spiritual love that transcends the physical body never existed. Those were the truths behind the purest and sweetest love. Those were the truths of my heart I had to acknowledge were not being honored. Those were the truths of my love that I wanted to enjoy in this life. Those were the truths of my authentic self-love found trapped in my heart behind my own walls of fear and doubt.

I sensed there would be something more profound with the concept of authentic self-love. Something that would be at the source of who I am. As uncertain as the notion appeared, I knew it was a necessary journey. My heart required it, as it has kept me alive. It was time to keep my heart alive, and love was the only way.

It was within the spaces of life where I had unknowingly carved the paths of deliverance. Once I opened the floodgates with writing, I had to choose to accept or decline what was on its way. It was only a couple of months into writing that the reflections, the awareness, the discernment, the intentions, and the latent felt emotions became the catalyst of an explosive culmination of my being, exploding throughout my heart and propelling me into the universe to return to wholeness. I could feel the powerful swell of emotion as I reigned everything in:

- Joy and love that filled my heart and the years...
- Choices made with meaning and intention...
- Gifts the journey has bestowed upon me...
- Miracles I see in the treasures of my children...
- Roles I had chosen to hold with my heart...
- Perspectives encountered along the way...
- Journeys that remain unknown and silent...
- Seemingly differences imposed upon us, among us, and within us...
- Preconceived constructs of faith, religion, and spirituality...
- Societal and self-imposed expectations, limitations, doubts, and fear...
- Tools preserved in my well-being toolbox...
- Passion my heart held and wanted to express and share...
- Optimism and positive intentions...
- Desire to live life to the fullest...
- Service to a greater purpose; a Divine Intention...
- Gratitude for every blessing in my life...
- Light to guide humanity...
- Spiritual gifts to heal humanity...
- My powerful love...
- The majestic song of my Soul...
- Your heart emulating the purity of our love...
- Being one with the light...
- All of my heart's desires in abundance...

Every cell of my being willingly participated during each culmination of breath, and within each present moment. I trusted that each meta-physical step I was taking backwards would achieve healing into the future by means of the love I was restoring in my heart. I could feel love was leading the way. All of me followed as love guided me back to love.

36

Connecting to My Spiritual Senses

I knew that I experienced life through my senses. For me, it is part of the human experience that makes a moment so enjoyable, sensually enjoyable, even in the absence of one or more of them. It even felt as though my senses were overcompensating for the lost parts of me along the way. There was also the only absolute dream I have ever held, a spiritual dream. It was the dream to hold the super senses, the spiritual senses, the clair senses - clairvoyance (clear seeing), clairsentience (clear feeling), clairaudience (clear hearing), clairalience (clear smelling), clairgustance (clear tasting), and claircognizance (clear knowing).

I believe the spiritual senses to be the most glorious gifts in this life, our human superpowers of this experience. Everything about my experiences were sourced in my senses, and although I did not believe I held the clair senses, I desperately wanted to experience the reality they would reveal. It felt like I was supposed to be in the world that used spiritual senses, a world I was journeying towards to connect to fully. It was a world that felt so powerful that I had to walk towards the strength required to hold it.

When I experience something, I want to experience it wholly and completely. I want to smell the smells, hear the sounds, taste the tastes, see the sights, and the most delightful is to feel how my internal world interprets the external world and, in return, impacts my internal world, a sense that can never go void. I wanted to experience the same in the spiritual sense so that I could see what cannot be seen, feel the energy that governs our existence, hear the voices of Angels, smell the scents of history, taste the sweetness of love, and know through universal wisdom. It is pure joy to experience a moment as all the senses come together at a single point. To sensually experience the world has always captivated my utmost attention.

I found that my sensuality, my primary source of enjoyment, had been quieted, hidden, un-nurtured, discouraged, disrespected, and ignored. I was either the one doing it or choosing to allow it by another. Either way, I was choosing to change. I wanted to allow my senses to guide me back to the purity within. If I was going to return to my heart, I needed to release my mind and surrender to my senses.

I had been practicing the management of my mind my entire life. I was used to believing all things are possible and keeping negativity and doubt at bay. I believe that our thoughts and emotions are critical to our self-journey, yet I somehow remained mindfully detached from truly feeling my own. I could openly and diligently walk through any thought and yielding emotion into dissipation long before it had a chance to be felt. I mindfully talked my way through the biological and physiological truths of my bodily reactions embedded in the psychological processes of the mind. I reminded myself of the machine of parts that we all are. I mindfully knew how I wanted to feel yet remained unknowingly shielded when my heart tried to feel. I could sense this was an opportunity to choose differently.

I vowed to remain as authentic as possible while following my heart. I had to learn how to allow myself to feel deeply when the emotional waves would crest while concurrently unlearning how I instinctively shielded my heart during the trauma of my youth. Writing caused me to connect to the emotions of the trauma so I could finally connect in love. My spiritual trauma was starting to have space and the means by which to heal. In reaching for my spirituality, I released what felt like layers of armor and false masks from my humanness, and I continued to experience physiological and physical changes throughout my body as a result.

I began feeling every aspect of growth. No matter the growth phase or lesson, there was a related physiological and emotional experience, a sensation. Everything became a sensual experience, and I felt everything down to the cellular level once I chose to experience it. It was messy and ugly as tears journeyed me through the emotional spectrum as they flooded my heart. The highs and lows fueled order into the chaos by blasting my heart wide open.

It was the space of my body that my heart had to learn how to love. I could sense my nervousness in allowing myself to feel my body. Due to the new sensations, I understood what I had been so afraid to uncover in the past. As I opened my heart towards my body, and every slightest change in sensation, I was walked through each experience as if to ensure I made it to the other side alive. Even each medical instance and dance with death felt more like an operating system upgrade that expanded my spiritual senses and stabilized my physical body with new abilities to integrate into my reality.

The deeper I grew into my body, it felt like each experience, especially medical emergencies, morphed my being, creating an authentic sensation of expansion into dimensions beyond this life experience. It felt like I was remembering and growing from lessons coming forward into my current life. I could see the veils from each life cloak me to ensure I embodied all that had been learned thus far, now expressed into who I am today; the very cloaks blocking my authentic light in the here and now. It was a whirlwind of journeys across dimensions filled with lessons that made absolute sense, yet I was a human mess.

I found I started to build the process upon a series of intentions and deep trust. The first was around the experience of thoughts. I believed that a thought would only come into my experience if it was of the same energetic essence and would serve my intentions in some way. So, I welcomed anything and everything that aligned with my highest good and believed that the experiences encountered aligned with that intention.

I decided that everything needed to be honored and explored if it came into my awareness. I have always deeply believed my thoughts are sourced in something. This belief allowed me to disengage from them when they did not serve me. I knew early on the process was about allowing emotions and feelings, and since managing my thoughts seemed doable, I felt prepared.

I aspired to incite positive thoughts and emotions within others, and while I did, I was also left feeling as if my misalignment was sabotaging something deep within. I believed that if I could discern if a thought was sourced outside of me, inside of me, and anchored in fear and doubt, I would be able to deconstruct it and release it. Only if it served my soulful mission in bringing about love and joy would I integrate my thoughts into the process. All I had to do was pay attention, close attention. It felt easy and authentic. I had not yet entered the depths of the journey.

Soon enough, I realized that experiences were leading me to the precise elements that resonated deeply within. The thoughts always came first and then I would seemingly stumble upon their presence in the world. I was led to the exact earthly experiences to connect the dots that had been collected and precisely plotted throughout the world of my reality. Dots within my mind that my soul had selected. A world my mind had been waiting patiently to understand. The experiences were subtle reminders of the truth in that you bring about what you think about. Even more so they emphasized the need to transcend beyond.

I entertained concepts that came to mind. I remained aware of the resonance experiences had within my energy. I listened to the whispers of my soul, and I allowed my heart to feel. I patiently followed my inner wisdom and connection to self as they both continued to speak louder. Every aspect of my mind continued to be the subject of analysis and deconstruction, while every part of my heart and soul came forward, vying for my attention.

With each unearthed step in precision and accuracy, my soul guided my mind through physical experiences, creating anchor points that allowed a cognitive involvement to make sense of the exposed metaphysical needs. I found myself mystically positioned in experiences, uncovering literature, entrenched in my own reflections, and finally beginning to understand the world within, now merging into the world without. It was freeing to start integrating my soul into my mind versus my mind trying to mold my soul.

Although the synchronicities presented before me created a clear path to follow, my mind constantly tried to intervene. I followed every sacred synchronicity like breadcrumbs on a barren path, all the while, my mind felt the need to direct, monitor, and analyze everything. My Inner Spirit felt annoyed that my mind needed a physical world label but indulged as it was part of the earthly journey. In the unfolding, I sensed a new deeper connectedness to everyone and everything in this human physical experience. I found comfort in discovering that I was not alone, albeit I never felt alone, more hidden, limited, and bound.

It reminded me of prior manifestations I had co-created along the way with my thoughts and if they were in alignment with my desires. It highlighted those that were not. The more I aligned with my inner world of infinite potential, no matter the thought, it was manifesting somewhere in the world for me to see, near or far, as distance seemed not to matter. I was left wondering, praying, and dreaming alike that it was my family of Angels on display, affirming I was right, and it was their way of calling me home. My humanness doubted that I would be worthy of such a connection yet knew I had to continue through the illusion to join with the truth I knew awaited. That alone sometimes left me feeling frustrated by my own humanness.

Through it all, I developed a focus that felt like a laser beam through the frustration; intense and direct. It sometimes felt unyielding in its organic support to guide me through the process. It was a focus that seemed familiar as it was the one I had witnessed my entire life within everyone's outward projection of self. It was a focus that allowed someone to almost tune everything else out, except for responsibilities. It was a focus I didn't recall ever experiencing before except for maybe in the hospital but those were slower, quieter times. It felt like it was just a state of being back then yet now the noise of the world required a laser beam to break through to my soul. With a growing trust in the mystical experiences on display, and a focus that I could not shift when I tried, it became easier to trust myself. I just followed the focus. The more I leaned into the focus on me, I was positioned around vital elements that resonated with my body and somehow grounded me in ways I still had yet to discover.

Nervous in my exploration, I continued to choose the elements that put my body at ease during whatever transformation was occurring within. It felt hopeful that it would sustain me. I chose what felt right. The routines that became a part of my continued healing are crystal-infused water, aromatherapy, Ayurvedic diet cleanses, green smoothies, and calm instrumental music instead of music with words, television and reading. When my mind was idle, my authentic and organic focus was drawn to my body, breathing, and feeling each breath throughout my body. It was a practice that previously felt forced or incongruent and became a natural progression that illuminated and connected me to my mystical world within. As I continued to incorporate these into my daily practice, the various parts of me worked with the healing potential of these elements to collectively heal my body. I could feel what was happening long before I had trust in myself to describe it.

Although there was a tremendous sense of peace, the organic evolution of this process was alarming at first. Still, as I relaxed and began to breathe into the expansive space that the growth provided, more and more peace and joy surfaced, and my body adjusted toward balance. I felt it in my heart down to my pelvic area, shifting as I moved through each passing day. Many times, this was more difficult than I would have hoped or imagined, which caused me to falter from authenticity, and question you, question myself, question everything within the unintegrated parts of me. Concurrently, I was acutely aware of the parts diligently integrating into oneness. Those parts of me found it fascinating that it was inner wisdom guiding me to the spaces in the physical.

I found bewilderment in my own experiences, torn apart by my own dichotomy, and trying to find stability within an emerging world. It was as if various realms were becoming visible, transposed upon and within each other. At the time I knew I was seeing worlds that others could not, and at a quantum level that few had words to explain, including me. I could see worlds coming together and illuminating in a multidimensional space with me at the center, shining light upon all the darkness, mine, and yours alike.

It felt like the more I followed the clarity within, the further it brought me away from the collective. It felt like the very source of our oneness held potential to be the very thing that separated us. I could not see past the universe's radiance nor understand who would want to or choose to. All I knew is that I did not, and a part of me felt like I could not turn away. I wanted to experience the magnificence in the unfolding and all its impending glory. I knew I was a part of it and wanted to feel that connection deeply.

As I deconstructed my mind and made it closer to my heart while living through the days of kids, family, work, and friends, I became hyper-aware of labels, of all kinds. The world relies so heavily on labels. We have labels for everything. Although unspoken words tend to speak louder, we act as though we need a label for our minds to process, find a cause and yielding effects, justify and resolve, and to know how to nurture our feelings. That is why we have language; to communicate and express ourselves and the world around us. Labels were the very reason I wanted to distance myself from western medicine.

Throughout every breath of our days, everything is approached with a need to be labeled and placed in a bucket. We then further attempted to place each other in labeled buckets with guidelines of how it should feel and how to navigate those feelings. We even have buckets for things that do not fit in a bucket, and differ, or vary in some way other than a generalized norm. I found that my authenticity had become jaded by waiting to discover the label someone placed upon me before responding and engaging.

Although I always navigated labels and the mindful application and avoidance of my own, I felt peaceful and fluid. Since I rarely labeled myself and was more so deciphering those of others, if a label was incongruent within my depths, it was not worth my time nor energy. I found more often, rather than defending myself, my heart would respect the other in silence with an acknowledgment that they too were on a journey of the soul traversing a plane of lessons and try to hold compassion for life experiences that molded them in such a way.

My mind on the other hand was left wondering what it was they could not see since life was rooted in choices. I could not understand the choices others were making. My heart often times shared in the comedic side of the universe, with the universe, within my silence. It was all fun in the game of life until those labels entered my home. Once within my home, they made their way to my heart and began building a wall of shame and doubt.

I had lived a life unknowingly not labeling any part of my being and could not understand why collectively we were unable just to let something be. Allowing my being to flow freely was the only way I knew how to exist, until I realized the flow was around my shielded and fearful heart. Since the goal was to remove the labels one by one, I was ready to embrace them as they were uncovered. The aspects of my life from the beautiful life in between, and the new experiences underway began swirling around, and within me. The more I wrote, the more my body transformed, and I could feel the changes deep within the cells that make up my body. It was as if my body was turning back on, cell by cell. I could see and feel the slightest energy sparks within me.

It felt like I had catapulted myself into a process that illuminated the sensation of a split self. It had been forever present yet became profoundly felt within, like a zig zag down the center of my torso at my core. At times it even felt as if my soul was seeping out through the jagged edges, half in and half out of my body. The sensations solidified the experience of me watching myself walk down the narrow cobblestone roads in Rome and the many that followed thereafter when my Inner Spirit floated above the physical to protect my body from the human condition of limitations which caused pain and suffering, the source of my rough edges. I was ungrounded and merely held roles of expectancy. I was left with a body trying to operate without all of its parts, mindfully sorting through the matrix seeking the exit. It felt like I understood that I needed to create a sacred space to reign my soul back into my body, a safe space to rest.

It did not take long before I began assessing and honoring the sacredness of my body, life, space, relationships, soul, and heart during this physical experience and the lessons to be learned. I had to figure out how to house and protect my sacred soul, especially with refined intention and assistance from crystals, aroma therapy, and a quieted world. I welcomed the illumination within my mind that would free me from my physical barriers. I wanted to live embodied so I could enjoy my bodily senses. I felt like my mind finally understood that it needed to be pristine and step aside so my body could rest in my soul's expression. Understanding was easier than doing.

To anchor the multidimensional sense of self, I wanted to understand better the vastness and rapid pace of the mindful expansion I was experiencing. It felt like my mind was expanding beyond the confines of my own ideas of what is possible while knowing infinite possibilities exist. It felt expansive and reached the depths of eternity, all the while only contained within my body. It was as though I could see layers upon layers of energy rippling from the various journeys traveled by those around me, including my own. All I could see was the matrix web of humanity, the interconnectedness of every thought and action, and the potential clutch of the spiraling silk made of fear and doubt, all traveled by weary hearts within sacred bodies. Profoundly aware that I was the most prominent example in the world around me, a humble projection of self.

It was very important for me to understand these aspects of my existence, so I could put them into action and do them with intention. I needed it for myself, yet my children needed me to do this even more so, albeit they never knew. I knew I would be exactly what I was intended to be in this life, and I knew they would too, for everything is always divinely perfect in spiritual truth. Yet, I also knew that we as humans are molded by our environment and experiences endured, especially in our youth. Knowing this placed a tremendous responsibility upon me as a parent to provide for them the best I could regarding both while countering a sense of shame for not being able to do more, and more timely. I knew in my heart I had always done my best, and my experiences continued to prove that truth in my reality.

I fully embraced the potentiality of our sacred human vessels, the bodies that house our souls, and that we hold the power to create our life experiences in ways contrary to prior teachings. And based on my own experiences, I believed it happened in the metaphysical space of our existence before it occurred in our physical reality. I also understood the laws of thermodynamics as it relates to energy and entropy, allowing me to connect with all the dimensions within me while anchoring in the truths of vibrational energy and the beautiful purity of crystals; the Earthly elements that took millions of years to form, vibrate higher than our carbon unit bodies, and naturally will sync with our energetic bodies through quantum entrainment thereby organically raising the body's vibration. At first, all I knew was that I needed to raise my vibration. The highest vibration is love, so I focused on raising my vibration to that of love—the vibration of creation.

I traversed the spaces in between life by following crystals that resonated with my heart, witnessing numbers speak to me in ways that danced in synchronicity, hearing songs that arose from the silence, and when quiet enough I started to hear the whispers of Angels as they responded to the inquiries of my heart. I knew deep within that following the organic shifts would lead to love. Even so, I was still learning that it was through my heart that I would sync my humanness with these truths.

Within every waking day of this process, I felt my dichotomous beings swap places like rotations of a double helix. It was as if all of the expressions of my light that I had been giving to the world were flipped and directed to me, and all of the expressions of dark that were directed at me became my expressions to the world. As I was returning my light to myself, I could see and feel every vibration of dark energy leave my body. It was an awareness that demonstrated that the manipulation of my light into dark had occurred within my safe space.

The transposition that occurred with the energy left me feeling as though my consciousness was evolving yet simultaneously descending into a foreign 3D dimensional state of existence, escorted, and guided by the force within my heart. It was a world within which I became everything I had been warding off throughout life. I became the very things that were silently being programmed into my being. The more I found my light, I could feel them being released only once my body expressed it in some way.

There were times while I silently rolled my eyes as my body played out the purging process. I was saddened by the illusions I left in my wake as they were contrary to everything I had chosen and wanted to become in this life. I sent so much love and gratitude to the recipients of my ridiculousness. I hoped their hearts would understand. I bashfully knew some would only know that version of me and prayed deeply that others would trust in me and would grow with me into knowing. I knew that my love would be felt within the hearts of those that truly loved me, especially yours.

At times I was ashamed of my own expressions of self. It felt like my heart needed to understand what happened over the beautiful life through a new set of senses, my spiritual senses. It was as though my consciousness had to descend, collect my body, and together bust through the darkness around my heart before collectively they could reunite with my soul in the cosmos, and it had to happen while humanly aware in order to rejoin into oneness. It felt like my soul had been soaring with the collective consciousness above me, and speaking to my human mind while pouring wisdom over my computerized ego outputs. I had no idea that I had often times left my body behind. I had no idea that I had to collect it from somewhere. All I knew is that it felt like my body was not embodied with my light and was existing among the darkness within humanity. Eventually I could see how I had left my body abandoned and unprotected while my light floated above.

My state of existence, the dialogue within, and the journey towards the light was deemed ordinary, therefore, I allowed the guidance to continue not realizing what was occurring with every inquiry. I thought that was what being human was like for everyone. The more I felt the voice of my soul quiet my mind, the more my heart became closer to love. I could feel the difference as I approached a space of light, unconditional love, understanding, and compassion, breaking through the illusions of the human condition and its cocooning fibroids of limiting beliefs, especially those around love and within my heart. I could feel I was getting closer to your love.

The more I could feel what was happening, the more I realized there was still tremendous work to be done. I could feel that I was not yet at my heart's center. This awareness only made the desire to arrive at the destination even stronger. I soon recognized that I had spent many years longing to be back in the space of just being me. I wanted to be back in the space of being connected with my authentic self. I wanted to arrive back to an ability of being authentically connected to my source of energy like I was in my youth. The space that I was envisioning with the white light was that space. I wanted to bathe in the glory and magnificence of that space. That was the space to BE. That was the space to be ME.

It took several more years to discover that the last time I was my most authentic self was in the depths of my most traumatic experience. Then, I had all of the space and time needed to be whatever I needed to become; space and time to find breath at the start of each new day. With my new senses I saw it as a space when I was still and quiet enough to manifest my heart's desires. Somehow along the way, I gave up the space and time I needed for myself. I gave it up to many people. I gave it up to the collective human heart.

Until I discovered those truths, I desperately yearned to return to a sense of self and wholeness, alongside the sad recognition that it was within the walls of a hospital where I felt most safe to be vulnerable, authentic, and accepted. The truths were accompanied with the awareness that it was also the space that I felt most at ease with being. Perhaps because it was often behind the walls of a hospital averting a fatality when I was most sensitive to the awareness of my soul and the souls of others walking through life and beyond.

I was always aware of soulful connections, but at a different level. Or perhaps at an incomplete level. I have always crossed paths with sacred and soulful connections, and my life was full of their guiding moments. They did so for a reason, and I am forever grateful for the lessons they brought into my experiences and how they grew me in this life through their love and light.

Even so, because of previous encounters over the years and interacting with a new level of energetic allowance, there was a different vibrational connection to them; powerful and unexplainable. I always knew that I was being guided and carried during certain times in my life. As this type of connection relates to my Mom, I feel closer to my Mom now, more than I ever did when she was alive. I feel like now that she is pure energy, we are able to connect effortlessly. Although I can only communicate with her in the vast energetic realms and no longer through our physical bodies within this physical experience, I am connected to her love which continually manifests into my physical existence. My Mom was helping me in ways neither of us knew I needed while she was alive. It was as if she could see my truths beyond this dimension and now able to guide me along the way. In my humanness I had no idea what was genuinely unfolding. I only knew that I eagerly and bashfully trusted in the energetic presence of my Mom, my intellect, and my heart. Her beautiful love and energy grace my path every day.

With those experiences, I had to embrace my ability and truth that I communicate with souls. I had to decipher that souls communicate in expansive, multidimensional, high vibrational energetic frequencies, and our physical beings are mostly familiar with communicating in less sophisticated, lower vibration means of expression not realizing that the heart is the translator by means of the vibration of love. The ego-protective experience of language gave me the courage to settle into my experiences with spirit merely because of the dichotomy between labels and the label-less. Being guided into this understanding allowed me to bridge the experiences of my worlds and left me at peace and into a balance I was beginning to feel.

Through my Mom's energy, I knew what it would feel like to connect to the light energy of Spirit. It was important because of the dark energy absorbed along the way, and because the younger versions of self had grappled with my own struggle in the dark while trying to figure out where my light was sourced. I knew of, and respected the dark energy that must exist to maintain energetic balance throughout the universe. It felt like there was a blanket of spiritual protection in the journey through my shadows that was leading me to my light. It was as if my Angels knew they needed to stay close and aid me until it was time in my journey to reunite my Inner and Physical Spirits, embodied as one, and could take back my power and autonomy. It always felt like I couldn't speed up time fast enough to get to where I needed to be, albeit I knew I was exactly where I was supposed to be and had to travel through my present to get there. Even so, my heart was often elsewhere in my reality. It was in the future finding you.

I knew my Angels were present, and I desperately wanted to feel them and to know them intimately. In a sense, I believed that if I felt them, I could rest in the knowingness that it was true and not just my egoic mind fabricating false beliefs. The intensity of the doubt was an impetus for wanting to heighten my emotional intelligence of self and connect to my soul family in assurance. I wanted to learn how to cultivate an energetic path directly to them, embrace them for the mirrors they hold, and the messages learned from their soul, especially that of my Mom. I had to open my heart to recognize my soul family's energy even in the absence of their physical beings. In time, some created a stronger presence and essence around me. Some messages were louder than others, some visions were clearer than others, and some reflections were harder to embrace than others. Yet, all of them impacted the progression of my journey. All were guiding me to the same truths.

During several junctures along the way, I recall reflecting on my Mom and how a butterfly is representative of her beautiful and graceful essence. At times it felt like I was transforming into a

Beautiful Butterfly within the cocoon of my own body. A body that had held me captive for many years, similar to how she felt within hers. I was in my cocoon of life, growing new skin and developing my senses until my transformation was complete to expose my truths. The unbridled power within me was burning to be set free. It was evolving in the forefront of my existence while quietly carving its path to escape. I was transforming my humanness yet remained a human, experiencing emotions of the heart, within an always-changing body, with a mind that had a mind of its own, all the while trying to align with my soul song. An experience that I felt my Mom was leading me through with her guidance and grace. I did know that she would not abandon me nor mislead me. I know of my love, and trust in her love. I honored her presence and protection.

The compassionate love I found in my heart and the light of my Mom created a quiet safe space to rediscover my inner truths; for my mind, body, and soul to reacquaint themselves in my heart. With silent yet energetic love and support, and with a compassion that felt familiar, I was able to construct my laboratory of alchemy, fueled by the remembrance of who I am.

For most of my life, I have known that my soul would require the strength of love that comes with the test of time, not just this lifetime but of all lifetimes. Yet, I never honored nor understood where those sentiments come from until now. There was a sense of peace throughout the journey of releasing the constructs of love associated with my physical body and the reckoning of truths that I was being guided back to love. It was the very constructs that took months to release that held the message in a song about the magnetic attraction of the physical body and the sensual shape of love; the song that followed me through the universe, repeating for months and months, everywhere I went until I finally heard the unspoken message.

I remember the exact time and space when I felt my mind settle into silence and my heart stabilize in love; at least for that moment since sustainability had not yet been achieved. In unexplainable ways, I felt a remembrance of who I am and my passionate love. I have rarely heard the song since that moment. The very release opened the pathway of the pure love that transcends the physical body.

Through releasing my mind with my spiritual senses, eventually a Spirit Guide graced my path. It was the first experience in my new connection to self, other than that of my Mom. It was the spirit of someone I knew from prior experiences through life and someone I held near and dear. There had been no communications for decades, yet before the growth was underway, their presence had always been very strong within, in spirit, where we initially met, which was what brought us together in my youth. I always thought I knew why there was a strong connection that spanned time and space. During those moments, everything felt genuine in what I believed about our connection. That changed once my spiritual navigation led me to the depths of my heart and the scope of my passion and found the soulful melody to which my love wanted to dance. It was where I left love burning upon my departure from Europe. I knew my Mom was involved.

Although it felt like my Mom guided me to this particular soul, or them to me, it was this soul that guided me to my Mom in the world around me. It was as if she was ensuring I knew she was everywhere to catch me in the moments ahead. Catch me in a way she never could have done alive simply because neither of us knew I needed it. I could feel them both, hear them, and smell them; I could sense every aspect of their energy absent a physical body. The difference was that my Mom was only a Spirit with the memory of her body, and this soul was still embodied as a human. It was his soul that guided me without any physical connection yet everything in the spiritual experience was reflected in his life experience. His reality reflected my spiritual alignment. I was mystified.

I knew I guarded my sensual love closely, especially when it felt it was no longer honored for what it is and for who I am. And albeit it was only through another dimension, it was the sacred gifts of guidance, patience, and soulful compassion that this soul gave me to continue and believe in the journey to release my passionate love. It felt as though if I continued, the journey would lead to the space where the metaphysical transcendence would play out in my physical reality; transcendence into a new love for self and one to share with another in my experience.

It was remarkable to experience myself albeit overwhelming and tiresome until I understood myself enough to care for my needs. I was fascinated and concurrently my mind felt compromised and fought through the mysticism, both experiences occurring within me. I felt the passion in my heart struggle with the thoughts in my mind. My mind was unable to process the experiences fast enough before the next was underway.

I could see and hear my soul orchestrating the whole event, but my humanness was stuck in amazing wonder with shadows of disbelief. The tension of thoughts felt like they were swirling in my mind in endless loops. I knew I was stuck in the mindful inquiries but simultaneously felt powerless to stop them. I recall praying and believing that it was occurring for a sacred reason and that it would pass once the lessons were learned. As strange as they were, all of the experiences continued to support the beliefs in my connection to spirit, yet I understood that I had to let the mind go and allow those connections to exist, if I so chose.

I had built up many false beliefs about how I would, should, or could love another. I even had false beliefs about how I would, should, and could be loved by another, all delicately balanced on the pivots of fear and doubt. In the months of integration, I was continually greeted by this passionate soul. His message was always unequivocally clear. Abundantly clear. This is home, welcome home, and you are home were the main messages delivered. There was even one in which we discussed if we would reconnect in the physical, and we were left acknowledging the possible unlikeliness yet acceptance of it all, similar to when my Mom transitioned. The peace came with knowing that arriving home meant home within self; and not home with any soul other than mine.

Those were moments of affirmation that whatever I was doing was aligned with my soul and that I should keep doing that. I did not feel at home yet, but I felt better than I had in years; every aspect of my being felt stronger and more resolved. I considered it a blessing to receive such clear affirmations of the authentic alignment underway despite how nervous I was about what I was experiencing. It was a world that was just as clear yet used none of my physical senses. I was excited to choose differently and experience the new world emerging.

In time, my Mom's presence was always present, and this soul was less palpable in my experience but very clear in my visions. For many months, there were appearances in meditations, yet mainly during waking moments throughout the day. My mind continuously tried to reconcile the experiences, but every aspect of my being found more comfort in taking the private journey alone in my heart. After all, it was an extraordinary journey of my heart and soul and uniquely mine. Everything was worth taking the journey, especially if love awaited me.

The experiences of the visions and the tremendously strong presence of this soul captivated every aspect of my being. So much so that it became confusing within my mind to separate the worlds. I struggled with accepting that the soul of another living human had communicated to me in the metaphysical space, which thereby played out in the physical reality by mirroring my divinity in their divine path. It was beautifully perfect. As it should be. Yet once again, my mind was trying to get in the way of soulful love.

I had to discover the strangeness of experiencing both the physical and spiritual realms simultaneously within and afar. I had not yet realized I was learning how to discern the difference between realms. Up to this point my experiences with souls had only been in one dimension at a time; this plane of existence or another. In time I learned my multi-dimensional truths and the multiverse within which I traverse in this experience.

I enjoyed the fascination of everything in silence. Life around me felt like an illusion, while everything within was captivating and perfect. It felt like a matter of time before love would be manifested before me, yet my parts were still scattered across the universe. I was still very much fragmented. I could barely link experiences, thoughts, emotions, and actions. The more I journeyed to deconstruct myself, the sloppier the coordination became. At times it felt like my body was expressing my deepest fears and doubts while my mind and emotions tried to make sense of my soul. Concurrently, I was rooting the intentions deeper to alchemize my heart and soul, the sentiments and spirituality of my being, the framework of my physical and spiritual DNA. I could sense the presence of this soul was preparing me for what was to come.

I found my mind eager to discover the purpose of the encounters. I did not fully understand what was going on. I never shared the experiences with anyone and felt slightly uncomfortable as it was not deemed a normal state of existence within my own mind. However, I admired it in others I had encountered and dreamed it would be so for me. Even with my dichotomous parts, I chose to believe in it all. I trusted in the experiences because they were beautiful, peaceful, and felt deeply healing. I had to figure out how to let go and continue believing the truths would unfold before me as they always did. It continued to prove more easily said than done. It was the hope in love that kept me going.

In time I started to feel the energy across space - feeling, receiving, and sending as much love and light energy as my being could manage. Sensations that I have felt most of my adult life were amplified as if to ensure I did not ignore them once again. The sensations throughout my body began to make sense as I felt differently through experiences. I could feel the energy moving throughout my cells as if they were purging and breathing new life into my spiritual wheels, now starting to spin. It felt as if I was finally syncing with an energy that I had felt was a part of me ever since I became ill. It felt like I was finally correcting my own misunderstood parts of self. I was still sweating throughout the nights from my chest. Yet, I could feel a sense of strength in the core of my body with every rising sun. My breath was longer, more full, and had gained fluidity; a broken breath now one. It was a source intention to know and feel this connection. I had no idea what that meant, I only knew I wanted to honor myself enough to find out, and I was starting to live the intentions I had cast so passionately.

It felt more and more that I needed a strong earthly balance for my ever-evolving walk somewhere; it always felt like a walk toward love; pure love and light. The more I journeyed, the more I knew I was headed home, yet not in the sense that most would interpret, and certainly not in ways I could have imagined. At some level, I still just expected to write about my medical experience, knowing I would be changed in some way and move on. I never expected my sensual connection with everything to accumulate energy of its own. Yet, just from how I began experiencing the world around me, I knew I was in for a sensual and pleasurable ride. My free will of choice knew of only one answer; I was on board and ready to explore.

It became about falling back in love with myself and life, and a continuously evolving love sourced in universal energy. That was all I was guided to do. Thankfully that was all that was needed. It was a journey that would require me to slow down, ground myself, and allow the time and space to calibrate with who I am and the space I hold in this experience. It was the perfect set of experiences to reconnect me back to so many aspects of myself and my dreams of passionate love. There was tremendous gratitude to be celebrated, especially with all that continued to transpire and intertwine into a oneness that was leading me to you.

Although overwhelmed, I continuously walked into experiences that affirmed that it was indeed a soulful journey guided by a presence much greater than myself. It felt like a magnetic, collective energy pulling, pushing, and swirling around and within me. It became very easy to honor, especially when it felt like the powerful energy had more control over my body than I did. It felt like the Global Wave of Healing Energy was fueling my spiritual senses.

I deeply felt that I was attracting everything unto me. I had set clear intentions to sync with the essence that was of me. To me, that meant connecting with experiences and people of the same vibrational energy that matched that of my soul. I was emitting my soul's sonar signal out into the universe. I invited the acquaintance through my physical world experiences. I could see that my energy was my unique signal for my energetic parts, and they were pulling me through the abyss just as I was pulling them to me. My parts were traveling to the singular point where they would come together as one and in balance with one another. The more I attracted the parts of self, I felt I was also attracting you. The more I pulled myself in, the closer your love became and the deeper I felt your love in my heart. I knew my energetic, romantic, sensual, soulful love would in time be manifested into my physical experience of love. My spiritual senses were bringing me to you.

37

Fueling My Passionate Heart

 It was unbeknownst to me that fueling my passionate heart would unlock my spiritual senses. I was still discovering my multi-dimensional self, I had not been taught about the meta-physical world, nor how to navigate it to the extent that was needed, and I was only just learning that it can only be done through the heart. All I really knew was that once I fueled my heart, and the Spirit world opened to me, it was as if I had finally stepped into the auditorium of my live concert. I still had to make my way to the stage, rehearse within and remember with pure intention, quiet the physical parts of me, and let my soul song sing, but I was there with my entire orchestra of self, ready to perform a masterful harmonic.

I knew it was my time. It was exciting, and yet incited tremendous nervousness for it was all that I ever dreamed of in life; to stand

and perform on my spiritual stage of divine purpose. The "what if's" tried to maintain their grip with each step I took down the aisle.

The slow and wobbly walk to my stage was an almost five-year process that unearthed that my heart did not believe all that my mind had convinced it were true. Each step shattered the fragile egoic discrepancies around my heart as my soul walked proudly towards the stage. It was a process that exposed that I trusted in the metaphysical world more than I trusted anything or anyone in the physical world, including myself. I even viewed science as a manmade interpretation of the truths yet to be discovered.

It was a walk that revealed I was discovering my own interpretation, an expression of my divine purpose, as each ideal of the world was left in my wake. This required me to reassess all that I had mentally believed in, and shamefully admit I was a walking contradiction to the stories my mind had told my heart. To balance the shame, I held gratitude that my sound mind had the fortitude to get me to the here and now, the time to finally surrender and let my soul sing.

I prayed deeply that I would one day feel whole again however never truly remembered the sensation as a gauge. A known fear was that I would feel the way I felt for the remainder of my life. I was not accepting of that fearful notion as a truth and trusted that I was being led through the choices that would lead me to embody wholeness. I was so determined that I knew I would either arrive, or perish on the journey to do so.

I wanted my heart to feel like I believed in its ability to find truth. I wanted to fuel my heart with the strength needed to put my mind at ease, like I was able to do during the trauma of my youth. I wanted my heart to know that it had been leading me through the very experiences and that its love was growing me into being. I wanted my heart to feel a fully integrated life. It felt like I was living experiences that I had to walk through, navigate the awareness of what they meant, what the experience was like, and even more so what that walk felt like. My heart is what drove every expression of self, especially once I invited my soul and my love to calibrate into a sensual dance to the song of my soul.

My heart has always wanted to share the most glorious, energetic soulful love with another. I honored the kinds of love that entered into my experiences, growing me into, and alongside the versions of love that felt healing and rewarding. It was always bittersweet when the time came for a temporary physical love to end because my heart continued to evolve towards its dream, and the relationships did not. Even when married and believed it was for a lifetime, I trusted that the most glorious version of our love was awaiting our arrival together. Expressing my sensual, passionate love has always lived within the depths of my heart, yet concurrently the opposing experiences were teaching me that the love my heart dreamed of was unrealistic, and that I was unworthy of such pure love.

It was the absence of feeling connected to my partner that made me assess the truths held deep within my heart. Just as my soul guided me to journey with him, I trusted that if my soul's destined love was within our marriage, and with whom I had raised a family, then it would present itself clearly. It would present itself in ways that it had not over too many years prior. It was the messages I received through my spiritual senses that exposed the truths of my heart that I had to accept or decline as I was presented with choosing who I wanted to become.

Once I allowed the dream of soulful love to return, and not bound by the life created around my heart, I was able to grow into my worthiness, thereby willing to explore the depths of love I yearned to feel. With the dream of the most amazing love, I remained open to whomever and whatever it was that would grow me in love. It was not until after many months of experiences that I was subtly reminded by Spirit that I had requested for an all in one. I was reminded that my tired and weary humanness was adamant in my fragile request that these would be the life experiences that would connect me to your heart for eternity. I deeply believed that the soulful and energetic connection would be the indicator of knowing. I believed that I would attract the perfect match to my energy. The ying to my yang; the unexpressed parts of my spiritual DNA brought forth to enjoy through the expression of our physical DNA. I held hope in your love which made it easy to honor the dream of soulful love to return into my experience. In doing so, I trusted that I would receive the love that was meant solely for me. I knew my heart would know love. I knew my heart would know you.

As I deconstructed the beautiful life in between I sat with the spaces empty of love and joy. I knew I had married a soul mate. I knew that truth the first time I saw him across the bar in the moment of those times. I had to consciously reflect on the truth that I had received the message from a voice within that governed our connection. Once I accepted that it was part of the journey of love, I also accepted the commitment to follow the guiding voice within, no matter what followed without. I knew that if I was to engage in anything closer than across the room, then I would follow wherever the journey led me. It was an unexpected notion to find myself contemplating such a declaration of love that had never occurred towards another person, and one I had never met in person. Perhaps within self for the attainment of objects and experiences, but never for a love with another person.

The minute I chose to engage, my heart was at peace for the journey. My mind on the other hand had a mind of its own. There were times that I recall reflecting throughout our five-year courtship that the physical expressions and experiences were not always necessarily what I had envisioned they would turn out to be, yet concurrently everything about the connection felt soulfully right and I was reminded that I was where I was supposed to be. I consciously chose to honor those feelings within, and it proved to be a beautiful, mystical life.

Along the way I noticed that my life continued to be unexplainable and magical as I grew through love and surrounded myself with the tools to heal the still beknown scattered parts. I journeyed through a marriage of love as we grew balanced into a family as our inner healing fueled the love for our children. We did so collectively until it felt lopsided. It felt as though the energy that my healing was generating was being absorbed by his stagnation. I knew he was on his own journey, as was I, which was a beautiful thing until his energy began impacting mine. I felt it energetically long before it manifested into the physical truths of our connection. I had very few words to describe what I was experiencing within the dance with his love, especially when met with the seemingly fearful, irrational, and angry energy that kept proving to be a shield to protect the loving and wounded light within. I wondered if that too was just another projection of self. Over time his love felt like compassionate narcissism; a strange expression of the dichotomies of the heart on display within my experiences not realizing how my heart was being manipulated in the name of love.

In time, circumstances encouraged me to honor the truth within the depths of my heart that there was an even greater love yet to be discovered. An unbinding love. An unencumbered love. A love that grows with my autonomy. Accompanying this truth was that it was not with the soul mate I had married. The time was clearly before me to allow the evolution of self in order to receive what my heart desired. Since I knew I married a soul mate, I had to tilt my perspectives to find the storyline of growth into a love that was even greater. Just the fact that it was the next transitional space of my journey, I knew it had to exist even if I could not imagine it. All I could muster in my extremely limited mind was that there was an ever greater love than what I had humanly labeled as a soul mate, which to me at the time, was the most kindred spirited connection.

I knew your love was far more purposeful than just serving as a kindred spirit. It felt like my soul was preparing for Heiros Gamos, the marriage of souls, albeit that meant it was within another dimension. In my humanness, it was the love of the Highest Order, in my spiritual eternal truth it was the merger of energetic bodies that would then manifest into a reality of love. It was unclear where it would manifest within the multiverse, but I knew I would experience it in this life. A marriage of souls by divine design and not by any human generated illusion. I also did not yet fully understand my powerful being. Although I could see and hear it unfolding clearly within, I was somehow still timidly trapped by my humanness without words and no means of expression.

While remaining committed to creating and allowing space to reflect and integrate only thoughts and sentiments that serve a life of alignment, my heart needed to uncover what aspects were not in alignment with my soul. This was one of the hardest aspects of self-healing that was endured, primarily because the logical mind did not always understand the sentiments of the heart. I had to recognize that my sentiments were no longer sourced in my heart and instead had become fragmented within in my mind. I had to accept the life walk that moved me out of my heart and into my mind to be driven by survival, protection, and security; a thriving love between hearts now jaded and manipulated with no space to thrive.

With some of these reflections, I noticed the direction of my love felt wrong; airy, and porous. When I felt my love, it felt like it was flowing into me, as if some cracks and crevices were never fully penetrated as love journeyed to the center of my heart, in some spaces not even reaching my center. It felt like my love was on the outside flowing inward. I left the center of my heart feeling isolated and hidden. I believed deeply that my source love should flow out of me and not into me. I knew love needed to do both, but my self-sustaining love needed to come from within myself. I knew I had to figure out a way to change the direction of my love and have it sourced within the center of my heart and radiate outward.

I believed that if I could flip the direction of love and have love radiate from within, then every space of my heart would encapsulate the purity of love before I emitted my energy into the world. Changing the direction of my love would leave my heart radiating a love sourced deep within; a pure and sweet unconditional love. That seemed much more enjoyable and pleasurable to experience. In order to change the directionality of my love, I found myself navigating to the space of what I have always known to hold in the depths of my heart, passionate love.

Even though I knew, acted, and created a life sourced in the truth that happiness comes from within, these reflections left me with the sense that I was somehow still relying on my external world to validate my sense of self-love. I recognized that awareness within me and was unwilling to accept that as part of who I was choosing to become. My mind was wiser than that, my soul knew the truths within, and my body was indicating it needed me to love it more. My heart pleaded with me to resolve its conflicts so my parts could live in freedom and ease, with love and the experiences of joy, and comfortably to enjoy this body.

It was discouraging to discover that in the background of life I had silently transitioned into living mindful love and not soulful love. It became abundantly clear that this was the source of the overall misalignment within my heart yet wondered why my path of love would lead me to such a place. Deep down I knew it was all linked and by design. I often chuckled when I uncovered the ways in which I had to learn lessons in life. I found myself having to forgive myself for the same life walk that once was whole, now broken similar to me. Even though it felt like the life walk had broken me again,

I concurrently celebrated that my soul song was approaching its release and was thereby creating space in my life. Knowing it was all a projection from within, it did not take long to identify that I needed to align with my heart so that my soul could manifest into my reality. It felt as though aligning to the reality within would organically align my physical reality. In my version, intimately sharing the ease of love with another, and with a heart full of eternal love was the outcome.

As my mind took its freeing journey through the matrix, it felt as though the two independent strands, my heart and soul, had bonded to form the unified energetic DNA double helix of my spirituality, fueled by the DNA double helix of my physicality: body and mind. My physical being was fueling the alchemy of my spiritual being, which would then require physical surrenderance so that my spiritual being could flow freely back through my physical being and live in my spiritual being's pure physical expression. These sentiments were linked to the direction of my flowing love and the need to source it from within. I could feel my body transform as I set intentions to align in reverence of spirituality and sentiments, further bonded by truths; my truths; our truths; the truths of the human collective; the truths in universal energy, God consciousness, and this miraculous world within which we exist.

I recall uncovering these truths within, and the peace that followed when I embraced the fear and doubt about certain aspects of my life and self. I also accepted them as part of the human experience as cognitive thinking beings. What I was slightly surprised by, yet completely accepting of the absolute truth, was the unbeknown clutch I allowed them to hold on my heart and soul. It was not until the release was felt that the degree of the grasp was experienced.

I had spent about five years reflecting on the journey of my heart in the background of life before starting to write and unearth my love. I spent many soulful hours assessing the truths within me as it related to the love for self and that to be shared with another in this life experience. It was the greatest desire of my soulful heart. It felt like I had experienced tremendous mysteries and miracles, and had so many amazing things in this life, yet love was still incomplete and unfinished within me. It was the one absolute I have always deeply known I would do in this life. It has always felt as if all I am intended to do in this life is love one uniquely beautiful, and divinely delivered soul designed only for me; for me to love wholly in the intimate truthfulness and vulnerabilities of who I am. This became the beginning of my secret love affair. A love affair with the universe. A love affair with you. I allowed myself to sensually experience such a glorious love with the fullness of my being in the silent space within. My heart felt free once I allowed myself to love you the way I dreamed you loved me.

Once the love affair began, I allowed the life experiences that were created within the partnership to lead me through the spaces of my soulful love. I allowed myself to dream of the most glorious love, while aware that I was living out a very different version of love with another. I was able to recognize when my mind was dreaming of love versus present in the relationship before me. I became aware of the limitations being placed on my love that I then deflected back out into the ethers of my faith.

It often felt when I would direct my love energy towards the relationship it was met with all things but openness and shared sentiments. I witnessed my love being blocked by fear and limiting beliefs; within myself and by my partner. I found that love was most often found disguised in the mishaps of the physical experiences whether rooted in keeping up a home, raising young children, financial stresses, or any of the myriad of life experiences that became the grout sealing fear within and around our hearts. I found that my heart compass had become tarnished with hurt, sadness and shame and no longer pointed to love in every direction.

The truth was that there was no honor. There was no vulnerability. There was no intimacy. The truth was that the love of my experience was not sourced in spirituality. It was not sourced in the energetic essence of who we are in this life experience. It was not sourced in the purest and sweetest taste of unconditional love. This was the soulful love I dreamed of experiencing. A love that transcends the physical body and defies time and space. A love that holds the energetic affinity that connects all creation.

My lingering essence of spiritual betrayal left me framing such a love in a much different way than a spiritual love. It felt like it could not expand within a framework. I was solely relying on my heart to feel my way through the journey. As I felt my way through my heart, it felt like a longing for a part of me once whole. My mind rationalized the feeling with the physical experiences and the parts of self lost and let go of along the way, acknowledging the truth in that wholeness is achieved within. My heart felt a yearning for unity with a part of me within the universe while overshadowed by the mindful considerations to the teaching of being human. My heart pulled towards a love that felt was infinite and intended uniquely for me as my mind intervened with convincing tones of others that I would never be worthy of such beauty. My heart knew otherwise by remembering the mystical perfection even embedded in my trauma and trusted that it would be equally present in the experience of love.

I was often amazed that even I could look at my experiences with trauma and still believed that the life journey has been perfect for me. These were sentiments that emphasized the grandeur presence of a force outside of me yet simultaneously knowing it was from within me. Silently, it remained a beautiful truth within every aspect of my multi-dimensional being which provided a deep sense of peace and tranquility throughout the process. It was a truth within me that felt like it was up against every opposing sentiment of the world around me. I was constantly left in a state of curious wonder as too how extreme trauma was an integral part of what made my life so magically perfect. Even in the moments when life did not appear to be perfect, there was still perfection in the chaos.

I felt fortunate to feel the infinite capacity of universal love burning within the confines of my chest, and sensed I had an abundant capacity to love, and to be loved. I walked the walk of my life with my heart in my hands as I felt my way through every step I ever took. Even when unstable and not sure footed. I held the faith that my soul would be matched with another that dreamed the same dream. Someone who dreamed the same passionate dream in the depths of their soul. My love affair with the universe assured me that it would be with a soul that had achieved the same existence of spiritual soul and physical body alchemy, enjoying the spiritual harmony within the physical experience. A beautifully balanced being similar to the balanced being I wanted to become. The balanced being I had already envisioned and knew deeply that I was on my way to achieve.

Within the sacred space created within and around me, I began to experience the bliss of my intentions to anchor the Heavens to the Earth. I deeply believed that we all have the capacity to become a Spiritual Warrior Poet representing the Heavens to the Earth, and of the Earth to the Heavens. I already felt like a Physical Warrior Poet, and it felt like balance would be gained by achieving the same spiritually. I believed if anyone could do it, I could. It had everything to do with me, and it felt critical to let my heart lead the way. I knew my heart would lead me to the most amazing love this universe has to offer. If it was contingent on my beliefs, then I knew it would be amazing. It would encompass all the beauty and magnificence that I dreamed it was meant to be. Plus some.

This is when my fondness for science, primarily Biology and Chemistry, influenced the molecular breakdown of my love. My deeply buried passion was found smoldering with just enough heat to stir up the chemistry in my love affair. The time had come to compile the elements needed for my soulful love. I started with the elements that I knew must be integrated into my love as part of who I am. I knew that if I would be blessed to experience such a glorious love, it would be with someone that was capable and willing to receive the authentic love I had to offer. Keeping in harmony, I held the opposing honor in that I had to be capable and willing to receive the authentic love from another.

In time and through life experiences, I casted my dreams of love into the cosmos and held the belief that I was attracting this glorious love unto me. In honor and respect to my partnership, I also reflected and believed that if this glorious love resided within our relationship, then the indicators would be there. I already knew how to spot them and continued to let my heart lead the way.

I was aware that I felt our relationship was lacking, and I also knew that I had allowed experiences to create that sentiment. I identified my desires and tried to incorporate them into the reality of my partnership. It became the foundation upon which I uncovered my heart. As I continued to act out the desires of my heart, I was presented with clear opportunities of why I needed to choose differently.

> I wanted to be authentic and vulnerable in honor of our existence...

>> ...empathize with the human condition and hold compassion for hurting hearts...

>>> ...help heal when I am graced with the privilege and opportunity to do so.

I was advised to mind my own business.

I wanted to celebrate the good in this world and remain positive in my spirit...

...believe in the good and act in kindness towards others...

...be of service with kindness and compassion, and to love with the purest of intentions.

I was reminded of the negatives, and the imposing limiting beliefs.

I wanted to integrate the energetic affinity of my essence...

...experience the heat of the kundalini energy as it harmonizes throughout my being...

...let the passion of love energy lead the way into the moments of alchemy with another.

I was deemed an unrealistic dreamer.

I wanted to share the love that moves my soul...

    ...a spiritual love that transcends the physical body...

        ...an easy love that suspends in the tranquility of time and space.

I was accused of wanting to live a life in the "honeymoon phase" of a relationship.

I wanted to share my sensual love...

    ...a love that engages all the senses and is fueled by the energetic soul song...

        ...the sentience of energetic harmony translated into passionate expressions in action.

I was encouraged that sex would stimulate desires and incite emotions.

I knew I had to make a decision. I was either going to accept, or not accept the dreams of my heart. If I was willing to accept the dreams of my heart, that meant that I would also need to be prepared to navigate all that I would be led through to get to where it would lead me. I had to decide if I was willing to accept any impending consequence of any decision I would have to make. I had to determine if I was going to fight for my heart, or for that of those around me. Deciphering the priority was the easy part; following through would require the focus and faith.

Molding life experiences through intentions is a skill that thrives on discernment and faith, but not so much so that the lessons in the journey are missed. The ebbs and flows of life will undoubtedly impact the journey, but it is within our reactions that the path before us is forged. If we become so focused on the outcome of our intentions and desires, we jade the authentic unfolding and the discovery along the way. I knew the journey of my heart would be no different. I knew I had to hold the intention and then enjoy the unfolding yet remain flexible enough to be nimble in the dance of love. My love was also naïve and childish and would have to grow in its strength.

Although I could feel love energy burning within, I felt disconnected from love and I believed that integrating myself back into oneness would heal the disconnect and restore deep, soulful love throughout my existence. It was all I had to anchor my heart. It was the risk I was willing to take for love. Love has always been the one constant that I have passionately believed in and dreamed of even in the face of everything within self and the world around me. I have always believed that love always win, and up to this point I had not been proven wrong, so I grounded myself in that truth. Love *always* wins.

As I honored the elements I wanted to integrate into my love, and those of the experience of love that I was living, I found that my spirituality was fueling my passionate heart. Still uncertain of so many things, in both my spiritual and physical worlds, I began exploring how to ground the spiritual senses of my heart so it could join forces with the physical experience to bring about the greatest joys of all.

To do so, I began caressing love in the purity of my healing white light. I began welcoming love to settle peacefully within my being. I surrendered my heart to my soulful essence, and I surrendered my soul to my passionate love. I let my heart and soul guide the way, and in a way that I had never allowed before.

Through the experiences, I learned where it really matters most. For me, it matters most in my heart. It really matters to feel the energetic and soulful connection. It really matters to honor one another with words and actions. It really matters to be co-creators sourced in unconditional love. Everything else, the possessions, the money, even experiences, if they are not sourced in honor and unconditional love, they become noise to my senses, blocking my energy; blocking the magic of the universe; blocking my love. Sorting through the details that led me to the realization about my heart was not nearly as important as owning and honoring my heart, and the depths it was craving to explore. It is my heart that matters most.

Putting my heart back in the forefront of my mission forced me to assess why my heart felt so empty and dark when my reality was seemingly surrounded by and filled with so much love. I even wrote to a long-time connection early on in the process and expressed that perhaps the journey was about tearing down the walls within. The experiences led me through the processes to learn that exact lesson;

and to tear down the walls within. I realized that the path leading to the infinite capacity of love that my heart is capable of holding, and the depths of passionate desires, may only be found through the journey to authentic self-love. The energetic love with another would be the reward for the depths of self-healing. Somehow, I knew that.

Initially, not even fully aware of the scope of growth underway, I knew I had to focus, yet I did not even know what I needed to focus on. Since I believed in the Law of Attraction, I focused on what I knew I wanted. And it was simple. I wanted my heart to swell with love and joy. Feelings that I had not felt in my core in a very long time. I was indifferent as to what would bring about those feelings for me, I just knew I wanted to experience them again. And deeply.

As I continued to meditate on having a love and joy filled heart, I had the most amazing experience one evening. It was an experience that connected my heart to the universe. It was an experience that provided an example of the physical manifestations that are possible from a simple intention. It was an experience that took months to process and integrate into my reality. Although I had experienced the power of the mind and manifestations, this one was different, the first of its kind and the first in a seemingly endless flow of whimsical and mystical manifestations. It was a glimpse into the fascinating world within now on display in my reality.

I had been meditating for years, so it is relatively easy to get into a deep, relaxed state fairly quickly. Even so, this time was different. There had been an interesting inner change occurring in the more recent practices. The sentience of the experiences had been heightened tremendously, as if to ensure I embraced the moment to the fullest to prevent my rational mind the opportunity to refute the possibilities of truth. This was also during the onset of heightened sensitivity to vibrational energy, and there was plenty of energy shifting internally and externally. Among many things, the self-growth brought about a beautiful, peaceful, and authentic honesty about every aspect of my being and existence.

My partner had accepted my journey albeit not always a beautiful and peaceful experience for him. Even in the moments when we were discussing the potential greater growth for both of us if we were to continue to evolve on our separate paths. Beautiful, loving, honest and hard conversations. In the depths of these conversations, we paused for a short break, during which I took a moment to meditate.

It was dark outside, the stars and moon were shining bright, and nature's creatures were signing in the dark. I was sitting in a chair, so I made sure that both feet were positioned firmly on the ground in an effort to ground and absorb as much energy as possible. While relaxed in the chair and eyes closed, with every breath I made the request to open my heart to love. Mainly self-love since it was I that was being drawn away from everything that used to make sense.

After a few deep breaths a strong visual appeared that transcended dimensions and connected with my physical being. It was a tunnel connecting my heart to the heart of the universe within and beyond the moon lit sky. Not only could I see it in my mind's eye, but I could also feel the connection on the outside of my chest. My heart was pulsing with every breath, and with every breath, my heart was connected to the tunnel, and the heart of the universe. Our hearts were beating in sync; as one. I could feel the heart of the universe in my chest, and I could feel that I was present in the heart of the universe. With each beat of my heart, the knowing and feeling of that truth intensified. It lasted for three deep breaths, and the oneness amplified with every pulse. My heart felt the most infinite openness. It was intense, beautiful, and short lived, but I knew that my heart was forever altered by the experience.

It was the first time that I had ever felt so infinitely and intimately connected to universal love. I knew and felt deeply that I would forever live from within the heart of the Universe throughout each day forward, and that I would forever hold the heart of the Universe within mine. The experience opened me to the sentience of infinite love, which in turn made me even more determined to continue on the path in order to sustain it. For in those brief moments, I learned what the experience of infinite love truly felt like and deeply wanted it to last for longer than three breaths. Simultaneously, I somehow knew that the path was only through authentic self-love, something I had yet to uncover that I did not truly hold.

During more cycles of looping thoughts, deconstruction of egoic constructs, and trying to rediscover me, buried under all the labels and expectations, I found something unexpected. I found that everything I had been taught and experienced thus far were only illusions of love. It exposed how love had been treated and taught to me that it is something to earn and can be withheld or used in some way. It felt like my love was busting through the very misuse and abuse of love and around love that painfully shackle the hearts of so many people around the world. The silent love that lives unexpressed within the roots of our heart's tree of life with branches that give us breath. I was saddened for love. I was drawn deeper in love with love, and when I found my love, it just exists. When I was able to finally see my love, it was just there, being love, waiting to be seen, shared, experienced, touched, smelt, enjoyed, and honored for its purity of source, and innocence of expression. Fueling my passionate heart made it easy to work towards the fullness of authentic self-love. With every breath of love I took for self, every cell of my body began to feel the truths in love.

38

Authentic Self-Love

Our physical bodies, primarily our minds, are designed to protect us. Furthermore, society often provides constructs to guide our logical, thinking minds through attempts to understand the world around us. So much so, that when a person undergoes self-reflection and what it means to live a purposeful life, a societal perspective has molded and labeled the process as a mid-life crisis. It was even suggested during moments when I was still trying to learn how to express the inner world I was experiencing, that I myself was experiencing such a crisis, or being tempted by the proverbial greener grass on the other side of the fence. The point in one's life when this pivotal moment occurs is generally at the perceived mid-point in one's life. Perhaps it is the timing, depth of reflection, the fragility of the egoic constructs, and the strength of spirit that determines the degree to which the process is deemed a crisis by self and society. The tremendous growth surely never felt like a crisis within.

Other depictions encompass how we spend the first part of our lives learning an education, then the focus becomes getting a job, earning an income, buying a home, getting married, having children, supporting a family in every aspect, and then what? Once those things are achieved, what comes next? This moment usually falls at the halfway point, at mid-life, providing a pause to recalibrate and realign with life's intention. A half-time break during the game of life to connect with Self to review the self and societal imposed expectations and belief systems, evaluate if the constructs we hold continue to serve who and what we want to be in this world, while remaining true to inner desires and passions. This resonated more with the growth I was experiencing. The graceful recognition, embrace and change in the areas of my reality that no longer resonated with my life's intention. This process felt right.

I knew for several years that I was in a state of misalignment. However, during those times I was unaware of the true essence of what misalignment meant, nor the impacts of such imbalances. All I knew is that I felt it. Later it was revealed that I was also perpetually fueling the imbalance. I was aware of some of the contributing factors, and I was also aware that changes need to take place. But the process began exposing the core causes of the imbalance, revealing all the contributing factors to be merely symptoms of the systemic disconnect. This caused an even greater desire to embrace the growth and change like I always do, head on, with optimism and faith. The blessing to be discovered was the truth in that the elements that caused the misalignment were the very elements that propelled me into the unexpected gift of soulful transformational healing and beautiful love. Just as with everything in my life experience, I would not be here experiencing the glory of today, without each step and breath of yesterday.

On the outside, life was seemingly perfect. I was married and together we were raising three handsome, healthy boys in a loving home, our jobs were secure, and life was good. It was the picture-perfect family that many dream of having. However, there is tremendous truth in that the world knows not what happens behind closed doors, the doors of a home and the doors of the heart. Life was good but it was not great. It was not great where it mattered most, within my heart.

There was a sense of knowing early on that the journey would commence the reunification of my Inner and Physical Spirits. The blessings were in the unimaginable depths and magnitude of growth that the inner wisdom had graced upon my life. It was the sentience of the experiences that provoked continued trust in the walk, which in time, divinely led me to the destination of my greatest dreams. The truths of my love.

I had spent nine months living out a broken physical reality between home and work life as I focused on deconstructing my worlds. There was a message broadcasted within everything stating that there was only one world within versus the multiple versions I had created in my reality. I was one person at home, a different version at work, and yet another version amongst family and friends. The version of me that showed up when alone with myself was rarely given space for authentic expression.

I thought that was how we all were as humans, all trying to figure this out. One of the greatest pains in my life was knowing that healing the spiritual space would manifest healing in the physical yet never knowing how to connect to Spirit. I could see it and could imagine it in every way while concurrently aware that each growing breath was needed before I would be able to do so. This is where the lesson of patience was practiced most. Until I was able to sustain breath, the physical world experiences played out to teach me and guide the way. This was no different, and I felt as ready as I had ever been when navigating through necessary experiences. Especially the ones that left me befuddled.

In October 2017, I had decided last minute to go on to a conference in Washington D.C.. It was one that I had intentionally negated in prior years yet this time I was being drawn to go for reasons outside of work. Nothing in particular other than a hunch that I needed to go. I took it as an opportunity to see the Nation's Capital. The first night of our arrival, our group arrived at the restaurant, secured the large round table being held for us and we all found a seat, reserving one space for a mystery guest that would soon be joining: a long-time friend and professional colleague of a group member.

The reserved space was directly across from me at the round table and within fifteen minutes after being seated she arrived, wisping in with her rolling suitcase in tote. Before taking her seat, she walked as far around the table as she could, greeting and acquainting themselves with everyone, one at a time. I was the last one she could reach before being blocked by an artificial tree in the corner. I remember feeling honored by the personal greeting and grateful that the corner tree did not interfere with the connection and shake of the hands. She returned to the reserved space and finished the introductions while seated, meanwhile, I was sidetracked with the sensations buzzing through my being from her touch. I felt a transference.

There was something about this individual that captivated my attention. She was whimsical yet demonstrated an unyielding virtue of strength. She was wise, yet there remained tremendous compassion in every word spoken. The restaurant was dark with softened lights, but the room seemed bright in her presence. I sat quietly, watched, and listened as she spoke and engaged those around the table. I was completely intrigued. I knew there was something about this sacred soul, I just couldn't quite figure it out. So, I embraced and enjoyed the moments. Or at least tried my best, since there was also a medical episode with an active bleed that was being monitored in silence.

After a while, she asked everyone at the table, "Have you ever been to the center of the universe?" Naturally that was enough to be curious to hear what would follow, especially given my journey thus far leading to the space of universal awareness, infinite love, and vibrational energy. As she continued to speak, she interjected a self-acknowledged transition from spiritual strength to universal intentions when speaking in terms of Einstein.

Universal intentions? And Einstein? Did she really just say both of those, in the same sentence? Speaking in terms of universal intentions is central to my authentic self, and I had just spent months living and analyzing the in-depth exploration and the energetic connectedness to all things past, present, and future, which cultivated a much more believable and realistic concept than that of time itself. All of which had been nicely rounded out with a surprise copy of Einstein's Dreams, mailed to my home by a fellow soul sister about three months prior. Please, carry on. She had my full attention. The universe was clearly speaking, and I was most definitely listening.

For what felt like minutes, that was all my mind could think about, and concurrently I was fearful that my thoughts would cause me to miss what could possibly come next. In the actual seconds of disbelief, my mind quickly accessed all Einstein and universal records I had uncovered, created, and stored in my mind along my life walk.

It was time to pull them out, review what I had acquired and then live the physical manifestation. The interesting thing is that there was still a sense of soulful disconnect which prevented me from embracing the magnificence of it all in that moment. It was all still just an amazing wonder and not yet truth. It wasn't until days, even weeks after I had returned home from the trip that the miracles began to unfold; a forty-month journey of unfolding, discovering, and integrating until I could finally hold the extraordinary truths that had been for ever present and now again on grand display.

She proceeded to describe the large bronze statue of Einstein and the accompanying celestial grid etched in the ground before him. It was stated that if you stand in the center of the celestial grid, which is representative of the center of the universe, and speak your intentions to the universe, your intentions will be repeated back to you just as clearly as you state them.

That sealed the deal for me. She had my attention with universal intentions and Einstein, then to proclaim that there was a space in the physical that represented the very foundation and demonstrated the very essence upon which I had based my journey? Universal intentions, the Law of Attraction, energetic affinity of all things and encapsulated within the iconic representation of energy itself? If I claim my universal intentions, they will come back to me? The energy I put out into the universe, I will receive? I knew and believed this to be true, but a representation of these concepts in the physical? I knew the universe was aligning me with the truths within.

As soon as she finished stating that they always take people at midnight whenever they are in town, I quickly asked if she would take us there. I knew I needed to go. I also noticed that perhaps I should temper my excitement or justify it to the table. I expressed that I was working on a project and had just read Einstein's Dreams, and that the talk of Einstein and universal intentions was profoundly resonating with me and my project. I also expressed that it did not have to be at midnight, and perhaps we could go after dinner. I also acknowledged that maybe not everyone would equally enjoy the visit to Einstein so I could get the address and go alone. After indicating that I would like to go even if they did not, it turned out that almost everyone had been to D.C. before many times and had never heard of, nor visited the Einstein statue. Everyone voted for a visit to Einstein without ever knowing the depths of my soulful mission. Collectively it was decided we would catch Ubers and head to Einstein as a group after dinner.

The moments after it was decided we would go, while finishing dinner, I felt my mind searching for the intentions that I needed to speak to the universe. As if it were the big moment of opportunity and I didn't want to mess it up. I could see my mind thumbing through the rolodex of fears, false beliefs, and constraints; the passions, desires and needs. I had to prevent my mind from becoming desperate for the right selection.

Instead, I somehow was able to quiet the mind, block out the noise and knew that I would know the intentions to speak when the time came. I definitely did not want to miss a moment around the table due to an overactive mind. More than any other moment in my life, the universe was pulling my sight from inward reflection toward outward enjoyment. I finished my meal while quietly rejoicing in worldly mysticism and grateful that I was being drawn into the world in a new and exciting way.

Dinner ended, the Ubers were called, and we stood on the corner in the D.C. night life. We were waiting on the curb talking, and the consultant commented on the interesting connection between my project, Einstein and their mystery guest friend all coming together over dinner. Without delay, my response was that it was no surprise as all aspects were part of my universal intention. In the moment of speaking my truth, I acknowledged that with my truth there was a lack in knowing anything about what accompanied the statement. I embraced that I was on the universal ride in a state of fascination and deeply wanted to trust the authentic voice of my soul.

In the moment of speaking my truth, my statement was acknowledged for the truth that it was, and I received the warmest, most endearing hug from the mystery guest. It was not a quick, thoughtful hug, it was a heart-felt embrace, as if taking the moment to deeply honor the truth of the statement. And while I was honoring them and the truth in the statement, it was only in hindsight that I was able to see that they were much more in-tune and in alignment with what was unfolding than I was in that soulful moment.

With the odd number count amongst us, we had to split up into three cars. Again, in my favor, I was blessed with a joint ride with the intriguing guest. Just her and I, headed to Einstein to speak universal intentions. Within the fifteen-minute ride, the synchronicities of their presence continued to unfold. Unexplainable and yet completely believable as most were sourced in the presence of my Mom; just as her butterfly presence graced the walk to the restaurant. She had studied in Bruges, which is a city near where I grew up overseas and was my Mom's favorite city in the country. She randomly spoke the words, "...something bones" when we were speaking of my "project" that I then had to disclose was a book about a traumatic medical experience with a title that included the word bones. They offered kindness, support, and love during the ride, and although I was equally as kind and loving, my mind was in a state of bewilderment. All the while my soul joyously played along with the divinely timed encounter. Hand in hand my physical and inner spirits tried to integrate every moment while riding through the universe to get to its center before Einstein.

We arrived at the magnificent Einstein statue, representing strength, wisdom, and infinite possibilities. It mimicked the same strength and wisdom I saw in the mysterious being, and the same strength and wisdom felt while admiring the architecture around the Nation's Capital. Everything about the experiences of the trip were so perfectly timed, soulfully glorious, and physically joyful.

While navigating through this very unfamiliar, yet peaceful spiritual self-exploration, I had trusted in my divine inner power and strength to be a co-creator in this universe. In doing so, over the months I had repeatedly set the universal intention to open my heart to strength, courage, and love. Every situation I had ever encountered required me to draw upon at least one of these within. As it related to the current moments of my life, the source intention was the same coupled with the circumstances of the present.

> **Strength** to complete the book and be vulnerable to the world...

>> ...**Courage** to trust my inner wisdom as I realign all aspects of my being no matter how challenging the path may be...

>>> ...and to embrace every aspect of my being in the light of authentic **Love**.

When it was my turn, these were the very intentions I repeated in front of Einstein. **Strength, Courage** and **Love**. In the majestic echo of the universe, I heard my very intentions returned back to me. The words strength, courage and love were amplified and projected unto me, as if to demonstrate that I would receive those very intentions through the universal Law of Attraction. I would receive strength, courage, and love, amplified, precise and in the direction of me. Time stood still as I stood before Einstein. A poetic moment as it was defied in his presence.

Once everyone was ready, we posed for a group picture, said our goodbyes, and went our separate ways for the night. The nine of us were spread across three hotels, two cities, and two Federal Districts, D.C., and Maryland. The next day was the actual conference that brought us all to D.C. in the first place. The conference turned out to be ridden with political constraints and apprehensions which prevented an effective engagement, so most of the time was spent reviewing work related matters as the conference played out in the background.

From time to time I would look around to see if I could spot the mysterious and whimsical guest from the prior night, but only seeing her across the room briefly at lunch, and then towards the close of the conference. It was not until the conference was over and while everyone was exiting, gathering, and discussing business points that we reconnected.

I had walked across the back of the auditorium to see if I could spot her, and to no avail I returned to my colleagues. Moments later I spotted her doing the same thing, walking across the back of the auditorium as if looking for someone. Just as I turned and looked to my side, there she was, standing beside me on the outskirts of our small group. I recall pausing in disbelief because I had just seen her moments ago off in the distance, then suddenly her presence was before me. Her whimsical essence overcame me once again as it did when she floated into the restaurant.

When I saw her, I took the opportunity to express my appreciation for her and the gratitude for taking us to the amazing Einstein. As I went to hug her, she reciprocated in kind while speaking the words, "there you are," and encouraged me to stay in touch. My first thought was that surely, she was not looking for me when I noticed her moments ago. This is when I recognized that with that thought alone, I was fueling the lack of authentic self-love. I already knew at a deeper level that the connection was greater than me, sincere and very genuine. I found I wanted to quickly let go of any apposing thought and to heartfully accept the sentiment, yet my mind tried to taint the experience. I believed that it would not have been spoken if it were not truth since that is the level of genuine honesty I command of myself.

We all left the conference and four of us prepared for a night of D.C. sightseeing. We returned to the hotel to freshen up and then hit the streets. We walked, took public transportation, and explored the beautiful sights in the night lights for five hours. Five hours! I cannot even remember a time that I have walked for five hours since my illness. That is over twenty-five years of mindful, limited walking. The most amazing part was that I did so without experiencing any physical repercussions as I would have in the past, and after a considerably less time span of walking. The experience taught me a lot, yet it turned out to also be the last time that I have walked such distances and with as much ease. A memory of pure enjoyment to take with me as my legs tire from the walk.

I somehow was able to walk for five hours, with my legs and feet, with only one working muscle to control the flexing and balancing movements required to walk and did so with tremendous ease and joy. It was exhilarating. It was an unexplainable experience that gently revealed the very beliefs that were perpetually fueling my inability to do such a task over the years prior. It brought to light that what I thought was self-nurturing love was inadvertently the very cause of physical ailments. Yet another hint towards the lack of self-love.

We returned to the hotel at around 12:30am, went to bed and prepared for our departure the next morning. While falling asleep, I reflected on the trip and how everything seemed so surreal; my Mom's presence starting with the beautiful butterflies, the mysterious dinner guest, the magnificent Einstein, the synchronicities of the whole experience and the resonance with my personal growth. I welcomed to receive whatever it was that I was to gain from the experience. It was evident that there was tremendous growth embedded, and I could feel the universe was delivering something glorious to me. Even though I was not sure of what it was, I knew that hidden within there was a radiantly glowing blessing to be uncovered and enjoyed. I could sense that it would be profound. It felt bright and expansive, just as I had experienced in my meditations. Throughout the night and following day, and as I began to uncover each layer of growth, I could feel the ascension in my awareness as my own vibrational energy was rising, while the essence was simultaneously juxtaposed with the sensation of going deeper within.

Once I returned home and was back in the office, I sought out the email address of the mystery guest, tracked down the group photo with Einstein, and emailed my gratitude with reiteration of my appreciation for her presence and the experience. I also wanted to share a little more as to why it resonated so much within my life. This was when the real authentic love and beauty began to unfold. This was when I began to see the light and the lessons awaiting discovery upon my path. This was when it felt like authentic self-love had the space to expand and be seen within.

In my correspondence I had expressed that it was an honor to have met her and that words were limiting in the expression of the delightful yet unexpected resonance and timing of her presence in my life. I expressed that it was all very powerful within my own universe. She arrived at dinner, shared her strength, wisdom, and light, brought us to the amazing Einstein, and then just as quickly as she came, she was gone, spreading her wisdom and light in the world. I provided a copy of the group photo around Einstein and affirmed that it was definitely an experience I would never forget.

I went on to further express why our encounter was so meaningful. I recalled a small comment that had been made at dinner about how people fascinate her. I explained that I too am very intrigued by people, their life journey, and meaningful connections. In a very unexpected way, she was an example of why; because every once in a while, you encounter someone that really moves, touches, and inspires the soul. I kindly thanked them for being that blessing.

I did also comment that I would cherish our Uber ride together even though I was still processing the synchronicities of her being and shared some book excerpts since we had spoken of the book and her expressed support in the process. My email was short and heartfelt, with no expectation in return. I genuinely wanted to let her know how meaningful the experience was, and how much it impacted my life. I held tremendous gratitude within.

Before the day came to an end, I received a response back from my email. I was eager to read what inspiration would deliver and was rushed by evening engagements to attend my son's football game. Although slightly behind schedule, I acknowledged the choice point and chose to pause for my soul to read the email. I knew the football game would be the perfect time to reflect on the response with minimal distractions. I could watch the game while deep in my heart.

The response was totally unexpected, completely welcomed, and tremendously gracious and loving. To a certain extent, it was hard for my cognitive mind to even comprehend. As honored as I felt, and as lovely as the statements were, my mind remained curious to know why she would have felt such a way about me; someone she had just met and did not even know. All projections and evidence of the lack of a fully integrated authentic self-love.

Her kind words expressed a great desire to acknowledge my message that touched their heart and soul before the day was over. She thanked me for being brave, vulnerable, and kind. She expressed an equal appreciation for our encounter and pointed out that it was not happenstance that we were the closest to the heart of Einstein in the group photo. It was true, we were the only ones near his heart when posing by his enormous sized body of bronze.

She continued to write that everything I had expressed equally resonated with her, so much so that tears of joy and blessings filled her eyes. She expressed gratitude for touching their soul with clarity and kindness. She also thanked me for trusting and standing beside her during the Uber ride and joint walk to meet Einstein together.

It was when she wrote about the thoughts that surfaced after reading the excerpts of my book that really impacted me at the core level.

She was thankful that I had shared my writing, and although she indicated that she could think of many things to say, she discerned that nothing was more important to share than that she had met me in the light of divinity. She proceeded to tell me that I was a true light being. She graciously invited the dialog and for our newly minted, divinely orchestrated friendship to continue and ascend. It was the most unexpected and poetic email I had ever received. It seemed surreal that it was sent to me, and yet divinely perfect that it was sent to me. It was the precise thing my soul longed to hear, or that of which I was yearning to experience in order to grow deeper. Both were very plausible, and evidently very possible.

Recall the night sweats that started about three weeks into the writing process? The night I received the email was the night my sweats stopped for my first reprieve. It had been 264 nights after my soulful sweats began that came to a temporary end with the receipt of this email. In those moments I was completely amazed. I had to practice patience until understanding surfaced. When understanding was revealed, and the blessing of lessons were unearthed, I was graced with a sweating reprieve until it was time to continue on with the next phase of lessons to be learned. When the sweats started back weeks later, I knew that the sweats correlated with the soulful lessons that awaited my discovery.

At the time I did not know how or why, but I knew the exact statement that stopped my sweats. A light being? I had never heard that term before, nor understood anything about what it meant to be a light being. My mind was intrigued and knew that my soul found peace in the truth that was exposed. Even given my experiences with Spirit and visions across what only appeared to be a multiverse of dimensions, I still had to humanly process what it meant to be a light being and find how to exist within the realms. For in this brief moment, I am alive in the human experience.

This was when I started to learn that I could channel Spirit through writing. It took three days of integrating the expression and shared sentiments that allowed the space for my cognitive mind to catch up to my soul; at least to a certain degree. It took almost twenty months to truly discover what that means to me in my life journey. In the moments that it was unfolding, it was as though it took three days for my mind and soul to finally join together in written expression in response. It was only through automatic soulful writing that I was able to understand that of which my soul had rediscovered three days prior.

My own soul was teaching me that through my universal intentions, this individual had been divinely delivered in a manner specific to my universe. She literally brought me to the center of my universe, and I have watched the continued magic unfold. The universe brought me strength, courage, and love through every encounter we shared. The love in her words incited emotions and thoughts within me, which resonated within the pillars of her strength and courage. Even reinforcing the lesson of authentic self-love that was still under pursuit. For it was only after deconstructing the ego that there was enough clarity to embrace the profoundness in that **we all see in others that of which we hold within.**

I trusted in what I saw in her, because I know and trust in what I hold within. Her compassionate words reflected what I saw in her essence, while concurrently mirroring the strength and divine light within myself. She was the spiritual grounding force in the physical exposing the very essence of divinity within herself; within me;

within us. For it is only once we recognize our own divinity that we are able to live in the full essence of who we are.

Not only did this individual's essence profoundly impact my life in a spiritual way by simply holding the mirror in divine time and space, but it was as though she molded the bridge between my Inner Spirit and Physical Spirit with strength, wisdom, and light. When she whispered the words "there you are" in our farewell embrace before my five-hour walking adventure, it was as if she knew she needed to infuse my Physical Spirit with the spiritual strength needed to enjoy a soul embodied physical experience. As that too had been a desire of my heart. To explore the world and not feel constrained by the limitations of my physical body. A gift reopened many times over since that day.

My spiritual fabric is woven with healing aspects from a variety of ideologies, and it was as if her soulful strength and wisdom had casted light and clarity on the blueprint of the masterpiece I was creating. Being closest to Einstein's heart was indeed not happenstance, nor is it that one light being finds another.

As I began to really embrace, I mean *really* embrace, the messages being sent to me through this being, I could feel the disconnect between my heart, mind, and soul. As if I could feel the light of my soul radiating from my heart up towards my mind and then blocked in the throat. I continued to invite the bliss of when the light would break through and my heart, soul and mind were an integrated being within my body. I could not help but to continue to honor the experiences that organically guided me through the authentic process.

The energy behind my soulful love continued to surface as a

passionate dream of my heart, which only lead to more experiences, support, and expressions that such a soulful love exists. Again, evidenced that the dreams of my heart should be honored because it is most definitely possible. I still knew deeply that it was only once self-healing and oneness was achieved. That was when I realized that I had been blessed with the very examples of strength, courage and love needed to hold the vision that was leading me to my destination, the soulful energetic love of my dreams. I could feel and see the bridge that would reunite my heart to love. I had experienced a beautiful, earthly representation of what the inner wizardry work would bring. My life was forever changed. I saw the future reflection of me in the presence of a beautifully integrated being of body, mind, heart and soul, a radiant Earth Angel. She was an Angel sent to me from the Heavens.

Early on in the process when the exploration was tremendously new and uncomfortable, I would often communicate with my Mom. In a moment of uncertainty and despair, a beautiful vibrant orange butterfly landed on the driveway beside me. It flapped its wings while sitting beside me as if in Morse code while it awaited my slow and cautious approach.

While observing in peaceful disbelief, I recalled hearing that if you touched a butterfly's wing it would kill it. I knew there was no harm in the transference of oils unto the delicate wings as I had been told and trusted that my touch would be gentle enough not to dislodge any scales on its wings needed for flight. I deeply wanted to touch a physical embodiment of my Mom and had always prayed that my love would never again harm another.

As I moved in closer, it remained still as I extended my hand and reached in to pet its vibrant colored wing. As I slowly stroked the delicate wing, I knew and felt my Mom present in that Beautiful Butterfly. I knew it was my Mom then, just as I knew she had played a part in the experiences in D.C. and starting the dance with energy. After several moments of gentle caressing and speaking from the heart, I stopped the interaction with the butterfly as I concurrently wondered how long it would have allowed the engagement. It was the poetic mystery in experiences such as these and the depth of soul in the connections that made my heart dance in joy and excitement. Butterflies remain a part of my daily experiences in some form or fashion, for my Mom is ever so present when I align with divinity.

Through the soulful transformation that brought on the quest for self-love, I felt every aspect of my being energetically realign and bring about more strength, courage, and love within myself. The very intentions casted before Einstein. Everything was full of love, and radiated love. The more experiences unfolded the more clarity was gained and I could see and feel the light of my love starting to radiate into the world around me. The more I honored the truth of love within me, the more love manifested into experiences in the world and into experiences of others.

In order to remain in a space to receive and embrace the experiences of love in the unfolding, I had to learn how to stand in my own abundant love. I had to learn how to command certain aspects of self. The first being that I would put myself before others. This did not mean that I had to become selfish, nor that I was not giving to others. What it did mean was that I had to consider all of me, my sensual body, mind, heart, and soul, before giving myself away to others. If it was not in alignment with whole body wellness than I would require myself to choose accordingly. This was the navigation to a fully integrated conscious awareness to be practiced.

I had to choose me. I had to choose all parts of me, even the parts I did not understand. I had to choose to finally embrace my hypersensitivity to the vibrational energy emitted by all things in this universe, including my own. I had to cultivate a new definition and level of honor when it comes to matters of my heart. I had to redesign the focus on my physical body with the new awareness that my focus had been sourced in the wrong energy; manifesting dis-ease. I was unknowingly self-fueling my physical ailments out of what I thought was self-love nurturing. I had allowed my mindful fears to overrule my soulful healing. I had to learn how to foster and allow my own spiritual superpowers to carry me through the remainder of this earth walk. I had to be reminded that these superpowers are within us all, and the more balanced, centered and fully integrated we become with our authentic self and our source energy, the more powerful we become as co-creators in our universe.

I believed this so deeply that the more I experienced the magic in life, the more reasons I had to surrendered and follow with all my being; with all my senses; with all my heart. I found I began living life versus just existing in the matrix. It finally felt like I was walking my own. I was unsure and sloppy footed, but it was my own.

As with all my spiritual experiences, there had been a prior physical world experience of my trauma that was of the same vibration. This one was no different as my essence was flooded with the remembrance of when I took my first steps in my recovery. The wobbly first steps that felt like the start of a walk into physical experience divergence, yet now I was taking spiritual steps to reunite my worlds, balanced between the physical world and the spiritual world.

My life's storyline was magically becoming less mystifying, and I was able to exist in truths within to my mind while concurrently gracing peace upon the depths of my soul. It was a love story with self; a love story with Source Energy; a love story with the forces greater than our beings; a love story I knew I was experiencing and was a co-creator in its existence.

As I continued to lean into experiences regardless of how uncomfortable, my heart and soul danced in the truth that what was divinely perfect in my life was also divinely perfect in the path of everyone encountered along the way. It is what maintains balance. It also applied a soulful responsibility that I have never been able to escape. I am always aware of which side of the contract I am fulfilling. These experiences where refining my ability to fulfill my responsibility when on either side - giving and receiving spiritual love.

It was as if I myself had become the Beautiful Butterfly that entered the lives of others until my presence was no longer needed as a grounding force of love. Similar to how my Mom grounded her beautiful butterfly wings while she infused me with her love before returning to flight to grace the path of another. Again, mirrored in the presence of the mysterious dinner guest that seemed to float into my experiences, align with my soul and then just as quickly off grounding the fireflies of the world. I was learning how to float and connect to Spirit so that I can live comfortably in my body and enjoy it while in love.

I trusted that in time, as evidenced in Einstein, that I would continue to experience the mystical physical reality leading me to the soulful dance of my love. As I began to fall in love with myself again, the more I fell in love with life again. The more I fell in love with life, the more interconnected I became. The more interconnected I became, the more love I manifested into my reality. The more I experienced love manifested, the more I fell in love with love itself. The more I fell in love with love, the more I felt like an energetic magnet attracting love. It was a beautiful self-perpetuating cycle of love manifesting love. Powerful and unsustainable at times until my humanness caught up.

As an interconnected being in an interconnected universe I knew that the soulful steps I was taking were the dance steps to the soul song playing within my heart. I could feel deep within that loving myself to my core was the gateway to a much greater and more glorious love than any encountered thus far in life. I bashfully hoped that Divine Love was making my acquaintance.

39

Angels Amongst Us

I received the gift of an Angel.

An Angel from the abyss manifested into my physical experience. A gift from the meta-physical space of my existence before me here on Earth. A gift from myself. A gift from the universe. A gift from God.

An Earth Angel before me.

I believe in Angels. I always have. Yet I had only ever conceptualized them in the spiritual realm, despite knowing that we are all angels of light energy here on Earth. Ever since my unexplainable survival in my teenage years, I have held a deep desire to meet and know my Angels, the Angels that have protected me along my life journey. Even though I had lived a life believing my Angels were present, I had never before met them nor felt their presence. I certainly had never met an Earth Angel, nor was I prepared to meet one. Even so, it was perfectly aligned with healing the unintegrated parts of myself. I felt my soul rejoice in a spiritual teacher, my mind sought out control over the bewilderment in the unfolding, my body vibrated and adjusted to achieve energetic homeostasis, and my heart was overwhelmed with a swelling fire that filled my body with light. I felt love beckon recognition from every cell in my body.

I was still processing the truth in my lifelong connection with the voice of my soul guiding my physical being through a life walk. It was as if my soul walked me on a journey to the purity of the Heavens and handed a sacred gift of divinity to bring back to my physical life, bridging the Heavens to the Earth. I could feel your presence in both planes, embodied in the physical, and knew that you were bridging the gap between the realms within which I existed yet had never fully integrated either to live the fullest life in both.

I knew my Mom was instrumental in meeting you in the physical form, and she subtly affirmed it throughout our connection. I found that I became spiritually drunk in your presence as you delivered divine messages from the realms beyond our physical existence that were designed solely for me. It was a gift for me to hear, see, feel, and smell you in this experience since my physical senses were fully engaged, and all my parts needed to catch up for the expansion of energy within me. I could feel my spiritual senses activated by your energy; a more powerful energy than mine yet very much in and of me.

Being seen as a light being a year and a half prior echoed throughout my universe from the moment I first read those words. The resonance of those words kick-started my body's vibrational transformation to ascend in order to be wholly present with you. For three and a half years, my body vibrated as I navigated towards a fluid and fluctuating balance. I knew my body would eventually have to reach a resting point, not the zero-point field it felt I had lived within my body, containing energy in motion, and appearing at rest. I knew there would have to be a moment when the energy within me would be still. I knew that would be my resting point within the universe. I knew those words were at the source of who I am.

The unbeknown truth yet to be discovered was so encompassing of every aspect of my being that it felt like I did not have a choice in the matter. It felt like my only choice was to do whatever was needed to honor the force within me. It was a life force that surrounded, pulled, pushed, moved, and transformed every molecule that made up my carbon unit body. I knew it was at the core of what I was learning about myself. Over and over, I was called to sit quietly to allow whatever was occurring within me to expand into my reality. There was only one thing pulling me into the physical human world, and it was the experiences of you.

For over a year, there was a collective spirit energy that traversed the meta-physical plane alongside me on my physical journey. They always presented themselves timely, and in the configuration needed for the moment to complete a trinity. Sometimes I was a part of the trinity, and other times I was the recipient of the powerful trinity formed amongst themselves, interchanging, and amplifying the messages and energetic vibration needed for my physical body to ascend towards them.

With all the experiences overlapping and intertwined, I integrated them as I settled into the truths within. I found myself discovering my inner light, finding my voice, and connecting to the energy beyond our life existence. The same elements of self that many great minds claimed were at the source of our true home, within ourselves. I found myself reflecting on what caused me to question why my home never felt like home, how I had allowed my light to dim, why I never had the words to express my soul, and how one truly connects with the energy of the universe.

I wanted to understand why reclaiming my space and being more intentional felt like a soulful prerequisite for every action. I wanted to understand why it felt like those intentions were draped across humanity like a blanket of purpose. I wanted to feel at home within myself so that no matter the physical structure, I would always be at home within my heart. I felt so peaceful, and at ease over the beautiful life in between that I wanted to understand why there was a new push for whatever it was I was feeling energetically within. I felt deeply that I had found peace in all spaces of me, less that of the true depths of my heart.

During the beautiful life in between, it felt like I was floating over my life while believing in the belief there was something worth believing in. Although I held those sentiments, there was an emptiness about them; a sadness for not being connected; a longingness to feel love deeply; a weariness from the patience. All the while, I remained uncertain of the source of what that truly meant. I chose to see it as a beautiful gift of faith.

Although I did not know what I believed in, I did believe that understanding would be bestowed upon me within my life walk when my time was right, and hopefully on a grander scale than the nuggets received thus far. I needed my balance to the trauma. I believed in divine timing and knew there would be a time for me. That was the deepest space of my faith. It was deemed the only true gift that offered peace to my mind, the most cumbersome aspect of any experience.

Writing opened the floodgates to the world I had experienced and observed while floating above life. It opened my heart. It became the bridge to integrate my soul into the physical experience by reconnecting to the source of who I am, love. None of this was clear to me in the understanding that I would later walk into, an understanding that continues to unearth during the voyage through life. I trusted that everything would occur when the timing was right, and the time was not right until my heart made it clear that it was the true compass of my experience in the physical. I was beginning to understand that I needed to connect to my heart in order to traverse the bridge and bring Heaven to Earth.

While building the bridge, a powerful spirit collective continuously walked me through the experiences that connected me to these truths that have been at the core of who I am for most of my remembered life. Even so, it was not until I took the journey of self-discovery that I learned the extent of my ability to navigate the physical and meta-physical planes of existence. Furthermore, connect to universal energy and flow with it by living from beyond my physical body while still embodied and alive. Once I was far enough along in the journey, I knew who the Spirits were without question due to their energetic signature.

Although I never had the words during the younger versions of self, the freeing release that came with the discovery served as the validation needed to honor that for most of my life, I have held what has felt to be that of the collective human experience. The sensation of holding that of the collective experiences and consciousness of the souls that walk this Earth. I attributed the sensation to my experiences which always allowed me to relate to others in some way or another.

Yet when I stepped into my truths, I could see my body from above and knew I needed to be within it. It was frightening when I felt my energy exit when embodiment was unsustainable. The more I connected to the powerful spirit collective, the more they exposed the truth of my existence. I discovered that after my illness, my body's energetic vibration was so low after coming back from death, that the high vibration of my soul's pure energy could not be sustained within my body. Not to mention the growing manipulation of my human heart throughout life while above and trying to ground into being.

My core energy source, my soul, remained connected to the collective while my body healed to hold its own. My energy was flighting in an out based on physical world circumstance and without my awareness nor control. It made sense in an odd way when coupled with the knowing that my sympathetic nervous system is compromised in how it triggers my fight or flight response. I had to forgive myself for the unbeknown limitations the low vibrational frequency of my physical body was having on my ability to embody my soul. I found breath in the discovery that my energy had flown above and with the collective, watching and trying to ground.

I am grateful that my humanness had your love to follow instead of fear. Your love was much more powerful and magnetic than the human fear my body could generate in defense. Once I could correlate my crashing platelets and my fleeting energy, I knew I needed to learn how to raise the vibration of my body in order to achieve sustainable embodiment. I held gratitude that the journey had already provided me with the new healing tools. I used them to ground myself and they somehow kept unlocking spiritual gifts within. After all, I am here to experience a joyful life, growing through lessons, while in love and embodied.

The unexplainable, intensifying, energetic connection between our human hearts was raising the vibration of my body with every breath of love. I was unsure how it was happening yet every breath that stabilized my heart grew me deeper into my energetic truths. The experience pulled me in every human direction, forcing me to reconcile my existence; conscious energy embodied in a human vessel; energy embodied in a carbon unit machine fueled by the energy that I am. With my light shining upon myself, my humanness could finally process a decades-known overwhelming truth that I, too, am an Angel here on Earth, a light being embodied.

An Earth Angel.

40

Sacred Orchid of Divinity

    Although an eternity in the making, this story began on January 1, 2017, the day I started writing this book. Every prior breath was leading me to the very moments of being and the experiences were resolving every confliction within my heart. The time was clearly before me and slightly disguised by the intentions of many smaller, progressive moments, and delivered by an Angel.

There were many communications with my Earth Angel that were sourced in writing for many months. This in itself was a blessing to my vulnerable and fragile being. It was these soulful expressions in writing that exposed a much greater purpose other than two people exchanging dialogue. One afternoon I received an email correspondence that began with a quote,

"We cannot live in a world that is not our own, in a world that is interpreted for us by others. An interpreted world is not a home. Part of the terror is to take back our own listening, to use our own voice, to see our own light." — Hildegard

While an Angel to me, and while doing my best to honor what felt like a delicate and sacred connection, I was still learning aspects of this individual's physical experience. I felt comforted by the truth that I had shared little about my own situation and yet the perfect resonating quote was shared. One of the few details that I had learned was that Hildegard was the name of her late partner. In the innocence of the experience, I asked if the quote was written by her partner, as it resonated so deeply within. I was hopeful to read more if there were others and available to share. It was expressed that it was not from the works of her partner, but from that of Hildegard von Bingen. Unfamiliar with the name, I quickly started researching the poetic and profound author.

Had I remained deeply rooted in the Catholic faith that surrounded me in my youth, I may have recognized the name, however, my walk did not lead me down that path, so I turned to research. I discovered writings and music composed by Hildegard von Bingen, and learned that she was a German Benedictine abbess, and among many things, she is considered the founder of scientific natural history (1098-1179). I also learned that she was canonized in 2012 by the Roman Catholic Church as a Doctor of the Church, 833 years after her death. In both expected and unexpected ways, the discovery of the Saint was already resonating deeply within me and reflected throughout my life experiences.

A few days after, one morning at work I began playing the music softly in my office while I processed routine reports. Within twenty minutes of starting the music, a long-time dear friend and soul sister, then coworker, entered my office on business matters. Before discussing work, she instantly commented on the music of Hildegard von Bingen by name. I sat in silence, and in amazement for several moments before asking how she knew of the composer by name. All she stated was that her father used to listen to Hildegard von Bingen's music all the time and that she knows it well.

We had to pause momentarily and reconnect to our own divinely sourced connection and found humor in one of the unique aspects of our shared life journey; the comedy in that both of our fathers were Brothers, and both of our mothers were Sisters in the Catholic Church prior to wedding and bringing children into this world. We laughed in amazement then sat quietly for a moment in the mysticism of our spiritual friendship before we continued to discussed work matters and went on with our daily journeys.

The next morning, I returned to work to find two books about Hildegard von Bingen on my desk awaiting my arrival and impending enjoyment. There was also a small tub of hand cream, labeled in German and clearly marked as being of Hildegard von Bingen and from her German abbey. I knew the treasures had come from my soul sister, but before inquiring of how she uncovered these blessed treasures, I opened one of the books to take a quick read. I thumbed through one of the books and fell upon page three where my eyes were instantly drawn to the center of the page. I obliged with my senses and read the following passage,

...become the blooming orchid... "and one does so by doing all things with good intention." - Hildegard von Bingen

This passage, along with two others on the same page, resonated so deeply within me. The other text that was quoted were expressions of encouragement in that "trust shows the way," and mention of her talks of the "sweating power" of the Earth and the need to stay moist, green, and good humored. If there was only one thing I held during those moments it was trust. There were so many uncertainties, and I was very aware that I did not always trust myself, but I did know that I deeply trusted that I was being led by a force greater than myself. I had stopped sweating during this period of time, but I certainly had felt there was a tremendous power behind my nightly sweats that kept my skin moist.

Coupled with the powerful force that was leading the way and the joy it was inciting, it felt as though I had been living her recommendations within me for decades. With these events in the unfolding, I trusted even more so that the universe was connecting my soul to powerful universal energy and to the Source of who I am. It was another spiritual experience that defied time and space by connecting the essence of me to that of this mysterious woman. A woman I had never heard of but inherently knew her upon every aspect of her being unearthed over nine hundred years later.

I was only able to read a few more passages befor I had to put the books down. The more I read the more intense the need to stop became. As I walked through the growing intensity, I learned that she experienced a life of chronic ill-health and endured a sense of death overcoming her physical body until she received the divine message to write. I surely resonated with those sentiments. She was forty years old when she found that her salvation was through expressing the voice within. I was forty when I began writing, forty-one by the time I received the books. The more steps I took through the discovery of self, the more it felt like my expressions were saving me. I have always known that there was a message within that was greater than me and trying to make its way out. I connected even more so to Hildergard von Bingen when considering how my physical body felt prior to and after I began writing. It was the state of my physical body which was one of the propelling forces behind my actions to change; change in what organically presented itself as needing change as it held tremendous potentiality to have a negative outcome otherwise.

I was also able to read about her earthly practices, gain a sense of her voice, and the graceful all-knowing love in her heart. Not only did we connect through the visions of the living light, art, and the voice of her soul, but everything I believed about the healing powers of Mother Earth was reflected in her ideologies and methodologies of achieving health and wellness. She used organic crystals, herbs, and spices to heal the ailments of the body, and nurtured Mother Earth knowing it contains all that is needed to nourish the sacred vessel of the soul.

She even emphasized and practiced the important truth in that good humor of spirit nourishes the soul, a refreshing and needed reflection of self. Even though I had been able to present the playfulness to the outer world, the true space of me held the seriousness of fulfilling my sacred role. My childish giggles that continue to travel with me through life somehow eventually found space too. I could feel the balance with maintaining the lightness in life; the seriousness within and the playfulness without were discovering how to hold space together. A balance was indeed needed for sustainability.

I was completely unaware of the accumulated energy I was holding within, and with each passage that I read, the more I felt deeply connected to this Saint. I remember the pause in my reality when I read about her and her documented works. I read how she expressed the workings within her own mind, how she spent a life holding it all within, and her connection to the visions, infinite knowledge and universal energy was explained in her words "as the reflections of the living light of God." I found myself within the beautiful white space of healing found within my own mind and it became increasingly more difficult to discern between us; her or I; her and I; it felt like we were one in the same. I silently honored the awareness of my own lifelong affinity to Saints and welcomed her into my being. I found myself captivated by the peace brought on by my own experiences. It felt like I uncovered a part of me.

After reading the few passages I was able to enjoy, I went to visit my friend to find out how she had come across the books, and to uncover the story of the hand cream. I knew I would return to reflection later that night before falling into slumber so I made my way through the office hallways to visit my friend. She was not surprised to see me approaching her desk.

She indicated that she was not sure herself, and that all she knew was that when she woke up, her eyes were drawn to a tiny bookcase in the corner of her late father's room, and on the bottom shelf, nestled in the middle of a shelf full of books, her eyes fell upon these two books, side by side. She said she instantly knew she had to bring them to me. She then came across the hand cream and wanted me to have that too.

She demonstrated the miraculous properties of the hand cream, and we watched the skin on our hands transform before our eyes into the similar softness and freshness of a newborn baby's skin; which to me represented the purity of divinity, unjaded by life experiences; the purity of a newborn child; the transformational power of divinity contained within the container of hand cream. It was becoming more and more evident that I was living an experience of divine intervention all over again and felt full of amazing wonder in the mystery of the beautifully synchronous experiences within my journey. I joyously followed.

That night was a whirlwind of memories once I connected to the force within that cause me to stop reading more text from the books. The memories had never left me, instead remained silent and patient as if waiting for my engagement. I suppose waiting for me. I always saw them in the background of my being. There were two experiences that came flooding back into the spotlight of my heart. One revealed my lifelong connection to spirit and heightened senses, and the other exposed the fear that existed on the other side of the same experience; seeing the light and dark that always exists.

It must have been the first time I tuned in and channeled spirit. It was not clear to me what had occurred for many years that followed until I was exposed to the language that explained it. What I recall vividly was what I experienced leading up to, the experience of looking out and speaking, and the reaction of the person to whom I was speaking.

It was a packed house inside and out, a football party of sorts, perhaps even for a Superbowl. I have never been a football fan, but my partner had always been. The house was full, shoulder to shoulder, mostly of people he knew, while I knew a few women. First, from across a crowded room, muffled with a blanker of uninhibited chatter, I heard my partner talking about me. It was so clear and precise it sounded as if he were standing beside me and speaking into me ear. I turned and he was across the room, the furthest distance possible, standing and talking amongst friends. I knew I heard him. It was not kind. I silently questioned everything about what happened as I assessed the physics and acoustical possibilities of the surroundings. And then I questioned him.

Not long after within that same night, on guard and weary of what I had heard and continued to hear, I stepped outside where it would be less crowded. I hope the outdoors would help dissipate the volume. I made my way through a different crowd of unknown faces eventually making my way before someone I knew. Long story short, she was my prior roommate, and turned out to be my only roommate outside of marriage. She had been introduced to her boyfriend through my partner's ill-hearted intentions, and in time they married, brought four beautiful children into the world, and created their own story. This was in the beginning, and it had been over six months since we had lived together but we had stayed in touch mainly because of our boyfriends.

Standing before her that evening, while dark outside, I started speaking with such fluidity. Words were flowing out of me like never before and were about my miraculous healing and writing a book and sharing my story. I had never spoke any of those sentiments and had already questioned many times over if that was part of the purpose. My heart was quiet in its inquiry yet that evening they exited me with uncontrollable ease. The most interesting part was that while looking out I could see that there was an intense light beaming from me. I was unable to see the source since I was creating it, but I saw all of the rays of light emitted upon her before me. I saw and felt the glow I was emitting. Once I spoke for several uninterrupted minutes, it was like the connection to light slowly closed up. Somehow the conversation organically ended, and we went our separate ways.

A couple of days later we were speaking on the phone, and I asked her about that evening. I asked if she noticed anything when we were talking outside. She knew exactly the moment I was speaking about. The minute I asked, she abruptly responded with, "yeah...it was like you were possessed." I felt my shield close the more it was displayed that I was unable to explore it further with that person. It turned out to be decades before I met people who could grow me into my life of experiences. Until then I was grown in a much different way.

I felt it. It did feel like I was possessed in some way, but more by something of me and not like something had taken over me. Everything I spoke was of me. It felt more like my own soul stepping forth. Several weeks later when I was unable to shake the experiences and the reaction, I decided that I would read the Bible. I had never read it from cover to cover yet had been taught to love by its contents my entire life. I truly felt in the depths of me that I had walked a life depicted within the covers and that I would find pieces of me within. I was in my early twenties and knew that I should have already done so, and it seemed like the time was prudent.

The experience I encountered that night when I attempted to read the Bible I was left even more spiritually conflicted. An experience that I was expecting to bring me peace and comfort instead left me leaning into fear and doubt. Using the expression of being possessed by someone who was raised similarly to me was jarring and shielding and was merely a representation of the voice among the world around me. Then, when I attempted to read the Bible, I experienced an overwhelming energy throughout my being. It was so powerful that the only way to stop it was to close the book. It was the same immense pressure I felt when I tried to read the books about Hildegard von Bingen. Her words had the same impact on my body that the words within the Bible had almost thirty years prior. I was afraid of it then yet there was a new spiritual love surrounding Hildegard von Bingen that invited me into and through the fear. Serenity was on the other side waiting amongst my words.

I knew they were linked in some way however it took the journey to recognize how I had chosen fear and doubt of self, instead of spiritual love. When I experienced the sensations with the Bible, and because the world around me enforced it in some way, I believed I was possessed. I believed that evil spirits, or worse the Devil, was in some way involved. It felt as if the spirits I had sensed were also a part of it and prevented me from reading the sacred words of the Bible; the very words that would save or heal me. Back then, I did not know what else to do other than to respect the contents, keep it closed and nearby, and abide by the message. It felt too powerful for my body. It did indeed scare me back then.

After deconstructing my ego and reconstructing my heart, I saw the memories replay alongside new experiences with the same sensation. My perspectives were different. I was different. The more I looked to the new words of Hildegard to discover our embedded likeness, the more the intensity grew when I tried to read the books. The same continued to occur when I tried to read the Bible which demonstrated that collectively there was a message being sent from beyond. Through a new network of people to provide safety and love I was able to weave the elements together. Even though my humanness was still very much in the way, I could sense that the new lens through which I was looking at the same experiences was with intent to find my voice. It felt similar to Hildegard von Bingen which was what prevented my discovery; as if I could not read our likeness until I first found my own voice, and discovered the significance of a light being.

Within three days of receiving the books and flooded with spiritual memories, my friend and I were scheduled to have lunch with a mutual friend, a fellow soul sister to us both. We had arranged to share in a Christmas lunch together before the holidays. When we arrived at the restaurant, our friend popped open her trunk and inside were three beautifully bloomed orchid plants. One for each of us.

I had spent seven months experiencing Sacred Geometry around me; numbers danced their significance during every day of the journey, but it was the sacred number of three that caught my awareness in the unfolding of Hildegard von Bingen and the beautiful orchids. The number three had been a prevalent number in my journey for many years. As time progressed on my soulful quest, it had become more and more pronounced in everything that was encountered. It was deeply felt that divine presence was centering my experiences in the essence of the Holy Trinity, the Father, the Son, and the Holy Spirit. For me, it became my God, my Soul, and my physical experience. When my friend graced us with our orchid plants, I sat in silence and gratitude in the spiritual synchronicity of all that had transpired. I felt tremendously blessed and became even more eager to travel the path before me. Together, my co-worker and I acknowledged the blessing in silence and honored the truths before us.

Christmas rolled around and amidst the hustle and bustle of the season with young ones, I allowed time and space for my journey to rest. I felt as if I was closing out the year blessed beyond measure but with a tired and weary body, mind, heart, and soul. Time was spent pouring love into my children, and into a broken marriage, while draped in the awareness that even with our continued joint efforts, the brokenness was not healing. I chose to continue my reconnection with self and spiritual healing. I continued to restore my spiritual strength that carried me through life, while revitalizing my very essence and connection back to the universe. I wanted to feel the source connection to love and joy, and not expend energy in constantly trying to not feel the sadness that filled the hearts around me, and sometimes within me; all sourced in a yearning to have a joy and love filled heart. I wanted to be joy so that I would feel joy. I wanted to be love so that I would feel love. By this time and space, I felt tired of warding off energy and deeply felt like I needed the space to emit my own.

With beautiful new members joining my soul tribe and my increased understanding of their presence, I closed out the year with a beautiful presence of all things purple on Christmas Eve and Christmas Day. It was not in the expected ways from the world celebrating with decorations and traditions. It was exploding from within and popping up in the most unexpected of places. I reminisced of my childhood bedroom painted and filled with all things purple. I felt safe in that room. I rested in purple as it represents the birth of Christ; a measure in humanity graced by God within Christian religions. I felt like I was a child of the same universe; love manifested. I felt the energy of creation within me trying to bust free. I felt the universe expanding into me, and I into the universe. I felt the infinite space and love within me, and they were clearing the pathways for emittance beyond me. I myself felt reborn. I felt like a child all over again in a field of flowers casting dreams inside my heart. There was a definite glory to be celebrated. Mine and God's within and around me.

While I rested in the knowingness of my truths, my physical world continued to unfold around me. It was a beautiful awareness that the Advent season of the Catholic Church was aligned with the experiential walk I was walking. In a sense, I had been fasting, purging, and preparing for the royalty of my rebirth before me; preparing for the reconnection back to the very energetic essence of who I am.

It was during the magical time of the Christmas Season, through the celebrations, laughs and smiles shielding the path within, that the brightest of lights was casted within my universe. It was as if I saw a glimpse of the blueprint of my existence. My inner light had grown so dim, and I had allowed the ebbs and flows of life to almost suffocate my shine, and then when I had done the work and the timing was right, I received just enough light for me to know what to do. It was as if I saw the pathway out of darkness into the space of light I had been envisioning. I was ready to continue the journey into the new year. I was eager to arrive at the divine and intended space to rest. I knew it was close and if I stopped it would take even longer to get there. It felt like I had already waited long enough, and I was tired and weary; tired of feeling tired, afraid, and alone. I wanted to continue on so I could truly rest and enjoy life; soulfully and sensually; all parts of me; as me.

I had also learned along the way that my body had been trying to intervene over the years when I did not adhere sternly to my own inner wisdom and the guidance of divinity. I had gained this awareness as my physical body stepped in again to provide a gentle reminder to slow down. I did not feel like I was rushing. I felt tired and weary but not rushed. I did not know what it was I was truly moving towards, nor how to slow down. I actually felt more peaceful than ever. It was all the years prior that felt like I had rushed through them. It sent me into a reflection on the pace through which I had navigating life.

It was true, I had rushed through them. Not in physical speed, but in heart and soul speed. The moments in years prior I had recognized the absence of soulful love in my relationship but accepted the love and commitment to the life we had created. Over time, there was less and less to honor within the relationship, and in the choice of acceptance in something that lacked soul love, I ultimately sacrificed a deeper part of who I am; I sacrificed me. As time went one, more times than not, my insides felt rattled, uneasy, and unpleasant. It felt like I was racing through moments for my next reprieve. The dis-ease within my body became a core reason to make a change. It was the catalyst for my heart to revive itself and pulse life back into my body. For once, it actually felt like I was slowing down and discovering the soulful reasons to do so.

My soul kindly showed its disagreement in good fashion through physical manifestation within my body. Once again, I found myself behind the isolate walls of a hospital room, receiving life-saving treatment for critically low platelets. Although demonstrated through completely new symptoms, my body was unable to sustain all the beautiful transformations I was experiencing within. Although I was enduring unfamiliar, soulful, energetic growth, it proved to be stressful on my body. Before similar medical experiences left my body feeling weak, frail, and afraid. There was an irony in that the source of the stress was from a completely different space, and the onset of symptoms albeit most common in others with ITP, had never before been experienced by me, blood blisters inside my mouth. There was definitely a lower energy of uncertainty through it all, but I was unwilling to nurture it with fear. I knew the treatment process, and if in the final hours it was my time and space, it would be my time and space. I was resting in the most serene and tranquil soulful peace; all was very well with my soul.

Generally, there was a misunderstanding in how my physical body felt before, during and after treatment. When asked what it felt like when my platelets were low, the best description was that I felt loose in my skin. As if I could feel a layer of fluid between my muscles and epidermis layers. This may have been fostered by the truth in what was actually happening; blood so thin that it seeped out of the veins and into places it should not be. During and after treatment my body felt solid and firm as it should, but it felt foreign and injected as it was.

The treatment would effectively increase my platelets to normal ranges and in a sense exposing a sensation of wholeness with blood full of voluptuous platelets. I would then become subject to weekly blood testing, bi-weekly doctor visits and at least ten months of medication weaning and observing my platelets organically stabilize with doctors eager to intervene more often than I. It was a cycle that I was very familiar with, but there remained the beacon of newness that lit my path, especially when I was dazed by the mystical tranquility within my reality. I deeply believed I could make this time different; somehow.

I remember feeling tremendously gracious for the notion that my medical incident and consequential hospital stay was in a sense my denouement; the final scene when the strands of the plot come together; the climatic point of clarity. I cherished the new perspective and intently worked on cultivating that truth into my experience. The four days spent in the hospital with the hours of the days and nights in reflection was ultimately the time and space that changed the course of my life; everything changed with the physical, mental, emotional, and spiritual space within me. It was the physical body platelet crash in the midst of my spiritual healing that indeed purified the alchemizing laboratory of body, mind, heart, and soul, solidifying the resolved clarity in truths. The windows of my hospital room once again became the lens through which I viewed my world yet this time there was a majestic kaleidoscopic beauty that casted the most vibrant rainbows of brilliance with each slightest tilt in perspective.

As the experience organically evolved, everything became organically different. It had been four years since the last need for medical intervention to save my physical life. That was the longest time frame over the past twenty years since diagnosis. Before the four-year respite, hundreds of thousands of individuals, and the science of western medicine have been saving my physical body on an average of every two and a half years. That is about eight times since my illness. All the while it felt like my soul was waiting to be saved by my physical body.

Just the required medicine alone relied on the gracious blood plasma donations from hundreds of thousands of donors; donors that once felt foreign, invasive, and unwelcomed in my body were now being integrated into my being. The purity of the desire to heal my body with that of the earth, was now yielding to the aid of my gracious healing tribe; realizing we are all from the same source which is love and love heals; love manifested, now manifesting love. This time receiving the treatment felt peaceful; this time felt graceful; this time felt pure and authentic; this time felt healing.

The change in perspective and the welcoming of modern medicine and the one hundred thousand blood donors tried to cause confusion within my mind but serenity was sweeping everything clean. Thoughts and fears effortlessly floated in and out of my being as I surrendered to the unfolding. I much preferred feeling peaceful and graceful during an experience that continued to try and incite fear within myself and in others, especially that of my children. My medical experience was even used against me as a sign of my own weakness and inability to stand alone in this world.

I was continuously reminded that those I stood before the longest, and believed honored and protected all parts of me, did not know the true depths of me. Instead, every aspect of me felt ridiculed, dismissed, ignored, and dishonored. It took patience, love and understanding to know that the actions and reactions were not personal, but the mere struggle of the human condition self-manifested by another yet before me. The journey of another before me, co-mingled in with mine perfectly as it should be, but needing tremendous space in the aware disarray of it all. The four days in solitude created the space needed to breathe. It allowed me to find my breath. My breath; not a joint breath.

Although beautiful growth within, it was a whirlwind. I was experiencing new levels of unconditional love within that kept sweeping me off of my own feet, while contrasted by the conditional love outside of me. There was a divine presence in every experience encountered, and noting it was not present anywhere within the relationship with my partner. I was literally falling in love with myself all over again at the dawn of each new day which caused me to fall out of love with my partner. The more I loved myself, the world around me fulfilled my intentions, dreams, and desires, while casting light and clarity upon a deep truth within - my romantic, sensual, soulful love no longer held space within our relationship.

An even deeper truth was that our relationship never held space for my soulful love which incites the romantic, sensual love. It never needed to hold space for my deep love. I never allowed for it due to my own limitations and limiting beliefs around love. Now that I was choosing to create space for self-love and soulful love, the relationship could not sustain it. There was no honor, compassion nor soulfulness; not in the sense my soul was choosing to align with. Once I chose soulful love, all of me agreed to follow.

Although the romantic, sensual love has always been a part of who I am, it had become lost, hidden, scared, vulnerable, nervous, timid, and felt tremendously naive. My soulful love wanted to dance and play in the energetic sandbox of the physical bodies yet felt trapped by mindful vulnerability. I found myself before a truth to either love myself and follow my heart or bridge the divide. It felt like the choice between mindful love and spiritual love. My entire existence felt like I was journeying towards your spiritual love. I was patient and gentle with myself as I sat in the sad acceptance that it could not be both, and I knew my answer.

It became clear that I needed my physical world to align with my inner world instead of trying to mold my inner world to my external world. It felt like my lifetime had been spent trying to do that, and albeit it was in the wrong direction, it served its purpose during those times in my life. But everything was changing. Everything was shifting. I felt it throughout my entire being. There was newness throughout my universe being navigated carefully and mindfully, all while trying to return to my heart and carry on in life, now behind the walls of a hospital. The irony was that hospitals had become like a home to me. It felt like I was at home, where it all began, now sterilizing me from the experiences of the past in order to start anew. I knew I was aligning with healing energy and universal abundance. I was connecting in new ways that created an even greater divide in the physical experience of love within which I was living and preparing to change.

The experiences in the hospital were always comical, which is where I found joy in the otherwise uncertain experience. There was never gloom nor sadness, at least not from me. I always felt fine, especially after treatment started. I was rested and optimistic because I knew I would have almost a year of high platelets, especially with the newness of everything and the serene stillness of time that I was perceiving. I would only ask for assistance if I absolutely needed it, which was hardly ever. I know how to restart an IV pump, I know how to maneuver around with caution, I felt fine, and I was really only there because it was an IV infusion that had to be started promptly and my vitals required monitoring. I did also have the heart monitor that now accompanied me through my medical experiences due to the diagnosis of bradycardia four years prior. The condition characterized by a low resting heart rate, also meant that experiences would be accompanied by a heart monitor, and possibly a staff with their uncertainties and unfamiliar experiences with the low rates of the condition.

My heart always created a comical space that balanced the seriousness within and around the free bleeding potentiality of my low platelets. Generally, this meant that the usually silenced joy within was free to be exposed and lightened the spirits of those around me. Expressing the joy within my heart outside of the walls of my home had unfortunately become part of the normal existence of my heart. When space was created between my partner and I, I had the space and freedom to authentically express my joyful and loving self and align with the truths that I am sourced in love and joy. It was not until I viewed my experiences through my heart that I felt the attempts of manipulation to feel bad for being happy. Bringing joy and smiles wherever I journeyed was not uncommon even when the space was within the confines of what is generally a sad and somber place.

Along with the joyful attitude that I brought within the sentiments of my heart, the physical matter of my heart also played a role in my brief stay at the hospital. Upon arrival to my room, my heart was greeted with a small blessing in the presence of a familiar nurse that I had met four years prior during a brief stay for the same reason; low platelet emergency treatment. That time I had been placed within the telemetry unit as it was the only unit with an available bed to accommodate the emergent admittance. The catcher was that anyone in the telemetry unit was generally there because of their heart, so I was treated the same and received a heart monitor for the duration of my stay. The familiar nurse had recently transferred from the telemetry unit which was where we first met four years prior when I was first diagnosed with bradycardia.

I know that my story and my physical body make for a memorable encounter. It always had and had even become part of the energy that I had difficulty connecting with over the many years in the beautiful life in between. I never wanted to be remembered and identified by my story and the truths of the story always felt too magnificent to contain within further conflicted with the knowing that it is my story that grows me into being. I would never be able to avoid my story, and for many years did not even realize that it was an integration avoidance that was causing a disjointed self within. By this time, I had already learned that and had been working to integrate all parts of me, which meant the unfavorable parts of the experience as well. It was important on my path to healing because my story is indeed me, and I am my story. It is all very much a part of who I am. It felt much easier to embrace all parts of me instead of feeling shamelessly powerless because of them and the energy that accompanies avoidance.

She immediately remembered me, as I did her. She was the lead nurse in the team of five that had come charging into my room during the first night of a five-night stay. I never thought anything of it when they hooked me to the monitor and placed electrical feeds across my chest, nor had there ever been an indication of any issue with my heart other than it had not loved wholly from the depths it desired to love and be loved. Although it would have been nice to have had a soulful love monitor to aid in the alignment with soulful love, that is not the purpose that the heart monitors serve, nor was it time for the evolution towards such a love. This was something much different. Bradycardia is a heart rhythm condition that holds a serious potential of causing blood and oxygen deprivation to the brain. When there is a lack of oxygen to the brain, a stroke becomes a very real and serious possibility. It was during the time of accidental diagnosis that I learned about the condition itself and the new delicacy of my physical body.

During the time of diagnosis, on the first night, just as I was starting to relax and fall into a peaceful slumber, I was startled by a team of five as they came rushing to my bedside to make sure I was alive and ok. Uncertain as to what initiated the alarming concern, they explained that my heart rate had dropped to thirty-two beats per minute. I was not concerned because I knew I was still breathing and more so because it was the rate of my usual relaxed breath. To them, on the other hand, a rate that low was an indicator of imminent danger and the impending possibility of a stroke.

The familiar nurse was the lead on the team that rushed to my aid.

After she explained what had occurred, and confirmed that I was alright, she maintained calmness among the staff as they witnessed my heart rate drop throughout the night, sometimes as low as twenty-seven beats per minute. Needless to say, a myriad of tests were ordered and scheduled for the next day to ensure that there was not an underling issue with my heart. After multiple tests confirmed that the circuitry of my heart was normal and that it was solely a heart rate phenomenon, I was left to rest despite the silent intermittent checks of reassurance when my rate fell below forty while sleeping. After that first night, it was her strong, courageous, and loving heart that tempered the fear in those around us.

When I saw her again, I knew all was well, especially in the new space of my heart. There was harmony everywhere; ying was being greeting by yang; light was shining on darkness; there was love instead of fear. It was another meticulously intertwined fragility of my physical body that I would have to defy along my earth walk in wellness while tempering fear in those around me. The experience of the telemetry unit happenstance turned out to be another blessing in disguise, and one that was guarding and protecting all aspects of me - my heart and mind embodied in my physical body housing my soul. Although before a new staff, I knew we would make it through.

Since the bradycardia diagnosis I always receive a heart monitor as part of any hospitalization regardless of the unit within which I am placed. It was the first hospitalization since diagnosis and I was in a regular wellness unit, now with a heart monitor. The main aspect to consider was that there would be staff members that were not exposed to matters of the heart. The staff within the telemetry unit struggled with maintaining composure and they dealt with the heart all day and night. I was now in a unit that was unfamiliar with treating the heart, yet I was bringing my heart right to the monitors before them in the nurse's station. I felt tremendous ease when I saw the familiar nurse, and I knew that she would have everything under control especially given the experiences that unfolded with her during the time of diagnosis.

While in the hospital for the treatment of the current episode of low platelets, as a unit we experienced and navigated the treatment and my heart with ease and calmness. I knew going into the hospital that the experience was tremendously different than any prior experience due to my own state of mind and intended transformation and with that came a sense of tranquility. The presence of the familiar and gracious nurse was a silent blessing that relaxed my being even more. In a sense, coupled with the temperament of my heart, and her understanding my heart, together we set the tone of the experience.

During the visit another unexpected event occurred but it was an inner experience navigated in the sacred space of my soul. I had already connected to my spirituality which was changing the molecular makeup of my being. There was a surreal and angelic essence to my existence which left me floating above my reality. My spiritual evolution had been grounded in an unexpected connection to my Catholic religious experiences, Mother Mary had made herself present throughout many moments of uncertain spiritual growth. Her presence came with a reassurance that everything about my experiences, within and without, were to be honored as real physical human experiences intended for my spiritual being while living out a physical reality. I had spent many hours in quiet reflection with Mary, Her life journey, and Her gracious role as a Spiritual Mother to humanity. I understood what She represents and signifies within the Catholic religion, and within me. I felt deeply connected to Her and there was a tremendous presence of Her within and around me during my hospitalization.

This particular medical situation was also the beginning of a new relationship with a new Oncologist. My doctor of several years relocated which meant that I was reassigned to her partner, and he would become the new person to trust. Since my doctor finalized her move only a couple of months prior to my hospitalization, and I had not required any medical follow-ups, I had not yet met the doctor that would become a new member of my treatment team. I was patiently waiting his arrival and introduction while receiving treatment in the hospital. I was prepared with my interviewing mind to ensure that the dynamic would support the type of doctor-patient relationship my experience required.

It was the second day of treatment and while waiting for the doctor to make his rounds I was resting in reflection in the purity of my spiritual being. I was reflecting on Mary and how She is associated with the miracles within the human experience. I also found myself reflecting on the statues of Her that have been known to weep tears of blood. While believing in the possibility of such occurrences, I connected to the significance in that tears of blood have fallen not only over the sins of the world, but also over the pain She endured in Her earthly life experience. There was an internal depiction that represented the Seven Sorrows of Mary and the seven swords piercing through Her flaming heart. I felt even more connected to Her energy through my burning heart.

I deeply knew that as humans we are non-perfect beings that inherently have sinned at some point in this experience. I knew I had more than once. Released from burden through my own pre-existing spirituality was a space of peace, acceptance, and forgiveness even though it was through a disjointed perspective and not fully integrated into the depths of my heart and soul. But what connected me even more to Mother Mary was the incomprehensible truths within the human experience. I knew deeply that I had struggled with the overwhelming truths of the many miracles that had filled and continue to fill my experiences. The pain associated with the physical experience was sourced in the same essence of disbelief in experiences that were absolutely and unequivocally real. The tears of blood signify the pain associated with the inexplainable miracles that graced our paths. Hers being Hers, and mine being mine, yet sourced in the shared miracles of life. I could not help but couple the notion of my low platelets and the potentiality of free bleeding with the idea of tears of blood. I certainly felt weepy, and my eyes burned slightly from my own tears and from the medication I was receiving. For a brief second there was a vision of me weeping tears of blood. The image vanished just as quickly as it surfaced, and I mindfully acknowledge the unlikely possibility of that unfolding in my experience.

I was reflecting in my bed and waiting for the next event to interrupt the silence, and in walked my new doctor. As we acquainted ourselves with each other and reviewed a life history of my ITP condition, his practicing style, and my personal involvement, he suddenly made a statement that froze time within my spiritual space of existence. He was sitting in a chair aside the bed and in the midst of the discussion he stated,

"...it's not like you are going to start bleeding from your eyes..."

Of all the statements he could have made, he commented on the very reflection within me just moments before he entered my room. It was a moment of divine assurance that the circumstances that

I was experiencing, and the choices being made out of spiritual healing were in alignment with Divine Intention. It was strangely perfect that he spoke those words, and it felt like a sacred shield of protection had been wrapped around me as if to shield me from further real-world suffering. Not in the sense that I would never experience pain again, but in the sense that I had been seen, and would forever be seen by my Spiritual Mother for who I truly am which is a spiritual being living a human experience and that my faith and connection to Her would protect my soul with the truths in spiritual purity. I was honoring, protecting, and nurturing my heart which at times felt as though it was fueled by flames of passionate, unconditional love. There was a sense of poetic peace that my heart, my beautiful and serene energy, my miracles, my blood, Mother Mary, Her beautiful and serene energy, Her miracles, Her blood, and the words of my doctor all came together to form a blanket of peace and grace that cloaked every aspect of my existence.

The rest of the hospital stay was uneventful in comparison, and before I concluded my stay, I somehow managed to view all aspects of my physical experiences of love through new sterile lenses. By the time of my release, I knew that my marriage was over. From that moment onward it would be about the choices to align with those truths. When my body was strong enough, I had to begin the processes to do so; file for divorce, move out, build a new life, nurture my children, and become separate from a version of love, and to do so with love and understanding. I prayed for peace as I vowed to reacquaint myself with the depths of who I am. My mind, heart and soul were undergoing tremendous transformation, it would only make sense for my body to join in to ensure all aspects of my existence were involved in the integrated growth underway, collectively and now sourced in love. I had to figure out how to sustain my body.

I knew that everything was as it needed to be, even in the blatant awareness when my own medically fragile state was used against me as proof of my inability to manage life on my own. That was when it was clear that the one person I trusted most with my heart had chosen not to know me at all. By the end of the week, I had stabilized and was released from the hospital with a new navigation to add to the journeys already under way. In addition to caring for my children, nurturing a broken marriage, maintaining a home, working full time, writing my book, and navigating the journeys of my heart and soul, I also had to navigate that of my delicate physical body. My hope in love held me together.

Within days of my release, another surreal and defining experience marked the onset of all subsequent moments that led to the experiences of my intention to sync with global energy and the essence of who I am. Love for self manifested, and self manifesting love. In one marking event, I felt the synchronization with global energy; the vibration of creation; the vibration of love. I was in sync with you.

I remember where I was, what I was wearing, the sounds of the space, the smells in the air, the colors of life. I remember the sweet purity within and around me as the porch chimes swayed in the wind resembling the summoning ring of church bells. Coupled with the church bell chimes signifying the presence of something greater, another beautiful synchronicity that presented itself was that I was at a location named the Blue Heron. Again, there was a sense of poetic irony in that the Blue Heron brings about a message of self-reliance and self-determination and signifies innate wisdom in the ability to maneuver through life and to be a co-creator of circumstance. It was all divinely perfect that the experience in the unfolding occurred in the light of perfection.

Time stood still in the moments that I felt the peaceful yet powerful energy flow into and throughout my body, throughout every aspect of my multi-dimensional self. As I viewed the world around me it was as if I could see the planes of vibrational energy superimposed upon the 3D matrix within which I was present. I could hear and see every movement and sound as it traveled through time and space. Life around me was in slow motion and I could sense the varying vibrations that were emitted by everything. I watched the energy move and swirl and transfer around and within me that day. I felt it deeply the moment the energy first entered my realm, and then before me. I knew I was being transformed during the very moments of awareness.

The most amazing aspect was that the initial energetic infusion occurred without the physical contact of anything nor anyone. It was between hearts. In those moments of our visit every moment of my life was converging into oneness. Just as I felt mine merging within me, I knew you felt yours merging within yours. It was the most sensual and energetic experience of my existence. I knew I was standing within the energy of Divine Love. I have not been the same being since that day and the resonance and warmth of the powerful energy still resides within my chest. I have felt it every day since that one moment in eternity. Even so, in the same moments I knew my humanness would struggle. I felt the energy pushing up against something within.

I recall attending a basketball game for one of my sons several days after which was the first public experience since feeling synced and connected to Divine Love. I felt mesmerized by the energy of the gymnasium; not the energy itself but in how I experienced the energy. The gym was large enough to hold two games at one time and seat supporting fans for both. I was very mindful of the pace of my walk as I entered the energy vortex of joy. I mindfully slowed down. It felt like my powerful surge would disrupt the energy if I did not continue with care.

I love basketball. Out of all the sports I have played, basketball is my favorite. There are some sports that I enjoy watching, but basketball was not one of them. I much preferred to play. That was until my sons started playing. I find tremendous joy in watching them play, enjoy, and excel at a sport that I also loved to play. Generally, everyone in the gym was there with pure intention of love and joy. That was a blessing because it made this experience what it was; and not something completely opposite, or indifferent. As I walked through the muffled hum of everyone's energy, it was as if I could see every energetic flutter created by every butterfly wing of every butterfly making up the Butterfly Effect rippling throughout the gym. There was a silent stillness of excitable joy that filled the gym that night; or me as I experienced the gym. I felt like I floated above the games, as an Angel in my own heart.

Over the next several weeks I effortlessly released any and everything that crossed my mind and felt my way into the awareness of it all. It felt as though I was walking up the stairway to Heaven. As I was growing weary along the path, I was continuously guided by Spirits through the last steps to reach my destination. Along the way I was graced with comforting and supportive words to encourage the continued journey.

It felt as though I was still being escorted, this time back into the illusion of the human physical experience protected by the love, compassion and understanding of the Heavens. I did not expect to be introduced to all my Angels up on my decent. The very ones that had been guiding me throughout my life. The ones I secretly wanted to meet. One by one they were exposed before me...

An Angel of Beauty...

An Angel of Grace...

An Angel of Joy...

An Angel of Peace...

An Angel of Purity...

An Angel of Serenity...

An Angel of Tranquility ...

An Angel of Sensuality ...

An Angel of Strength...

An Angel of Courage...

An Angel of Love...

An Angel of Hope...

All guided by a Divine Angel of Light...My Earth Angel.

I grounded myself in the profoundness once again in that we see in others that of which we hold within, creating a vortex of Angels within and around me. I felt like an Angel floating throughout the universe anchored in my heart by your love forevermore. I could feel and see my Angels within and around me everywhere I went. It felt surreal and magical. Everything in my being was slowly floating into its universal space of clarity.

Through it all, I found myself staring into the eyes of love. For the first time in my life, I knew and felt deeply that Divine Love had seen me.

Love had seen me in the purity of my essence.

Love had seen me in the authenticity of my emotions.

Love had seen me in the vulnerability of my heart.

Love had seen me in the joyful experiences of life.

Love had seen me in the sensual expressions of who I am.

Love had seen me in the humor through which I see the world.

Love had seen me in the nakedness of my physical being.

Love had seen the depths of what makes up beautiful me.

Love had seen me and loved me. All of me.

Love has seen me and blasted my heart out into the universe once again, yet this time it was to retrieve my parts and return to wholeness, and this time in the presence of love. Love has seen me and was guiding me home.

I had already prepared for the actionable choices that were pending in order to realign my heart to love. It did not take long after my hospitalization and immediate recovery for me and my partner to create the space we needed to finalize our separation. It was not always easy but eventually we created the heart and mind space to work through the respectful and understanding separation after twenty-two years. I became focused on outlining divorce petition details as a self-represented litigant, finalizing arrangements to move out of the only home my children have known, and learning how to love myself again within the freedom of love and joy. With the unexpected timing in the connection to global energy and the radiant resonance of love that was now embodied within me, I felt deeply that all was as it needed to be, and I was becoming exactly who I was intended to be in the unfolding of the changes.

The unexpected occurrence was in the crash endured in the final stages in my decent from the Heavens. As if energetically the purity of the Heavens could not descend to the depths I needed to return to in order to purify my life. I felt the energetic dissonance between my internal and external energy, shifting as I returned to the lower energetic vibrations of my reality when compared to the high vibrations above. I could feel the energetic difference so deeply that it was clear where the misalignment was sourced. The term light being made even more sense, especially after I experienced such energetic shifts within, and seeing light and dark so clearly.

The energetic difference was felt between the Divine Love of the Heavens and the loveless state of my reality that I was in the midst of realigning. Now I understood what I was aligning with whereas before it was merely a dream of the unknown. It felt as though I had floated so peacefully and gracefully through the realms to purity, approached the Heavens and found myself before love. Then suddenly crashing into opposition within my reality. The clash between the high vibrations of the Heavens when met with the low vibrations of the love in my reality would inevitably take many more months to equalize back into the purity of Divine Love. It was a jolt that led me to, and through, what felt like the final purging of accumulated negative energy, clearing the pathways of deliverance of everything that was not in alignment with the purity of my love energy. My physical experience would have to follow as it was time to let it organically align with my being as part of my Divine Intention.

It was in those moments and before the eyes of love, that I felt my disjointed self-struggle for cohesiveness, and achieving only an awareness of the oneness my soul was yearning to experience; especially while staring into the sacred eyes of love. My essence had been exposed. The sheer vulnerability of self, to self, and beyond self, became a multidimensional matrix of self-doubt through which I knew I had to feel my way through. It was something my heart had forgotten how to do purely, or perhaps never knew how to do authentically. I sensed that it was something that was needed in order to sustain the purity of the most glorious love before me.

During the moments of the energetic collisions within, I recalled a comment from a sacred soul tribe member that had been made many months prior. She was another individual that appeared to have been pin-dropped precisely into my experience, perhaps for this message alone. The words floated into my awareness as I felt incapable of stabilizing the energies within. I had been gently advised that I was not ready to receive the kind of love that I was attracting. In the moment that the statement was made I chuckled in disagreement for Divine Love was an intention from the depths of my heart. I believed that I would most definitely be ready to receive my dream of love when I found it before me. It had been a soulful dream for such a long time.

Although I was elegantly introduced to the many Angels that guide me, everything was further experienced by a deeply felt absence of your soulful guidance except for in my heart. I could feel you within everywhere I went and no matter what I did. As I travelled through the days, I could sense that the vibrations that I had to clear were too impure and I had to take the remaining journey alone, unguided and with the faith I held deep within. It was the ultimate test of my faith for the path to Divine Love had been exposed. It remained my choice of free will to journey back towards it. Or not.

In the presence of this choice, everything that had been obtained along the walk towards you and the guidance towards our shared love seemed to vanish before me. Gone without a trace. I had nothing to go by but the memories of written and spoken words, the presence of my guiding Angels, and the trust in their continued guidance from within our new intimate connection

While mystified and drunken by your love, I felt lost yet found. I felt confused yet everything was clear. I felt abandoned yet knew I was not alone. I felt lonely yet fulfilled. I felt every emotion that accompanied the mindful thoughts that I had masked with my own beautiful stories of self. Most of them turned out to be mere attempts to convince myself that I felt anything and everything other than what I was actually feeling. I felt betrayed by my own emotions and thoughts as I synced every aspect of my being into clarity. Humbled by my humanness while simultaneously grateful for the experiences to cleanse my soul.

While sourced in the purity of love, I was humbled by the truths of what I was experiencing. I became hyper-aware of my own sense of surprise, shame, embarrassment, naivety, and inexperience when in the face of real love. As I slowed down, found my breath, followed the soulful dance, and while love continued to heal, I found that...

>...In the face of love, I felt as though I was falling apart, when in actuality I was integrating into oneness.

>...In the face of love, I felt inferior to the purity before me, forgetful that it was the purity of my heart that attracted the purity of love.

>...In the face of love, I felt humbled and unworthy to receive such sweet, pure love, aware of the truth that it was a sacred love designed for me.

>...In the face of love, I felt shame in trying to compare love and trying to conceptualize the infinite capacity of love when there is no such thing when it comes to real love.

>...In the face of love, I felt judged, when it was judgment upon self and my own physical body experience.

>...In the face of love, I felt myself fighting the forces of the human condition, acting in fear, desire, and the uncertainty in so many truths before me.

>...In the face of love, I felt confronted once again with the clarity in awareness that I was holding all those sentiments toward self.

I was distraught to discover that in the face of love the work I had done through the walk to self-love was the mindful release of the constructs that clinched my essence, and what I was experiencing was a deeply felt energetic release of the human condition and the limiting constraints around love. I knew they were mine, but it felt bigger than me. It felt like the energy of the collective human experience contained within the scope of my experiences.

My soul patiently observed the physical experience. It was as if my heart, mind, and body had to go through a metamorphosis process to catch up with the deep truths of my old soul. I became increasingly more aware that every experience was divinely part of the experience and that of my own creation. I was learning of my ability to manifest my reality as I experienced the inability to stop a creation already in motion.

My physical body experienced moments of jolting convulsions from what felt like the collisions of energy; high vibrations of love with that of the lower energies being released, once cocooned by the mental constructs being cleared. I felt lightning bolts of energy sourced within me travel throughout my body, leave, and extend outward into the realms of others and witnessed them react in some way. I was emitting and releasing energy everywhere I went; especially when I stood before love. Love electrified my being.

My mind felt trapped in a desire to understand the deliverance of divine truth and the disjointed challenge within me. I held onto the desire for a fully integrated life experience but was unsure of what was unfolding. I could see the energetic circuitry of my mind intensify to the point of surrender so my heart could regain energetic control to lead me to wherever the experience was leading me. I knew it was glorious and magnificent. I knew it was healing me. I knew it was calibrating me back into balance. I knew it was intended for me to experience. I knew I had to make it through even though it felt like I was being ripped apart all over again, yet this time it was my spiritual being and not my physical being. Your love in my heart was holding me together.

My emotional compass was recalibrating into love while every unuseful emotion raced to leave my being. It was a jarring energetic collision that would take years to calibrate back into peace. They were all familiar emotions that were being cleansed by divinity as they were filtered through the new experiences of the heart.

All before the eyes of love.

All before the eyes of a love that energetically felt closer to purity than mine and felt inviting for me to allow the cleansing wash of divinity.

All before the eyes of love that reaffirmed it was all within me.

It was a truth that was then delivered through the beautiful presence of my Mom. Not within me, but within your human expressions, shielding the sacredness of the truths of my love that I honor within the depths of me. I was not ready which meant you must not have been ready either. Our collective human heart was not balanced and ready. Humanity thereby was still balancing to receive an example of Divine Love. I hold tremendous gratitude for my Mom's presence, protection, and guidance.

Even so, I was humbled and saddened by the message, and although I was encouraged that my spiritual growth was complete, I knew it was not since I was not able to sustain the purity of love. I could feel it deep within. Not to mention my body was vibrating. I sensed there was something more, something deeper I still had to heal and learn before the calibration was complete.

My Mom affirmed there was more to come and relayed those messages as my sense of divinity spoke through the physical experience. It felt like every engagement presented an infinite knowingness of me, beyond my own awareness. Much like my Mom unknowingly presented herself to me throughout life. It felt calming and peaceful within my soul, yet my bodily emotions felt nervous and apprehensive. They were all indicators that I did not yet feel balanced in energetic, soulful love. I then found myself in a sensual navigation of my heart, mind, and soul to the awareness that...

> ...before the eyes of the purest, spiritual love, I did not hold spiritual strength, courage, nor love within. I did not hold within for myself the same love I had dreamed of for so long and knew had been delivered unto me.

> ...before the eyes of love, I did not know how to love myself in my physical body. The same body that is perfect in spiritual truth yet a truth that was not yet felt within my heart.

I should have been prepared for it was a known fear that I held within and had deconstructed within my jaded ego. Just as I expect my dreams to be realized, I should have expected nothing less for that of a fear, especially given the truths in the natural affinity of energy. Although I never once felt afraid of being face to face and looking into the eyes of love, the silent subconscious fear had existed long enough to make its way into my manifested reality.

I knew this, so I journeyed through the experience in order to release it for good. For in the face of fear, there is no love. My fear was before me. In the face of love, I did not know how to love myself wholly, and be me, while in soulful love. I acknowledged the truth in that my fear and my love cannot exist in the same space. I continued to choose love and was dedicated to doing the soulful work to make my way back to the purity of love that was burning in my heart.

Love saw me for all of the truths within me for I am those truths. And when I saw love looking at me so purely and seeing the truths within me, my mind took over. I then found myself experiencing the magical, soulful bliss alongside the mind's curiosity. I found my spiritual mind and my physical mind were navigating the same experiences differently. I had finally unearthed the space of the dichotomy within. The split sense of self was because I was straddled between worlds; suspended between dimensions.

While all this took place, my physical experiences played out much differently as a result of me trying to mindfully connect to love. As my soul bathed in the glorious love, my physical experiences were full of words and actions that were reflective of me *trying* to be love, be funny, be sensual, be vulnerable, for those were the very parts of me that manifested love before me. It was only through *trying* to be those parts of me, with the old patterns still energetically present, that I understood that it was the essence of me that manifested love, not my physical body. So just be love and love will continue to manifest. Let be and be me. I wanted to rest and just be, but I could feel my body still calibrating to the newness. I could feel my essence was still evolving. It was daunting and lonely yet joyous and liberating. It was awkward and vulnerable yet felt truthful and authentic. It felt sacred and honored. It felt soulful and pure.

After these experiences and acknowledging the many paths before me from which I could choose in reaction to the realizations within, before and of me, I knew the purity rested within and that I needed to continue to focus on me. The positives, the dreams, the joys, the purity of Divine Intention, and all that makes up the radiant essence of who I am. I allowed space to discern why it felt challenging to just let go and be, while trying to honor the emotional crests that would flood my being in the most magnificent spaces of self. I found myself in a space from which my wise soul watched my childish body play out an experience in order to catch up. With my sensual connection to energy, I honored that I was willing to relinquish mindful control in order to feel my way through every awkward moment. Knowing the truth and holding faith that there was intention behind all of it; everything. My intention. Divine Intention.

I began to feel energy flowing more and more within me. As if my spiritual wheels were finally able to rotate freely and approach sustainable alignment. I was committed to more self-love, so I started choosing differently. I chose differently with my creations now rooted in the expressions of love energy towards self and those around me, all driven by you. I chose differently in the noise allowed around me so I can experience you wholly. I chose differently in relationships because my heart is now one with yours. I chose differently in nourishment to my body for it needs to hold the vibration of love. I chose differently with everything. I was not always graceful nor successful, and still felt misunderstood, but there was more love for self, and therefore it felt like there was always understanding.

I had moved out of the family home, was working tremendously hard to settle my children as alternating week schedules began, I was working full time, monitoring my medical journey as it played out in the background and creating sacred space. All parts of my being felt a deep need to rest in the tranquil moments it all created. I knew I needed to continue to cultivate the new sense of serenity into in my new space of being. It was a beautiful gift as I witnessed my body respond to the new, very welcomed path to wellness. The more I honored and balanced self, and the more I weaned off medication, the more my body was capable of sustaining a healthy balance, especially that of my platelets. In the twenty plus years that I have had to manage the condition of my platelets, my counts have never risen when I wean off the medication. I was witnessing and thanking my body for responding so kindly to the efforts I had made.

In one particular experience, I sourced myself in strength, courage, and love, tried to temper my utter vulnerability and scheduled a massage. I had probably received two real back massages in my life, and definitely never a full body massage; modestly rejecting the qualification of the many massages received on my skin grafts all over my body. I even scheduled the appointment while trying to convince myself that I only wanted a back massage out of fear and vulnerability of my scars and my seemingly different physical body. Astonished even in myself that I had allowed such a grip on my spirit for so long.

I was saddened to experience my own timid vulnerability as I considered and vaguely attempted to talk my way into only a back massage. It was a ridiculous notion after after explaining the very energetic experiences that brought me before my masseuse, yet there it was. Shame tried to keep me from the experience. There was gentleness with my vulnerability as collectively we acknowledged the understanding, need and sacredness of the entire energy body, and the trust woven into the experience. As I unclothed my body, I was reminded of the many hands that had touched, healed, repaired, and mended my physical body out of love. I found myself again bare and exposed before the eyes of love.

I was blessed with the beautiful gifts of my kind and compassionate masseuse waiting with a heart wide open to help me navigate the new energy shifts I was experiencing. Although gifted with energy healing, it was not a practice that was offered to the public anymore. They found that there were too many people with wholes and gaps in their energy bodies leaving them drained and depleted as their energy was drawn out of them to fill the gaps in others. However, through our encounters they invited the energetic experience that I brought and organically offered the service. I invited the unknown experience if it would help stabilize my body.

They expressed feeling powerful energy flowing into and out of me, so much so that they had to disconnect and stimulate the sensations within their own body. They commented on the vibration of my body and how they could feel my body vibrating by touch, something that was never disclosed but was a reason for scheduling the appointment. They continued to invite the growth I brought into both of our experiences, while remaining compassionate to my eroding vulnerability. They were continuously guided to the precise spaces of resonance upon my body the more I released my energy; one appointment at a time. They in essence became a tuning fork; a tuning fork for the tuning fork of my body that aids in keeping the energetic pathways open and energy flowing. This was when I felt the need to find a Reiki Energy Master to join my treatment team.

I looked for other ways within the world to feel more comfortable as I stepped into more self-love. Although pushing my exposure in familiar uncomfortable ways, I looked to the offerings of the world through new perspectives for ways to integrate my truths into the world instead of the world upon me. I never realized I had allowed the misdirection in so many ways. The ones that I was able to identify relatively quickly were pretty fundamental to my every day navigation. I knew if I took action towards improving them my being would feel a sense of greater ease.

The first identified related to traveling and going through airport security. It did not necessarily hamper my air flight travels, it did however make it extremely uncomfortable, vulnerable, and often times embarrassing. The flight to D.C. highlighted the need to make a change and assess why I had not done so prior. As I tried not to dwell on the holds from the past, I moved forward to change by obtaining pre-check approval with the Transportation Security Administration (TSA) so that I do not have to experience what feels like trauma upon trauma albeit small and seemingly insignificant.

When traveling, I just want to get through security as quickly as possible, as does everyone. In addition to not wanting radiofrequency waves blasted at my body, I also have to take off my shoes off, which again everyone does, yet without them walking is very painful. It has always been this way. I am always wearing shoes if standing. I need my shoes to walk as comfortably as possible. Even so, it is my skin grafts that cause the hold-ups.

While walking through the full body scanner and images appear on the computerized silhouette that identify areas of detection, the agents look back and forth between me and my clothed body and their monitors. My skin grafts light up in the full body scan leaving agents left with only one option, ensure security. I approach them as they prepare to advise me with instructions and announcements of what is to come - a full body pat down, private areas included, metal wand scans, and palm swipes for traces of dangerous explosives. The long line of people waiting to be cleared also get held up in the fifteen-minute ordeal with an array of reactions – patient, distracted, curious, rushed, and frustrated alike. By showing myself some self-love and getting cleared by TSA and issued a Known Traveler Number, I get to bypass all of it and go through the simple metal detector, fully dressed and bags packed. I gift to myself I get to reopen every time I travel by flight.

It was interesting as I watched the world come to me the more I opened myself to the world. This one in particular. I always held a deep desire to return to the travel lifestyle of my youth pre-illness; dreams that felt harder and more vulnerable to achieve with this body. Yet suddenly the world was coming to me in unexpected ways – movies of personal voyages, access to global artisans and crafts, and other means that incited a sense of remembrance of explorations. There were memories of a past within new times that were somehow blossoming within and around me. The most profound were the memories that did not feel like my own yet were mystically released and caused an unexplainable dissipation of a sense of need to see the world. In some way it was calmed by the global energy I was syncing with and linked to you.

The second and third changes I made towards more comfortable daily living were more contingent on State laws. The first at the State level was getting approved with the Louisiana State Police

Department to have darker tent on my vehicle windows. Not only is it recommended by my Ophthalmologist to wear sunglasses and would satisfy the general photosensitivity cause for request, but my Primary Care Physician also agreed that my skin grafts and UV exposure increases my risk for skin cancer. With the doctor signed affidavit and approval from the State, I am able to legally drive more comfortably with dark tented windows, darker than legally allowed. I could drive at ease without concern of breaking the law. I felt confident discussing the circumstances before a judge, I just did not want it to get to that. That held true for the other series of choices I was making for the sake of comfort in this life.

The other also had to do with choices I was making that had legal consequences. This one, however, had much more grave consequences yet ones that I was willing to make for my bodily comfort. I had access to black market marijuana for years. I had used it intermittently for medicinal purposes yet struggled with the legal consequences, especially having children. I knew it was helping me in indescribable ways. Even now humanity is still struggling with the acceptance of natural substance healing, and has been ever since pharmaceutical companies entered the healing space. Deep within I had to find a way to reconcile my actions with the world. I monitored humanity's progression from the sidelines for years.

Then, in alignment with my journey, Louisiana finally signed into law the allowance of medicinal marijuana. There were a lot of restrictions, paths to follow, approvals to get and limited access to products, but it was legal. I could write a short story of the ridiculousness behind the journey to get there, comical yet not surprising. Once navigated and approved, it felt like I could finally provide my body with a substance that helps without being bound by a law. Now, me and the law were in sync and my body has access to natural medicine that my body responds to and well, whether topical or ingested in some way. I eventually felt my endocannabinoid system relax, and could work with unencumbered assistance in regulating critical bodily functions such as pain control, inflammatory and immune responses, and even eating. There were likely other benefits for PTSD yet I never saw myself in that way. I did however always feel the physical body pain relieved, balance against the steroids, and my stomach tempered to allow an appetite. My body was feeling more relaxed in ways I did not know it needed.

I also participated in several vibration bowl healing sessions and was gifted a session in a saltwater flotation tank. All of these, coupled with your physical world experiences around the world, were perfect and precise pieces in my experience to sync with global energy. I did not mindfully know it, but I could feel it taking place throughout my body. My mind made me frightened but was constantly at battle and overpowered by a greater force. I felt the energy between my internal and external worlds converging, transmuting, synchronizing, and harmonizing, eventually stabilizing into peace and love.

While all of these events transpired, my orchid plant remained beautiful and in full bloom. Then, in correlation with the experiences that left wanting to align with love, and while making the choices to realign my physical reality, my plant began to experience the same energetic shifts. Or were the shifts in the orchid causing me to shift? It felt like the energy that I was bringing into the space around me was altering my beautiful orchid plant. It appeared as though my orchid plant was syncing with me.

At the time I knew I was still not in full alignment as I felt every pulse of love you sent rippling through my heart. I was not surprised that my realignment was taking time. It was overwhelming in the awareness that it was the same global energy that I intentionally wanted to connect with; the same healing energy that saved me; the healing light of my meditations; the living light of Hildegard von Bingen; the unwavering love energy burning in my heart. Logically I understood that it was all one and the same, and my soul knew these truths deeply. I sensed that I was integrating these soulful truths into my heart so that my mind, soul, and heart would collectively be in sync with the magnitude of the energy and its forces contained wholly within my body.

Then one by one, as I worked to clear each emotional block, the beautiful and healthy orchid blooms began to fall off the plant's thriving stalk. They were perfectly healthy blooms now tainted with the less than perfect energy in its presence, preventing continued growth in their vibrant magnificent; just as I was unable to flourish in the less than pure energy within me. The blooms fell off in the fullness of their beauty to be found detached from their once nurturing life source. It was a very sad awareness yet completely understandable given the energy I knew I was purging and emitting into the spaces around me as everything in my experience was syncing with the purest of energy now dancing within me.

My co-worker friend and I had decided that since her plant and blooms were thriving in her space, that she would take mine and nurture it with the same love and light. Time proved that those efforts would have no impact on my plant. My friend later decided to take it to her home with the same nurturing intention to restore the balance within the plant for there was clearly still life, just no blooms. Those efforts also yielded no change for my orchid plant.

Once I was settled into my new space and I became more balanced within, I reclaimed *my* plant to bring to *my* home and to nurture it with *my* love. I did so for several months as I continued to follow the journey of my heart and soul. My heart had led me to love by the guidance of my soul, but there was still something impending for my fully integrated being. I knew I deeply wanted to know this life's intended purpose. It was the essence of wanting a sense of knowingness that I had lived with for so long. It was a knowingness of arriving when I saw you before me.

During this time, my orchid plant continued to change. It was not growing new blooms, but it was evolving and growing just as I was. It was as if my physical reality was being portrayed before me through my orchid plant and in the sacredness of divinity. As my courage and strength in spiritual growth continued to evolve, my orchid started growing a new spike. There was a new energy breathing life into a seemingly empty and barren plant. Just as my spirituality was breathing new life into me, a new spike began to grow in the opposite direction of the still very alive stalk. It was poetic that every aspect of my journey was mimicked in the growth of my orchid.

The new path before me was in a completely different direction and was being fueled by the foundation of life experiences at the source of who I am. The barren spike that held the original blooms now gone, just as I had realigned and cleared my path to make way for more abundance and beauty. I found it difficult at times to contain the excitement and overwhelming sensations within. It was the same sense of overwhelmingness in perfection that often brought about a silent level of pain; pain only because of the glorious magnitude being trapped by the inherent limitations of being human and the inability to articulate and express the experience in the fullness that it deserved.

The new spike was growing longer and stronger, eventually forming new buds that would bloom when they became full of vitality, just as I was nurturing every aspect of my being in order to bloom into the radiance of my being. There were seven buds reserving their space and maturing into the moment of a blossoming flower, just as I was growing in purity in the reflection of the Heavens above; mirroring the seven rays of God and the vibrational healing of virtue; the seven swords piercing the flaming heart of Mother Mary; the sacredness of the number seven as the foundation of God's word representing completeness and perfection in both the physical and in the spiritual; the same number seven associated with the creation of all things. Given my divinely blessed journey thus far, I knew deep within that the buds would bloom in divine timing and in sync with the profound spiritual growth that I felt was still flowing unto me.

Over the months that followed, in the slow progression that is life, the buds began to expose their strength and courage in the warmth and love of the golden sun. One at a time, each holding space for the other, the buds grew closer and closer to opening, reserving the time that they would begin exposing the vulnerable and authentic beauty possessed within. Just as I was nurturing the flowers within the garden of my heart and the vulnerability that accompanied the new sense of self, the buds continued to grow closer to blooming, as if they were about to burst in the excitable joy for life. Just as I remained patient with self, the orchid plant was patiently waiting for the perfect time and the buds remained as buds.

Each of the seven buds on the nurturing spike held tight as the they bathed in the daily sunlight. Again, representing the very essence of self as I remained reserved and vulnerable in the unknown spiritual world that awaited my acceptance and acquaintance. Timid in the light of day and protected within the cocoon of transformational growth.

Several months had passed and in my daily interactions with my plant that only seemed to swell with life yet not enough for the buds to blossom, I continued to believe deeply that the timing would be perfect just as the experiences along my path continued to be. The more time passed, and the more experiences unfolded before me, I continued to hold the deep sense that they would bloom alongside profound spiritual revelations. It seemed as if the slowed duration corresponded with the time needed to integrate the unexplainable magnitude of growth within.

My orchid plant sat on my kitchen windowsill as life continued to unfold. Around this time, I had planned a trip to visit a soul sister from high school. This is a soulful connection that is acknowledged yet rarely discussed in our physical experience. They know how I feel, and I know how they feel, yet for them it is uncomfortable to disclose the depths of our connectedness and the love that exists. I would be joining her, her parents whom I know well, and her partner for a weekend trip together at a football game. We spent three days together except for during the football game. I visited with her Mom, partner and friends that happened to be present at the local restaurant, while my friend and her father went to the game, all reconnecting as a group afterwards.

This trip quickly turned into a very spiritual experience for me, beginning with a moving piano performance by my friend's uncle who was a former Juilliard student. While visiting his home prior to weekend activities, he played a self-composed tribute in remembrance of 9/11 which set my soul soaring while tears effortlessly drowned my essence. It was the weekend of a football game between our alma maters, the Louisiana State University Tigers, and the Auburn University Tigers, so while everyone was getting physically drunk, I became spiritually drunk, soaring above the football excitement. It was perfect since I am not a huge football fan, but a tremendous fan of my friend, her family and of my evolving spirituality. Their beer goggles and my Angel eyes both experiencing the same moments in authentic love and joy.

While talking, laughing, interacting, enjoying, and socializing amongst new and old friends, the silent journey of my soul remained ever so present in the experiences in the unfolding. Just as they always had throughout my life, but this time it seemed integrated into the experiences like never before. I was simultaneously living and experiencing both the physical and spiritual spaces within me as every moment passed. It was a very new and interestingly exciting experience. Although a little overwhelming because the rate of spiritual growth still felt accelerated, but it was beautiful, invigorating, and joyful.

I uncovered so many truths within myself while on this trip that it felt as the final pieces were finally falling into place. It was on this trip that I realized that my déja vu moments had changed. Throughout life such moments always triggered a sense of remembrance; as if I was being reminded to remember something deep within. What used to serve as precise affirmations of where I was supposed to be, and doing what I was supposed to be doing, they had changed in precision and clarity. What used to be exact in every detail had changed to only contain portions of an exact portrayal. This weekend trip was full of a variety of altered versions.

I had never before been to Auburn, nor had I met any of the people that were sharing in the experience except that of my soul sister and her beautiful family. Sometimes it was the place and the events that were familiar, yet the people were different. Other times it was the spoken words and the place that were different, yet the people were very familiar. The ones that occurred the most, and were the most profound, were the familiar people in familiar places with almost familiar statements yet not exact; the difference being in specific statements that were alarmingly unfitting to the circumstance, yet perfect for that of my inner journey. I was inwardly aware of everything, and many things did not make sense, but I had surrendered to the unfolding for there were divine messages being heard and seen within everything. It felt like I was becoming aware of when I had chosen differently in prior lifetimes. It felt as if I instantly knew where I had become stuck in those lifetimes and what it was that kept me coming back into the physical human experience for lessons of love to be learned. It was on this trip that I walked into the knowingness that this will be my last lifetime provided I am able to recalibrate back to the purity of Divine Love and fulfill my Divine Intention.

I knew I was in alignment with Divine Intention, and it would be the choices of free will to follow. I knew my choices brought all of this forward into my experiences and knew I always chose in love. It was on this trip that the premonition of Divine Love connected me to lifetimes where the unevolved love had been shared with another and why we both had returned to the illusion; to bridge the differences, heal our hearts and reunite in unconditional love. I was as if the trip to Auburn in the physical world corresponded with a trip of my soul throughout the infinite time and space continuums within which it is sourced. It was unexplainable with the words that my lips were incapable of expressing yet flowed from my soul within the infinite energy of vibrational thoughts and awareness.

I left the weekend driving in six hours of silent reflection and concluded that the essence of self that had been discovered could only be described as walking into my Divinity. I didn't know how else to describe it. It was like I walked into the knowingness of where I come from, who I am, and my life's Divine Intention. It was so much more than favorite color, passions, and desires. I am speaking of the core energetic essence of my existence, the energetic contracts of my soul, the truths in my beliefs in this life experience and in love, and the glory that follows when you have been touched by and embody the abundant light of universal love energy.

It made sense as to why so many things that had been perceived as hard, were now easy. It explained why there was a sense of soulful knowing in how to navigate life situations. It made sense as to why everything seemed like a memory, even when it was experienced for the first time, or even through the life of another. It made sense as to why there was an inherent wisdom that came with the discoveries along the way. It made sense as to who I am. It all made sense because I am one with Universal Energy, God, and the God consciousness. I had either done the work in prior lives or was connected to infinite wisdom of the collective, or both. I was in a space of newness, and connected with the depths of my soul in a way that surpassed any prior lifetime. It was a growth that restored the connection back to the Heavens never before achieved, anchoring Divine Love within the earthly experience as intended through the creation of me. It was all a beautiful blessing of discovery to my soul.

I returned from my trip knowing that not choosing my divinity was the choice in prior lives that prevented the fulfillment of Divine Intention to anchor spiritual love in the physical experience; bringing the Heavens to the Earth, and the Earth to the Heavens; anchoring Divine Love by bridging the seemingly differences that exist within humanity and restoring love to mankind. The most magnificent awareness was that the intention is fulfilled by just *being* me; by *being* the sacred love now embodied within. Just as I knew that I had never chosen my divinity in prior lives, I knew that I would succeed in this lifetime and by doing so it would be my last. Every moment and everything from throughout my life made sense. When I say everything, I mean everything. EVERYTHING. Everything most certainly does have meaning. Divine meaning in the masterpiece of Creation. The Creation of Love. After almost thirty years I could finally feel breaths of meaning.

Upon my return home, I quickly peaked at my orchid to find the buds still holding their space and waiting to bloom. As I settled into the evening with my children, I rested into the night feeling as if I was finally home; home within myself and at peace again. It was the same sense of peace as before I started writing this book and my heart and soul unraveled my reality. The difference was that there was a fullness within; there was a new warmth within my heart that was sourced in Divine Love. There was a spiritual strength that was growing with every day the newness was navigated. There was an excitement in the unfolding. There was tremendous love and joy blossoming in the garden within me. There was a celebration in the perfection in all that is.

All of these were truths even though I was like a newborn child trying to stabilize my new steps along my walk. I was sloppy and clumsy and was repeatedly falling many, many times along the way but I was determined more than ever to continue on the path. For although I was home and believed it to be so, I had to honor that my mind and heart were not yet operating at the same pace. My heart was still healing, and it took much longer for me to *feel* the truth that my soul and mind had found rest. I patiently waited for my heart to integrate the truths.

The following morning before getting out of bed, I read my weekly spiritual newsletter that over the prior year continued to yield messages of affirmation in my alignment versus guidance on how to achieve it. I read the newsletter and the opening paragraph started with the phrase,

> "...this is where you went wrong last time..." and that "it is so important to embrace your own Divinity." - © 2017 Simone Matthews

I was amazed and found tremendous peace in my inner work now complimented in the physical. It was another affirmation of the truths I had just walked into the day prior after concluding the spiritual and self-illuminating trip with members of my soul family. Although I was still in a space of being amazed by divinity when it was so unexplainably perfect and precise, I could feel that my reactions were changing. As I continued to walk into these experiences the amazement was slowly being transformed into acceptance of the truths in divinity.

When I got out of bed that morning, before waking my children in preparation for school, I walked into the kitchen and stood before my orchid plant. Amazed for the second time that morning, I found that the first of the seven blooms had fully opened throughout the night, and I found myself before a single, beautifully full orchid bloom. It felt as though I was illuminating into the mystical seven rays of divinity, completing my rainbow of seven colors, one bloom, one color at a time. It sensed I had begun the final steps and was concluding my journey home; nearly complete in the achievement of perfection in both the physical and spiritual spaces within further signified by the sacred seven buds, now six remaining to bloom. I was proud of the inner work completed and the alignment with the essence of a Spiritual Warrior Poet I was beginning to feel within. It was magnificently radiant in the light of the morning dawn, and in the bright white purity of the single bloom's essence.

I stood before my orchid and wept in deep gratitude for I knew deeply, even more than before, that the remaining buds would begin to open in divine timing. And they did as I slowly embraced my own divinity. I found myself throughout many moments of the day pausing in believable disbelief in what had occurred, often ending with weeping tears of gratitude. They were beautiful tears of purity, washing my soul clean in the truths of a faith I had held throughout my life now connected deeply to my heart and soul. It was the greatest gift yet received along the path to wholeness.

Several days later I was speaking to my Angel, the very one that had sent the quote from Hildegard von Bingen weeks before receiving the orchid plant from my soul sister. I shared the continued story of my orchid plant, my spiritual trip and settling into my divinity. After portraying the sequence of events that spanned over nine months, I concluded with the first bud blooming in magnificence throughout the night, discovered on Monday morning at the break of dawn. With a very confident and unwavering response they calmly stated,

> **"Of course, it would bloom when it did. It is befitting that it would bloom on Monday.**

I was intrigued by the statement as I sensed there was a deeper meaning embedded within that I was eager to discover. Without pause I inquired as to why Monday was a befitting day for my orchid to bloom. Again, to my amazement, they proclaimed,

> "Because September 17th is the Feast of Hildegard von Bingen. That is how Divinity works."

I found it overwhelming to accept that there was no understanding to be gained in how it could be so. It was yet another perfect culmination of physical world events exposing the truths in Divinity. The orchid that had been gifted to me immediately after being introduced to Hildegard von Bingen whom emphasized that the path to becoming a blooming orchid is achieved through good intentions. I was mesmerized by the manifested experiences to sync with global energy, the Divine Love found sourced within my heart, the collective human heart, and the heart of the universe. I was mostly mystified by all of the growth endured in my experiences found mirrored in the growth of my plant. All of the beautiful and unexplainable events were so perfectly interconnected that the final bud opened on the same day that is reserved within the Catholic religion as the day of celebration of her divinity and as a Doctor of the Church.

Again, I was left weeping in deep gratitude, and was tremendously humbled as it was within that precise moment that I experienced the soulful and energetic transition from **believing** into a **deep knowing** that it is within divinity that the magic of life occurs; it is within the heart of the universe, and that of God from which the physical world is co-created into a joyous life experience. I had experienced the very magic throughout my life, but it was intermittent, inconsistent, and lacked a trust in knowing these spiritual truths. It was in that precise moment that I fully surrendered to the mystifying mysticism of universal interconnectedness that had been at the source of every prayer and intention ever casted, even in the unknowingness of my beliefs.

In the many months spent removing every aspect of a jaded self to get to core of who I am, I found myself in the heart of universe. The very center from which I stood before Einstein. I found that I was never broken, nor lost, but my heart and mind were wounded from the perceived disconnect with my Source. I had just walked nine months into the mystical and physical manifestations of the divine wonders of the universe to find myself doing the best I could to be one with myself, and to let that be enough. Each bud busted wide open with every breath I took for myself.

Divinity was exposed yet again as the seventh bud opened into full bloom during the night after expressing my deep and dear gratitude. Embodying sacred geometry with the seventh bloom signifying perfection. There was a sense of completeness in both the physical and the spiritual realms. I knew I was finally home as I finally felt it within self, as it should be; love manifested and manifesting love.

The final awareness that graced my essence was when I found energy itself before me, represented in its sacred trifecta brilliance. The spiritual energy and divine presence that had been most present throughout the journey back to wholeness were that of my Mom, my Angel, their late partner Hildegard, and that of Hildegard von Bingen, of which both Hildegards were brought into my experience through my Angel. The truth before me was...

M = Mom

C = The first letter of my Angel's physical life name.

Hildegard **Squared** = two Hildegards both brought into my experience by **C**.

M C ^{2}

Energy itself.

Imagine the sense of surprise encountered when I revisited the text of Hildegard von Bingen that was the impetus of everything and discovered that it never mentioned the word orchid at all. Instead, it was the blossoming orchards that were used to reference the spiritual growth blossoming within us all. Even so, to keep the balance with divinity, I rejoiced discovering her connection to orchid flowers through other experiences and representations of her. Through the misunderstanding, she taught me how to find my own connection, and that I will indeed be a co-creator in the experience.

41

Understanding Love, My Light Language

I knew I needed to uncover my heart. It felt like my passionate love for you needed to be set free from within the confines of the physical body. By tilting perspectives through my spiritual senses, I discovered that an unbeknown shield had been erected around my heart. Furthermore, as I looked within with intention to heal my way to you, I unknowingly opened my heart wide open, only to experience the instant and uncontrollable retraction back behind the shield once before your eyes of love.

I was confused and saddened by my inability to stop my heart from shutting closed. More so embarrassed and vulnerable in how my humanness responded to the experiences. It was as if every silently judged observation within humanity made its way out through uncontrollable expressions. Despite knowing the truth in the illusions, and that our hearts beat as one, it was still hard to trust that your humanness knew the same. The difference was that this time I was aware unlike in my youth. This time I understood how to make my way to you.

Even with the awareness, my heart remained the one space of me that I was not connected to intimately and sensually. It was a humbling surprise of shame when I learned I was so deeply afraid of real love. It was the one space of me that I held shielded in the depths within, and I found it was primarily out of fear and doubt over my physical body. It was the one space of me that became buried by the human experience, so much so, that the light in my heart was no longer shining bright enough to guide me through my days in peace.

The only truth I knew to hold about understanding was to understand myself completely. It felt like I had spent my life trying to understand the various parts of me. It was as if they all had a different response and storyline to tell. This often left me feeling misunderstood in my intention to understand. Generally, the conundrum presented outwards as thoughtfully composed intentional questions, whereas inwardly was presented as a myriad of never-ending questions about anything and everything to self and my parts.

First, I felt it with others, as if understanding was perceived as a mindful action that I was choosing to engage with a seeking mind that was detrimental to my happiness. I knew that was not my truth within, albeit admittingly my footing would wobble and at times cause my mind to seek, especially when your humanness challenged my sense of knowing while discovering the truth in my sensing abilities.

In the moments of choosing to understand my reality, I could sense when I would get looped in a thought. I would see it flapping in circles like a finished movie paying from a vintage film reel. The tension that the looping image created was a sensation around and throughout the brain as a humbling reminder of our humanity, the dreaded headache. Instead of medicating with pain relievers, I chose to connect to your love between our human hearts and allow the mind to rest. I trusted in the calm that would surface by yielding to my heart as the compass of my soul, and I knew my soul would never mislead me in the physical experience, especially if I followed your love. It felt like my soul was an ancient teacher that knew exactly what to do. My humanness on the other hand had a lot of growing to experience.

Although I tried to not let my mind guide my soul along my walk, it was a very intended and mindful practice of keeping it at bay, and I worked hard at not allowing ego to rule out of fear. It felt normal given my experiences. There had been plenty of opportunities for fear to overrule. It was an intended practice ever since fear made itself known in my youth. During my transformational period, I found myself wanting to choose differently. So, I began acting out of intention to change that practice. I chose differently whenever there was a choice to realign with love. I wanted my mind to rest. I believed life should be easy. I knew that love was easy. I deeply believed that nothing in this life would ever be harder that what I had already experienced and I wanted to rest in that truth. Deep within I knew I was growing into something unique and special that would flip my reality into the truths within.

It was the lack of understanding during certain experiences that at times prevented my mouth from opening or stunting my ability to articulate clearly when attempts were made to speak the multi-dimension changes within; divinely stopping the unnecessary expression as a reminder to let it all just be. Almost as if my voice was withdrawn yet not by me. I was acutely aware that I sometimes became robotic, flopping from realm to realm in response to those around me. The struggle was that I had not yet learned that I was flopping between realms. It just felt like I was bouncing back and forth between something and vibrating within boundaries. I felt like I never understood how to operate the physical body with ease, especially amongst the presence of others. I have felt this incongruency for all my adult lived life. I felt it was an inescapable outcome given what my body had experienced.

Somehow, I continuously fumbled in the presence of your sacred love only to learn that it was due to my own lack of understanding in my spiritual strength, my meta-physical space of existence, and the powerful example of our collective similarities. I didn't understand who I was, that was until you manifested before me, a creation of me, me before me, mirroring all that I am while simply being you. I simply wanted to be me yet there were no words to break the silence while my heart experienced a burning love.

I knew I held a deep desire to understand certain aspects of my life experiences. As I walked through experiences, I could feel the energetic waves ripple through my head and then flow down into my heart. When this occurred, I was very aware that my mind space was holding and utilizing energy differently. I found myself seeking understanding of what had transpired because I felt everything in my head space change. I found myself eager to understand the newness.

I could feel different spaces within the physical structure itself, as if it was utilizing different resources to access the same spaces. It felt lighter and calmer within the deep recesses that once played the memories of my past, maps of the present, and projections of the future, now still shots still there if needed for retrieval. Unfamiliar yet beautifully peaceful and at ease. My mind felt empty, quiet, and wise, while somehow grounded by an intellect of the soul. It was a new navigation with a new mind being led by my new heart. It was then that I felt the difference in sensation when I would accidentally slip into egocentric living, letting my mind try to lead the way and seek out understanding; failing to honor who I am and allow wisdom to float into knowing from my soul.

When I have the time and space of allowance, in the quietness of my mind, the understanding that comes from wisdom floats to the surface, defying gravity by floating upward into my mind from the depths of my soul. There is always the moment of awareness in truth and a deep sense of knowingness, despite not always understanding the source of knowing. It had unknowingly developed into a tool of discernment in how to move forward; whether or not there is a need or opportunity to choose differently. This was the only practice I have known to walk and believed it to be a part of the human experience.

When my truths within were uncovered, the truths and understanding in humanity were also revealed. While communing with your love and the expressions through art, my heart quietly heard through wisdom. I understood how and why heart centered living had been replaced with mind-driven focus as a means to navigate the physical experience. I saw how in doing so creates distance between our hearts. I understood that emotional, intimate, and sensual living had become taboo and a sign of weakness and sin, yet without them we create powerless human robots living the life of, and for others. I understood how any degree of perceived trauma almost instantly shields the heart out of protection. I saw how not knowing a shield is present protects the heart from enduring more pain and suffering albeit triggering a simultaneous forfeiture of the true sentiments within. The second time around I saw my shield close up as if in slow motion. It was then that I learned that my heart had lived behind a shield while my light energy had remained wide open throughout life, unprotected while emitting and absorbing energy along the way. A strange dichotomy to feel a closed off heart with energy wide open and suspended between the pull.

I saw how the heart balances the worlds, yet it is the emotions that clear the pathway. When the heart is shielded, we become emotionally incapable of living our true self, for our highest good, and from the love sourced in our collective human heart. Instead, we are taught to conceptualize and intellectualize emotions while becoming numb to the sensual experience there is to live in this life. We find ourselves navigating illusions created by everyone and yearning a love that will shatter them all. Instead of celebrating and enjoying the juiciness of life, humanity is fueling the disconnect between the true source of our existence as unique souls in sacred physical vessels, traversing the physical plane for a brief moment in eternity. I understood how light gets transformed into dark. More importantly how I am of light designed to be a beacon in the dark.

At times I was hastily looking for validation that the energetic shifts, the connection to energy, the life spent ignoring and fearing the spirits around me now invited in for healing were real experiences. Everything made sense and fell into place, the memories, the visions, the premonitions, the prophecies, and manifestations alike. I knew it was real merely because I am here and alive. I wanted it to be real because it was the only reality I knew. I dreamed it to be real, and even so, I needed my physical senses stimulated in such a way to integrate the truths my soul was teaching me. My ears needed to hear validation in order for my body to undergo the same vibrational experience, so the realms could merge into one. Seeing your humanness, and experiencing your voice, touch, and smell did the same. I could taste the sweetness of love.

As I struggled to find my words, and my body told a story of its own, I settled in the truth that a voice has many forms of expression. Finding my voice in only spoken words proved to not be needed, nor worth my energy. I was rediscovering my sensual being and through a tilted perspective uncovered the untold sensual story of my body. I held my truth within and had to grow strength in knowing that was all that mattered in any moment of engagement, especially when I found few could hold space to grow me. I have always held the strength within but felt compromised when trying to stand in my truth before others.

As I worked to balance my strength between my internal and external worlds, certain moments would unfold in unexpected ways that I would then find myself unable to scurry a reaction. Most times I replied hastily, fumbling a response causing me to act out of alignment with the voice of my soul. I had to practice slowing down and allowing more time to honor the slower, more sensual processing that my being authentically experiences and enjoys. I had to learn that when I had faith, the understanding would come with grace as long as my mind remained at ease. Seeking understanding is what caused misalignment. Seeking understanding inferred I held fear. Seeking to understand out of fear implied I did not hold the faith that grounded my authentic self. In moments when I lacked faith, I became misaligned with love. For without faith there is no love.

I found that my truth was that my voice had not yet finished evolving. The voice to express my soul was still expanding and morphing into its unique language. It was a growth into a voice that I was painfully aware of ever since I awoke from the coma. A voice yearning to be set free as it pushed me through to the next phases of my physical human experience of soul embodied navigation. It was pushing me through to love. It was pushing me closer to you.

As I was learning and realizing that I never lost my voice, trying to speak my truths seemed less important. I had always struggled with the mere limiting labels that words themselves become and was often disgraced by the carelessness of their use when spoken from the lips around me. I myself became sloppy with words as I tried to live through experiences while navigating, coordinating, and integrating newness into every aspect of my physical and meta-physical beings. Something that I had to find the strength, courage, and love within to swallow my physical world pride and keep on moving with the purity of my soul's intention to serve our collective highest good.

I had seemingly lived in silence, and my awkward behaviors would often take over when I no longer felt grounded in my navigation. As if the actions and words to express my authentic self would lower my body's vibration as it personally felt and sounded like attempts to convince others of something no matter the topic. Unsure of what there was to convince. My existence? My journey? My reality? My soul? My truths? My opinions? For what? To pass time playing into the illusions being created for a myriad of reasons? While trying to reconcile all this, I was led through experiences that I was unsure how to navigate. The most vulnerable were those in the presence of love; the only space that truly mattered within. Once before the eyes of love, I was exposed to the meaning and the purpose of what my humanness needed from me. Through my spiritual lens I could see how I had failed in the past.

Among many things, I was forced to acknowledge that being sensitive to those around me often times caused me to navigate in silence, to hold space for their being to experience life in whichever means they were choosing to do so. I chose to be a part of allowance, instead of being the voice of another opinion, in a world full of them in mindful opposition of each other. I chose silent observance and compassion over trying to stand for something in the game of life. Deep within it was the passion for love that held the strongest voice; a voice designed for you. My silence was waiting for the time and space for my words to flow so they could dance within your being.

When I integrated the truth of my heart, I realized that my life in silent navigation was in graceful acceptance, that I knowingly made and honor, and I realized that I had never lost my voice at all. There were many, many times I spoke my true voice; perhaps too boldly to be taken seriously. Even more patronizing and belittling were the notions that I was uninformed, uneducated, less than or inherently lacked something others expected me to hold. I generally felt annoyed that I was unable to summarize the universe within me into spoken dialogue that exposed the vastness.

The notion of losing my voice was a narrative of the collective, and not of me at all. The idea of losing my voice was merely the space to which my mind had led me; an overreaching attempt of sabotage to prevent me from discovering the truths behind my existence. My heart held every word needed for expression. I held trust in knowing that when it was time for me to understand out of the intention of love, I would know, and my soul would have its voice. Honoring every sacred representation in the physical experience continued to guide me to the bliss in my heart. Step by step, I continued to walk into the understanding of what it was I was supposed to learn.

Once I embraced that my voice was still evolving, the universe magically presented me with opportunities to discover elements of my true voice. I was journeyed to and through experiences that connected me to various elements that had been woven into the energetic cloth of my soul. Through the guidance of my Mom, I was led to a community through which her voice had evolved. In the moments of my experiences, I felt gratitude for her growth as it was the groundwork for my entry. I was embraced by a community of like-minded and like-gifted individuals that bridged the gap between my Mom and me; between me and myself; between myself and the spirit energy around me; between me and a God; any God; hopefully my God; between me and you.

It was within this community of individuals that I was exposed to the angelic tones of light language; sounds similar to when someone speaks in tongues. I was exposed to opportunities to connect within and identify and release remnants of illusions clouding my connections to spirit energy. With only intentions to follow where experiences of love were leading me in order to stop my body from vibrating, I allowed myself to walk through the discovery of prior lives which began the release of unbeknown karmic energy buried deep within. In the safe space of this community, I also experienced events that highlighted the susceptibility of the human psyche to take on the ideals of others when boundaries are not maintained, especially my own as a hypersensitive being. The experiences shined a light on just how sensitive I truly am beyond my physical body and senses, and into the worlds that exist beyond.

All of the experiences were a beautiful gift to the voice of my soul, primarily that of the light language. I found I became hypnotized by the sounds of the label-less language and was mystified as to how my soul rested in the sweet sounds, almost an innate knowing of what was being transmitted. My mind was captivated by the sounds that soothed my soul while my heart began to trust in the maturation of its own voice underway. I knew in those moments of the experience that I was hearing the authentic language of my true voice; vibrations of color projected into my heart as my humanness was paralyzed in a state of serenity. I saw a collective of light beings calling out for me across the abyss, celebrating that I had found my way and motioning me to come closer.

As I continued on the journey that proved to still be underway, I had to find a different way of navigating. Everything was new and changing in unfamiliar energetic ways. By this time my mind was exhausted and desperate to release and let go yet there was a force still holding it back. Part of the practice of surrenderance was to accept whatever was delivered unto me. This was always easy to do until I met you, manifested into my physical experience, furthermore, connected to my human heart. There was a force on my body that I could not release.

Standing before your love exposed every possible contradictory dichotomy that existed within my human vessel; the good, the bad and every minute space in between. It was when my heart energy united with yours that I realized that I lived in a very non-human space of existence while creating a very human experience, one that did not ground my soul. The discovery was that it was a mindful creation of what I thought it was supposed to be. The light that was casted upon my humanness revealed gut wrenching and shameful shadows, when at my core I aspired to only emit balanced love and light.

It was your love that allowed me to see who I really am, and exposed the choice to step into my truth, or not. It was your love that exposed that it was within the meta-physical realm that I had always lived, progressively dancing with more spirits throughout my entire life. It was your love that taught me I had left my body behind and needed to retrieve it in order to ascend back wholly. Your love presented me with an opportunity to bridge my reality into this human experience. It was your love that guided me to Earth, grounded me as I journeyed back home to self, and patiently waited until I returned to our unity within both planes of existence. It was your love that guided me through the experiences that gave me a language of my own to bridge me to my reality, my light language.

As the days passed, it became easier to follow the images that my soul was projecting in my mind versus my mind trying to interpret them into something that proved to be different. The more I quieted my inner and outer worlds, the more I saw with clarity all that I needed to know in my humanness to trust in the events to come. It felt like my mind was finally able to rest as my soul took back control over my vessel. All of which was now beautifully connected to your love on Earth. All I had to do was follow. All I had to do was follow love. All my heart knew how to do was follow your love being led by the compass of my heart. I had to learn how to feel my own heart in order to clearly follow yours. Since your radiant white light was all I could see, and my body continued to vibrate, I allowed the experiences to teach me about who I am while in alignment with both. Nervous, anxious, and overwhelmed, I carried on with only an unexplainable meta-physical love that felt like it was magnetizing and tuning me throughout the universe. My perception of time and space continued to be defied with every breath.

The more I looked within, the more the physical world began to display a language, as if it was responding in kind to my journey within. I had noticed this happening in small experiences and on a much smaller scale throughout life, and I used to coin these as coincidences or serendipitous occurrences that generally ended with a lingering sense of wonderment. This time it finally felt in proportion with the powerful force within on the cusp of freedom. Even so, during the process of writing this book, the frequency, the intensity, the precision of everything was all very alarming to my human self, frightening at times. It was all very new and different as I grew more authentically connected to what was unfolding, leaving behind the façades and mindful assertions of yesteryears. This was when finding my voice took its true meaning. This is when I found out who I really am, and the truths of my infinite potential.

There came a point when my mind felt as though it understood enough to be quieted in peace; forever. It was as if every inquiry I had ever casted into the abyss about the journey of my soul as a human had been answered. There was a sense of relief when I was taught that I could chose differently within what I had always perceived to be a part of who I am, and how my mind was designed to work. It was relaxing to know it was by choice to understand and I could choose differently. I most certainly wanted to release the type of life experience that caused me to walk with a desire to understand; it felt like a life of waiting once there was a comparison. I would much rather just instinctively rest in truths, with understanding or not, and with acceptance of what shall be. If I changed that sole intention to understand, it would change the way I experienced life. I felt inspired to choose differently to see how it changed in the experience.

There was a mental tightness that was released once I was able to let go of the desire to understand. Living became more fluid, bountiful, and easier to navigate, with the most surprising gain being that I was able to rest in the abundance of memories, knowledge, and inherent understanding of many things that are innate to my being.

It was one of the greatest mysteries of self, to self, and drove much of my desire to understand the fascinating world within which we live while being human. It had felt like everything uncovered throughout life was a long-lost memory to my humanness refreshed to enjoy anew. The more I understood myself in this world and the quieter my mind became, I was able to connect to your love, feel your love energy pulling me through the universe, flowing me with the river of infinite wisdom so that I could find the words to express my love, my light language.

42

The Realms of Existence

When I looked through my meta-physical eyes, I saw and felt us as one, with a light chord splitting and descending into your human body, flowing out of your human heart and into mine, and pulling me down into my body here on Earth. A triangle of light.

When I looked through my physical eyes, I saw the light of our souls shining through our human bodies, blinding me from seeing our humanness while concurrently vibrating into the fluidity with that of which we both exist. A prism dispersing light into rainbows.

I tried for many hours to find those words. The words that describe what I was feeling and seeing. It was only through meta-physical experiences that I found the thread that strung the words together into what now seems so simplistic. I desperately wanted my body to stop vibrating so that I could enjoy the experiences that were before me as I discovered who I really am while connected to love. I wanted to be done with the journey for it felt like my heart had finally arrived at the place it had dreamed of being, not just in this life but for eternity; connected to yours.

I recognized throughout the journey of self-discovery that the world did not have what I needed to convalesce after my illness. The language, the actions, the support did not exist beyond my profound recovery, perplexed medical professionals, my human abilities, and my meta-physical state of being. Hidden within history were many scientists that experienced alternate worlds, yet their truths never intertwined with the western medicine and modern science that saved my physical being. Even so, almost thirty years later, science is still evolving into acceptance and exploration in the possibility of life beyond our human existence. I suppose my youthful entry into alternate dimensions occurred in such a way that I did not recognize that was where I landed. I had not yet grown into my humanness in life towards embodied ascension.

Instead, I was disembodied, walking a life towards descending into embodiment. There were no depictions of what to expect in a life experience after surviving death and dancing closely throughout life; each layer in the veil of ascension being shed from my humanness. It took many decades to realize that the experiences with death left me dancing within a world no one could see. Throughout life, everything felt like a vortex, clouding my visibility into the external world around me while my inner world depicted a much different reality. I knew I was growing into a language that would decipher what was within. I had traversed the world growing into the very moments before me.

As I continued to journey through life to the source of who I am, I encountered much of the same; a world that did not have a language for the space within which I existed. If there was a language, I had not yet encountered it, and the more I journeyed through the experiences, I wondered if it was because no one else had the language to express it either. I felt a deep pull that finding my voice was part of my purpose of adding to the perspectives of our existence.

I went into the journey with a lot grounding me from this life experience. I was extremely cognoscente of my bashful avoidance to engage in discussions centered in and around religion, and it was not until I allowed myself to explore my own sense of self that I now thoroughly enjoy those centered in and around spirituality and the expansive universe within which we live. To me there is a deeply felt distinction. I am not religious, but I am very spiritual. Even so, most of my beliefs were anchored in the teachings of Christianity and the Roman Catholic Church.

I believe in Mary's immaculate conception, Her blessed son Jesus Christ and His life journey, the word of God and all the prodigious teachings that guide many of today. I also believe in the Holy Spirit, the Holy Trinity, and the sanctity of what walking a life of Christ is intended to be and represent. I hold sacred my protected connection to God, my Angels and Spirits of past, present, and future, and hold gratitude for the gentle reminders that we are all indeed real in this experience of life.

Concurrently, I believe in Siddhartha Gautama, the Buddha, and that the path to peace is through mental discipline and the journey to self-enlightenment, all which is strengthened with a deeply shared Hindu belief that the nature of the human experience is not confined to the body and/or the mind, yet extends beyond both and integrates the spirit, or the light of God within our soul. I believe that we are all this divine spirit full of peace, joy, and love, and that refining the mind and senses allows us to feel this truth and experience this divinity within and without. It was not until after my soul had a sense of intended fulfillment that my walk led me to the depths of the Hindu Jnana Yoga practice depicting the very journey I had walked of self-questioning, reflection, and conscious illumination.

I believe in metaphysics, the laws of the universe, predominately those supported by Pythagoras and Einstein, and Sacred Geometry as evidenced in nature through the Fibonacci Sequence. I respect and appreciate the philosophical, psychological, sociological, and scientific intermingling of life experiences that create the human condition, in which we then find ourselves turning outward with the faith that there is something bigger and greater than us.

I found tremendous healing power behind the vibrational frequencies of the original Solfège Scale at the source of Gregorian chants, and experienced this beautiful Earth provide so many natural healing resources such as nourishment for our bodies, oils, herbs, crystals, and its place in the astrological space within this universe, not only for medicinal healing, but perhaps more in spiritual healing. I honor and hold tremendous gratitude for the Gods sourced all over the world for guiding souls to the One, and I remain open to weave the truths in pedagogical experiences into my spiritual cloth during my earth walk. We are all on a journey in a human experience, and everyone, everywhere is a beautiful example of the unique journey that we all walk, and the means that have and continue to support us along the way. The notion provides an opportunity to pause and truly reflect upon the means by which we journey throughout each day.

In the very intense moments before me, a connection with my sense of divine self had my undivided attention. It was an authentic and organic presence within and was in the forefront of every breath. The eclectic designs and intricate details of my spiritual fabric illuminated the unconditional sourced love, the unexplainable beauty and indescribable mysticism of this universe. I found myself connecting to the energetic, magnetic, and magical forces of the universe that are so vast and encompassing that it is challenging within my humanness to accept a label or categorization; in doing so simultaneously feels as though such an act dishonors the purity of intended essence.

I sat many nights quietly with the sacred truth that we are all on a journey and we all believe in something. Whether it is a God, or many, the Divine Universe, a Magical Manifestor, or an Orchid plant. I found myself for many years only believing in myself. Even the Atheist believes in something; they believe there is no God. I honor and celebrate the numerous and magnificent spiritual, energetic, and cosmic forces that have guided humanity since eternity. In time I found more comfort within to refer to the infinite capacities I was experiencing as only the deliverance from a God; surrendering to a label I had allowed to block the receipt of universal magnificence.

Your God, my God, one God, many Gods, we are all from the same essence and that is love. For the first time I felt connected to the truth in love, exposing the illusions around the stories of love within my reality. I wanted to live the truth that we are here to be love. I wanted to act in the truth that we are here to give love. I wanted to be healed by the truth that we are here to receive love. We are here to simply love. When there is love, there is understanding in the time of darkness. When there is understanding, there is compassion for the hurting heart. When there is compassion, there is empathy for the seemingly differences amongst us. When there is empathy, there is harmony within humanity.

I held onto all these sentiments in my heart while realizing that I am no different, and we are all light beings, energy vibrating to form matter, light dispersed from our true home in the energetic cosmos of the Universe, embodied temporarily while here on Earth. My body felt Einstein's truth that we are all interchangeable energy vortex's forming physical matter. I very much lived Carl Jung's examples of understanding and healing the human psyche. My heart rejoiced in Shakespeare's unyielding love for another and felt sorrow in Sartre's existentialist hell of societal and self-imposed constructs.

At our core we are the Apollo's and Artemis' of this Olympiad experience, and most profoundly, we are Socrates within asking questions to uncover our truths, and that of this mystical existence. I deeply felt the truth that we are the very fruit of the Earth from which we nurture and grow, within ourselves and into the world around us. And somehow as we exist in a lifetime as who we are, we are concurrently of those that have come before us and of those that will come after us. I felt the interconnectedness throughout every cell of my body as it found its space in the universe yet stifled by an inability to express it as my own.

Deep within I knew I was not done because I could feel it. I knew my body would eventually come to a rest and it clearly had something to do with my soul being grounded to this Earth. Until then, I had to shamefully walk a messy human journey as my parts fell further apart to rebuild back into wholeness. I could feel that I was vibrating my way through the universe to be where I needed to be, before you in my authenticity. You were escorting me with the love and light of your human heart. Even though you were everywhere it was through your human heart that I was grounded while I completed the journeyed throughout the universe. I had to carry on, not only to make the journey have meaning, but also to live comfortably in my body. My body was clearly finding its way, and all my parts were falling into your love found nestled in my heart.

I continued to experience a swelling energy around and within me that was constantly seeking to dance with my body. It was an energy that was flowing into my body from you, through the space of your meta-physical existence, and through your human heart, colliding in my heart space and purging my body clean. When it entered my body through my heart, it flushed my cells of all energetic vibrations that were not in harmony with the purity of your love. When it entered me from beyond, my vibration heightened, swelling with intensity until I found its outlet. Many times, the pressure valve was only released when my humanness could express my love to, and for you, between our hearts.

The spaces in between were filled with artistic creations and self-nurturing. Since none of my parts were in alignment, I fumbled on my words, my emotional intelligence was skewed, and my body was awkwardly engaged in unintentional motions not representative of who I have chosen to be in this life. It took many days, months, even years for your light to wash my cells energetically clean. Until then, I felt foreign in my body as it broke free and played out all the illusions around love that had been programmed into my cells.

My human actions and words were utterly sloppy and embarrassing while the meta-physical space of my being rearranged into the next phase of my existence. This was the space that I was very familiar with yet perceived distant from due to my perceptions of everyone in the world around me. When I felt at home, I did not feel human. I could relate to the tragedy and trauma of being human, and I could relate to the struggles embedded in the human condition. Yet, authenticity I saw the playground of life, light beings with costumes of flesh projecting stories sourced in experiences. I naturally saw the inter-connectedness of our collective human heart like a blanket of circuits wrapped around Earth. I could not relate to the expressions being used to describe what it is like to be human, especially the expectations of mine.

Organically I could describe what it felt like to see the world beneath me. It was natural for me to see my body as a machine that had four realms of energy converging in a single vessel trying to achieve an integrated fluidity to operate as a human. I discovered my self-proclaimed ordinary mind was actually experiencing the visions of an astral traveler, and the memories of lifetimes lived, and the souls encountered along the way. My soul was teaching my humanness that I had lived for a millennium. My soul was teaching me that my human wisdom is within physics, quantum energy and metaphysics specifically, and our space in the energetic cosmos within which we exist while living out that physical reality. It had become easier to tune my clair senses once I realized I had already lived life with them. When I could breathe into all that I discovered, there was a mystical reveal that exposed I was experiencing the same unseen worlds within and around us all.

Once I was able to reduce myself to the life force at the source of my creation, my body found peace. Once I was able to express my experiences as a photon of light, my body eventually stopped vibrating. I still had to take the journey to my resting point, but I saw how light dispersed into its wavelengths as it travels to reach Earth, and how the wavelengths interact with the matter that is our bodies, anchored in our spiritual energy wheels; vessels absorbing, transmuting, and emitting the very energy that forms its existence merely by varying in its frequency of vibration.

I felt the energy wheels within my physical body resonate and unlock as I used vibrational therapies to tune my body with that of the energy around me. It felt like I knew more how to live in the truth of energy, the infinite potential of a soul, and the purity of spirit, versus that of the human condition and the heaviness of its labels. I could organically see the magical precision in everything, even the horrid tragedies of our experiences, versus dwelling in the sorrow that eagerly awaited. I could see everything as it was in its pure existence and could authentically celebrate the mystical worlds that our God has created; the celebration of our existence compared to the sorrow that felt expected and was being created by humanity to be so. It was difficult to bridge myself into the experiences that I lived when there were few that could see it the same. I could sense that your humanness was misunderstanding me as I was growing to better understand myself. I trusted that your powerful energy needed my experiences to balance your powerful truths. It was purpose that pushed me to find my words so that together we could grow into the world.

It was not until I met you in the physical that I realized that this was how I navigated the world. I could see the soul and light of our existence, and not the humans we had grown to become in this life. I could not see your humanness, which merely exposed that I could not see my own. It was your light that exposed my human shadows so that I could grow into my purpose in this human experience. To do that, while anchored to your Divine Love through our human hearts, you gently took my meta-physical hand on a silent journey through the discovery of the scientific truth at the source of our spiritual love.

As my spiritual senses expanded, my physical reality required a quiet and safe space for expression. During this time, a conversation replayed without my request, yet I knew there was a message embedded. It was a conversation that halted every cell in my body that was in motion. I felt my body freeze in time when I realized it was revealing discrepancies within the human experience I had created. I was asked a simple question that held the expectation of something I had been unable to express in all moments prior when asked about any circumstance of any experience. This particular instance was regarding my marriage and the circumstances that led to its ending.

The two simple words of "what happened" froze my body as I saw the two realms of my existence blasted before me providing a meta-physical realm explanation and a physical realm explanation. I felt vulnerable to expose the meta-physical explanation that my heart always chose to accept as my reality, versus the physical world explanation that no matter the situation everyone else always seemed to choose. I felt naïve to trust in an explanation that could only be proven by faith. I felt shameful that I could not find the human expression of a physical reality that everyone around me expected to hear, even your humanness. It exposed how I had chosen the physical reality to navigate life in order to achieve the dreams of my heart, trying to impose my desires and perceived needs unto the world. Instead of speaking my meta-physical truths, I acted with an effort to sustain an illusion of love that unknowingly blocked the truths within that aligned with the spiritual love I desired.

Although I clearly saw, felt, and knew the meta-physical truth of my marriage, I stumbled terribly in my expression as I chose to relate to the obvious physical reality of broken love. I saw my own limited humanness walk through the process of discovery. I stumbled terribly because a physical world expression was not my truth. The meta-physical reality within which I lived was my truth.

Although my truths were exposed over time, I knew that I had been called upon me to marry the precise person to grow me through love and father my children, just as my soul called upon me to part from love; to grow deeper. My heart trusted at the youthful age of twenty that it was a calling from beyond and chose to follow in faith. My truth was that I walked patiently through the marriage knowing that it would walk me into your love. My truth was that love awaited me beyond the relationship of my marriage. My truth is that collectively we created the perfect space for us to grow; for me it was so that my body could ascend in vibration until my soul could descend into its temporary home. My truth was that my marriage was a karmic soul contract that needed to be fulfilled in the advancement of my energy in order to unite with your love. My truth was that the contract has been completed and it was time to move on; move on to meet you. My truth was that the physical reality that played out was a mere consequence of the contract our souls were fulfilling; a contract that would allow us both to continue to learn in this life experience, and to grow into love; a contract destined to end upon fulfillment.

In every moment that followed, both planes of explanation appeared before me. The paths were illuminated, and I could see not only my own, but that of those before me when a heart was opened and shared. The difference in my experiences was in the choices I was willing to make to follow love. The meta-physical plane was aligned with the fire in my heart fueled by yours, while the physical plane was aligned with a human heaviness of fear and doubt. As in my youth, there were clearly two planes to choose from in the walk that followed. After my illness, I lived within the physical plane explanation ridden with meta-physical wonder, while spending a physical life being programmed by fear and doubt.

Even so, all along it felt like I was living out a physical reality due to a meta-physical explanation. It was an explanation that I waited patiently to receive for over twenty-five years. It was an explanation I waited to receive from any of the sixty-one Gods that had witnessed my suffering. It was an explanation I prayed that a God would step forward to deliver. It was the explanation that I protected in the silence within knowing one day I would receive the golden light of truth. It was an explanation that I had to discover was within me all along if I was willing to do the work to uncover it. I had waited long enough and doing the work felt like the only choice worth making.

I knew deep within I had to resolve the meta-physical and physical plane discrepancies that I believed were at the source of my platelet instabilities. I deeply believed that if I resolved the imbalance within my meta-physical being, my physical being would follow in kind. I also knew my deep belief was creating it into my reality, yet it was so deep the only way to stop the momentum was to ride it out shifting, healing, and transforming out of a zero-resting point and into my true resting point.

I could feel that my body was forced to stop; stopped by a force much greater than mine, your love. I could feel my own internal relative zero velocity and acceleration yet stopped by the external force of my body. The force caused me to appear at rest albeit still containing the energetic force in motion, vibrating my body through the experiences. It was a very familiar sensation yet different, morphing into something new and powerful, something that I knew I could not escape; an unstoppable momentum; potential, kinetic, and chemical energy alchemizing into one. Every step that grew me into the strength and courage to choose the meta-physical explanation, the more forceful the pull became. The more I grew into myself, the more my energy tried to expand beyond my body. The more my energy expanded, the more clogged my body felt, where the energy could not flow through. The more trust I held in the meta-physical explanations, the more everything in my physical world transformed, unclogging my body with every vibrational pulse.

Since I had opened my physical being to receive the explanation from my meta-physical being, I trusted that in doing so I would be exactly who I was indented to be in accordance with my divine purpose. It seemed like an easy choice to make, and most certainly one I was willing to make given an unexplainable knowingness that all things are experienced first in the meta-physical plane of existence before it materializes into the physical. I was never sure how I knew this truth and was left curious in the discovery of how it could be so, even more so how to align in such a way to live that truth for the remainder of my life. All the while not realizing that I had lived that magical truth through the recovery of my youth, and in all that followed.

Ever since that simple question was asked, I knew I would forever choose the meta-physical explanation to navigate my physical world experience. I did not however know at the time of choosing what that would further require of my physical being in order to align with my meta-physical being; my soul; my true self.

Within the meta-physical realm, everything made absolute sense in contrast to the physical experience I was living. While my soul kept me focused on your expanding love within my human heart, my meta-physical being experienced everything needed in order for my humanness to learn and understand how to clear my energy in order to sustain yours. To my consciousness, this was wizardry work of meticulous perfection as both the meta-physical and the physical paths unfolded and integrated into one. It was the energetic merging of my universal and infinite soul with the energy of my human body; a journey of high vibrational light and the human expression of its wavelengths; acquiring my angel wings while facing my human shadows. The fragility rested in the discovery that my power intensified as long as I remained in alignment with my heart and your love.

This is when I saw the entire experience of my youth replay through a spiritually tuned lens. This is when I felt the entire experience replay in the meta-physical space of my being, mimicking a journey in modern times, yet this time I clearly saw where I could love, instead of the fear chosen in my past. This is when my meta-physical world illuminated the universe within my body. The intense vibrations triggered equally as intense emotions that my mind tried to rationalize. All the while, as more light balanced within me forcing every altered wavelength out, I unintentionally manifested all the programmed ideals into my reality. It felt like the energy being pushed out of my body was uncontrollably manifesting into my reality, beauty, and beast alike, love and fear alike. There was a new energy vortex being fueled around me yet this time it had been my choice to participate. This time I chose to be an active participant versus responding in stubborn accordance. This time I chose love. If for no other reason, I chose love for the love that I was feeling in my human heart. Your love made me want to be, do, feel, love, speak, see, and understand love. Your love was anchoring every wavelength of light within me.

I wanted to simply rest in the deep, magnetic love that my human heart was experiencing, especially once we were connected as one. I could feel it when you connected to my heart, and I trusted that you could feel it when I connected to yours. I found a deep motivation to quiet every aspect of my life so that I could be quiet enough to feel, hear, see, and experience you when the choice was made to connect to my heart. The choice was ever so present, and I could feel that choice within every passing human breath; mine and yours alike. There were even days when I cried for you to connect to my heart so I could love to my fullest capacity in the physical, while admittingly knowing that my human yearning was ultimately a reflection of self and an inner desire to connect more spiritually to you. You always appeared when I returned to balance between the realms of our existence.

In time, I learned that my Socratic approach through life had created the very experiences designed to answer the questions I had posed in the abyss of my faith throughout all lifetimes I had ever experienced. No wonder it felt overwhelming until I grew into the ability to hold these truths. As a result, I made my final metaphysical inquiry. I wanted to know you, and what it was like to experience me in my humanness, so I could love you more fully by loving all vibrations of me. I knew that in knowing you I would learn to know myself. I could see the clear mirror we serve to each other, further connected by the human heart, living out separate experiences as one. I am you and you are me. I knew I would find me when I looked to you, just as you were finding yourself when you looked to me. To know you was the most glorious and fruitful inquiry I have ever made in all my life experiences. It felt like once I knew how to love myself purely, I would know how to love you.

I knew it was you all along. There was great comfort in knowing I had finally found you, manifested before me. With every human word you spoke, I felt the meta-physical vibration reducing me into the smallest element of my existence. The answers left me never needing to pose another mindful question again. I knew.

Although we are already united as one, until I was before you again, I faithfully requested for the deliverance of experiences designed to grow me deeper into knowing your love. I found you everywhere; within and without. When I felt uncertain or unstable, you gently reminded me to follow love, quietly illuminating that your love rests within and I shall never feel lost nor alone again, and I am forever loved in your heart, just as I am. As I followed love, I watched every energetic constraint vibrate away into resonance with the purest vibration exposed; the vibration of creation; the vibration of love. I felt like I was naked in the universe with only our love energy as my guide, escorting me through the universe until I stabilized into my own; suspended between the realms of existence.

43

The Scientific Truth of Spiritual Love

The physical experiences were always playing out, and ever so clearly in response to the meta-physical storyline which was on grand display. As both realms of my existence were continuously illuminated, it became effortless to acknowledge that the meta-physical world was my reality. It was increasingly easy to find my way in the mystical interworking of the universe as long as I followed the light; my light, yet it became yours when I was unable to see my own exposing our oneness in the dark.

The most painful and frustrating aspect of my life journey thus far has been the overwhelming awareness of misalignment with my soul, heart, mind, and body, and not having the words to express it. Much the same as to how my physical world had played out, yet never realized I did not have the words in my youth or the decades of healing that followed. I internalized everything about the experience of my youth, processing big brain events with my youthful brain within a forced navigational fluidity. I had every single word I ever needed within my heart and heard the guiding messages on how to follow the path. I never knew I did not have the words since it felt like I was conversing with you every step of the way.

Before I had the words, I had the feelings albeit not emotional feelings. I had unknowingly navigated life through my sensory feelings, the same spiritual senses that I knew were being fine-tuned. It took life experiences to teach me those truths, and even more surprisingly to teach me the human emotions that blocked my spiritual sensing potential. While I journeyed towards words, I had to learn how to communicate with energy which requires no words at all. I had to quiet my world and feel my way through the energetic experiences trusting that the words would follow, sometimes even yearning for an expressional escape. I felt like Lady Justice, navigating blindfolded and balancing energy until my resting point was sustainable; until every cell of my body was at rest and still with the vibration of love.

It felt like I was flying above yet thought we all did so it left me perplexed about our human existence, connections and actions of others, and the world within which we live. I was connected to the truth of a greater collective purpose just not uniquely connected to my own, all the while everything contained a storyline that was seemingly in opposition to my own, and being expressed by the collective walking alongside me, especially when it came to the illusionary stories of love; the only storyline that mattered.

It felt like I was flying above life trying to land within my body. It felt like when my body was most healthy, generally after a platelet crash and rescue medications, I felt most alive, grounded, and present in life. Then slowly, as my body filtered out medications and left to its own accord, my energy slowly ascended out of my body, my consciousness traversing across planes, watching my body struggle through the days yet simultaneously echoing a guiding voice within on how to navigate my humanness. I could see how I had left my body behind, unprotected, and absorbing energy.

I knew that I was elevated in some way, only because I was me, above me, watching me figure out this human experience. It felt like I didn't understand how to live within this body. It felt like the voice within was wiser than my body could sustain while concurrently creating frustration with my own humanness. I was overwhelmingly aware of my human limitations, and the continued ascension of my vibrational energy, including the expansion of my consciousness, both leading me to the transition of my energy into the next phase of my existence, the afterlife.

I felt a contradiction between the infinite potentiality of my energy and the finite limitations of my human existence. I knew that I did not experience life in the same way. I felt so different than anyone I had ever met. It felt authentic and organic within yet unnerving and anxious in the world. I was trying to be human. I knew I was human, here, and alive. I knew it was for a greater purpose that was now being revealed. If we all held a perception of reality, I wondered what was real for I knew I was just like everyone around me; especially you. This led into a lifetime of growing into the separation, longing to understand the differences, and the deep desire of my heart to know and share myself intimately with someone who lives in the same realm of existence. That is why I dreamed so intently of, and for you.

When I began the journey back to wholeness, it felt like I had to travel back in time in order to retrieve certain parts of me; primarily my heart full of emotions frozen at sixteen. It felt like my soul was guiding me into the past before I could heal myself into a joyous future. During the process of collecting my heart, it felt like I walked into the past, secured by a rubber band anchored in the present as if to ensure that I would not rest there, for the present is where I needed to be. It was a welcomed sensation that created peace as each step into the past secured the pieces of me that make me who I am today.

Although there was genuine resistance countering the powerful force within, in time I understood that during the process, I had recreated the entire experience of my youth, yet this time it was a choice to participate. I chose to walk my way to your truth versus being blasted and asked to believe; jolted and required to trust. The gift of taking the journey was that I was not called upon to experience the trauma in the true sense in which it originally occurred, instead I was called upon to choose differently; to choose love. I was called upon to revisit the experiences in the light of spiritual love, which also existed in the meta-physical realm of my existence back then. I was just too young, afraid, naïve, and doubtful to connect after thrown into the catastrophic nature of the physical experience, and understandably so. This time was different. This time it was a choice. I no longer wondered which realm was real. I no longer questioned if I was real. I could feel that love was real and electrifying my heart.

With every step backwards I felt the accumulation of energy from a life walk, gaining momentum from my human deconstruction, releasing force from constant pressure, and unearthing myself from within. It felt like my body was creating an electrical charge the deeper I journeyed within, stirring up latent heat, releasing pressure from the illusions programmed into my being; the night sweats mirrored in the physical realm. It felt like the piezoelectric effect was occurring within my mechanical body and the crystalline characteristics of my energy, producing electricity from compression, the compression from misalignment from my true energetic self.

Once I collected my fragile and timid heart and was being pulled back to the present, the force felt so great and uncontrollable that it felt like the rubber band propelled me into the cosmos, like a sling shot with a trajectory to reach the stars, or returning to myself since that was where I lived. It felt like I was returning home. I discovered it was where my consciousness had lived during the beautiful life in between.

When my soul and heart were joined out in the universal abyss, and I felt my oneness with the universe, I discovered that it was the same space I knew as before yet now I was connected through the physical experience and returning with my body. It was clearly understood why my body began vibrating once I returned home embodied. As my energy sped through the universe, there you were, standing before me now manifested into the human experience bridging the worlds into one. Albeit extremely confusing, I clearly saw you in both.

My energy had such a forceful momentum I could barely slow down enough to humanly see you, even though I tried with everything in my human might to do so. It felt like you had floated into the meta-physical realm when my energy plowed into yours; a collision of divine design that entangled our energy and thence became one. I understood why it was your humanness that embodied the energy now connected to mine. I understood it long before my body could sustain and hold those truths; even longer until I found my words to integrate them into my being. I discovered that it was the same space where I was connected to you yet felt separate because I had not yet travelled through life to discover you.

I had to learn how to navigate life within a new energetic realm of existence. I was a beginner in the same world yet a new means by which to navigate, explore, and experience. My vibrational energy was higher than it had ever been in this life, and any life prior. I was witnessing and feeling the universal connectedness that I had achieved and felt deeply that universal light energy was flowing through me.

The more I honored and nurtured that connection, the faster the energetic manifestations occurred. There were times when it felt my energy was moving so fast that I needed processing time; time to linger. Sometimes even choosing to linger was an attempt to avoid the journey and create space for fear and doubt to plant itself in my vulnerability now exposed. Some experiences even felt like tests to see if my faith in divinity held the strength, courage, and love needed to stand before you once again, while left trusting in my new purity and fullness within. My life had led me to believe that the magic occurred when the heart leads the way, and I was willingly choosing to walk with that intention with a heart now connected to yours.

Intimated by the power of my thoughts as their masterful perfection was manifested within the life experience of another, I became fearful since the experiences had never before occurred in my awareness and before me combined into one. It was always afar for observance. It was the blatant awareness in that my divinity was connected to the same source of humanity that caused me to sometimes pace the hallways of my home while reminding myself not to think. Even aware that the very statement was a means to focus on anything other than a floating thought. Unnerved that it felt intrusive and unwelcomed when my thoughts manifested into your human reality without expressed invitation knowing that your soul called me in. I had to trust that the choice of free will protected us both from the experiences of each other. I had to settle into the truth of the responsibility that comes with the power to co-create and manifest into reality. The reality of a true light being, especially when two come together.

I recall once stating to my Dad that I could not discern if I was creating my experiences from my thoughts or if I was receiving premonitions of what was to come. His response was intriguingly simple. He asked me why it mattered. Although neither of us knew at the time, he was teaching me how to navigate energy. Somehow his response allowed me to see it as both; sometimes I was manifesting and sometimes it was a premonition. Over time, I was able to clearly discern the difference.

It mattered because the energy that was creating my thoughts had a direct reflection into my reality and in an alarming way. It mattered because my energy shifted with the truth of origin, something I could feel and needed to understand how to manage so I did not get thrown off my center and jolted into imbalance like before, often times manifested into platelet instabilities. The perspective was needed in order to healthily shift into experiences which further taught me how to hold energetic space, shapeshifting in an energetic sense. It was a very long and sloppy process to endure while swept up in unexpected energetic lessons and learning and growing.

I felt the challenges of my mind while my soul released emotional, mental, and physical blocks that muted my connection to universal source energy. I knew that the process would take time. I had already tried to broadly conceptualize what I believed the process would look like and failed tremendously in comparison. I knew when I had to surrender to the unknown and continue to hold faith. I remember even going back and revisiting intentions since they seemed to manifest so precisely and quickly, and even became fearful of thinking at all. Fearful of the truth that I manifested the very thoughts into creation when connected to divinity. There was such precision that at times the only comfort was to fall back on my Dad's words of wisdom that it did not matter in the presence of perfection.

It was clear there was much to learn. I felt a human shame overcome me for not knowing my own powers within now exposed and uncontainable. It was a frightening and unnerving process to unleash a power that propulsion fueled my energy into orbit. I knew I was crossing paths with your energy, both of us uncertain of the information now shared. I could feel your energy merging with mine exposing visions and truths, perplexing to my human mind yet held an unyielding truth of wisdom in my gut. As my body vibrated me through the cosmos and we transferred timelines, my humanness struggled to stay the pace, displaying a brokenness never before exposed, un-edited and genuinely human down to the cells of my bones.

Once our human hearts were connected, the real work began, the human work. We both knew that I was a teacher of energy, however I needed you to teach me. During the process, my energy begged your humanness to teach me so I would know what I was doing, and in turn your love guided the way through our collective human heart. You guided me with your unconditional love so I would feel that love, and when I felt that love, I was able to feel my way through the navigation since it is the only way to be one with energy. It felt like I had been zipped up so high, and so tight, trying to keep everything together that once I deconstructed my humanness, I had unzipped my human body and all my powerful love energy oozed out into the world; like a tsunami flooding busy city streets, finding its way between structures and into every possible crevice; engulfing the collective human heart, your heart. The force of the Global Wave of Healing Energy once contained now its power unleashed unto the world.

While journeying throughout the cosmos, I found everything needed to live a sustainable life in my physical body. Through the energetic conduit transmitting love between our human hearts, within the meta-physical and physical realms alike, I found exactly what I needed to sustain me for my final round in the human experience. I found my home in the meta-physical realm of my existence. I found the energy of the cosmos, the photons that travelled millions of years to reach me here on Earth, and the wisdom of the collective consciousness brought forth from the journey. Finally. I found all the components that create my sustainable life. I found my home. I found my boss and place of employment, I found my educational arenas, I found my library to wisdom, I found how to nurture my body, I found my playground, my garden, and space of serenity, and the most beautiful, I found the source of my infinite love. I found you.

Even so, all the meta-physical experiences with energy were wearing my physical body down. That was the premise of the very intentional journey in that the physical realm is a mirror to the meta-physical realm. I needed my meta-physical being to fall into place, so that my physical being could rest. Even so, my meta-physical being had to deconstruct further to its source, just like I had done with my physical being to get to the source of my soul. Now that my soul was naked in the universe, my physical body had to follow, broken down once again.

I was gently reminded that my physical body was catching up to the wisdom of my soul; a voice of past and future now merging with the present to grow into the future as one. The reminder included a reassurance that it was part of the process and to remain in love and light, for my human fear and doubt was still be eradicated. The love between our hearts was the only energy keeping me grounded on Earth, otherwise it felt like I would have floated away into the abyss leaving my body behind. The love between our human hearts was a reminder it was with purpose.

Not only did I need my body to stop vibrating so it could rest and be comfortable, but I also knew that every energetic ripple I was emitting was throwing your human heart off balance. I could feel my frequencies jolting your system as both of our bodies recalibrated into harmony. I knew I had to become pure in my human vibration of light in order to maintain the purity of yours. I was unwilling to become the human experience that kept you out of alignment. I trusted that you felt and knew I was doing the work to heal myself, especially when my humanness was a sloppy mess of realignment.

While looking towards you, I found me which then allowed me to see you more clearly. You helped me see myself, and since we are one and the same, I knew that once I saw me, I was also seeing you. I was feeling everything so deeply and knew you felt it the same, in your own way. I felt every vibrational wavelength emitted from my body impact you in some way. When I aligned with my truths and brought peace within myself, I felt that peace transmitted to you, and could feel you grow deeper into your spiritual love, whatever that meant to you. It felt like I knew what that was too since it was the same story as mine when simple labels where applied. I could sense that I had to heal myself in order to not disrupt your peace. I had to heal myself in order to love you with purity. It was through these discoveries that I found a greater purpose in the journey to achieve balance. Doing it for myself was enough, yet once a greater purpose was on display, it changed everything about how I wanted to navigate life. Every choice became an intentional alignment with divine purpose; an intentional alignment with spiritual love. I wanted to bring spiritual love into my physical experience. I knew this was the only way for me to sustain breath moving forward.

Since there was the corresponding physical world experience bonded and attached forming the universal DNA of my existence, I knew this would be the journey I longed to travel so I could rest in love. I was embarking on my explanation and the truth of my existence; my meta-physical and physical realms rotating at the source of who I am. Repairing my DNA went beyond the physical body; my soul needed to be repaired. My authentic energetic signature needed to be restored. It was overwhelming to think about how all my physical world experiences altered my energetic signature. There was so many variables that altered my human being; the experiences, the trauma, the medications, especially the breath sustaining immuno-globulin therapies containing the energy of millions of humans carrying their own meta-physical and physical energetic implications. It was an overwhelming embarkment of total restoration.

Before the journey could continue, the physical realm experiences needed to catch up so that I could continue processing the meta-physical experiences; my spiritual senses and my humanness needed to be in sync. I had collected my heart and had returned to my true home where we finally met, yet the warp speed propulsion into the cosmos required warp speed physical experiences for balance so my human senses could catch up. I could barely keep up with myself. You likely noticed.

Once I had learned enough, the meta-physical experiences subsided for a while so I could take care of the physical world reality. During those times, while feeling more humanlike, I experienced intermittent energetic surges that could only be described as downloads. I would get a tremendous influx of energy, extreme fatigue, and a message to lay down. Similar to the experience of the onset of crashing platelets during all the years prior yet with a newness that I could now adhere to the calling. As I did, I could feel a transference of energy occurring; the living light; the same living light as before now engaged and controlled. I rested with my eyes closed with peace, gratitude, and welcomeness, and knew that I would unpack the wisdom in the days that followed. It took quite a while for me to discover, correlate and integrate this routine into a way of life, yet I honored it just the same. It felt like a sacred calling, and I was beginning to understand the magnitude of my experiences and my expressions.

Throughout 2019 while I was learning about my soul, my body tried to stay the pace with its sloppy coordination of parts. I was a year into relearning how to live autonomously, and my children were happy and thriving, and were the purest joy in my experiences. While they shared time and space between me and their father, the boys were growing me along the way of uncertainty, just as I was doing for them. We grew closer and closer the more I shared in my experiences, and I witnessed them understanding themselves as a result. The new spiritually sourced relationship I was able to nurture with my children was a dream realized through messy and hard choices along the same journey of choosing self. It was a dance of discovery in the meta-physical realm the child within wished I had received in my youth while concurrently understanding why it was not part of my design.

The other influential space of my existence was the workplace, my second home. I had navigated within the same workplace for thirteen years. It was the place of employment that had grown me through some of the best and worst times in my life, as I did for many in return. The family of connections meant so much more to me than any career growth potential or even monetary gain. Even so, similar to me, the company experienced rapid growth. Different than me, it evolved into an increasingly more toxic environment for my own health sustainability. Both were thriving yet only one could sustain me; myself. I had fought against the shifts felt within over several years prior while simultaneously trying to construct a departure. My orchid had mirrored it was time to let go of perceived beauty and trust in more growth to follow. As I navigated the ending of my marriage, each attempt to separate from the workspace fell through leaving me aware that I needed to handle one at a time. Separating from the workspace would be one of the last areas of my life to transform. My heart was still the priority.

At one point I did not even realize that I had become impatient and began mindfully interjecting my will which only manifested through experiences and a perception of self-sabotage. I was trying too hard. It felt like I knew too much of self and I was unable to just relax and let things be. I knew once I could just relax and be, my exit path would appear, surrendering to how me and the universe dance as one; the same dance that brought me to you. It was an opportunity to let my body vibrate through the physical realm freely in order to align with the meta-physical gifts that awaited. This is when I fully accepted that as one, your will is my will.

I still looked for your humanness to guide me, yet during those times it was as if you went silent, stepping aside for me to sense my way to your love. It felt like every time I dipped into the physical realm to take action to realign my reality, you energetically could not descend any further. I could feel me pulling your energy to the Earth and the inability for it to lower in vibration. It felt like a tug of war between the dark and the light as the light chord pulled me through the veil of ascension. I begged you to send me clarity of mind and grace of navigation to help in the balance if you were unable to descend low enough to aid me.

After meeting and merging with your energy in the cosmos, it felt like I was falling back to Earth at what felt like an alarming speed; crashing to Earth and bouncing back into the abyss; back and forth until an equilibrium between the two realms was achieved. The energetic conduit between our hearts was the only thing keeping me in orbit, yet it was the very thing bouncing me between realms. It felt like my consciousness was traveling at the speed of light while my body was bound to Earth. It was too fast, it was too much, it was too overwhelming for my physical body to sustain. My inability to stay embodied on Earth became ever so prevalent during each attempted departure which was prevented by an anchored force in my heart; you.

Each time my energy tried to uncontrollably leave your love pulled me back into my body by the means of a light chord connecting our hearts. I could see and feel the energy conduit reigning me back in, conflicting with the energy of my body, trying to escape, and being dowsed in light to stay. It was your love that raised the vibration of my body that allowed my body to hold my energy. It was your love that taught my energy that my body was a safe space to stay embodied. Once our hearts connected, my energy illuminated the universe for me to discover how to find balance between the realms of existence. This was necessary to ensure that I do not leave my body behind on my final walk towards you, mimicking when it comes time to transition fully into the meta-physical realm. I had to learn how to stay embodied so I could live this life while learning within this body what is needed for the next.

I did not take long for me to remember that the descent to the Earth was a sacred journey intended for my purpose in order to learn all that I needed in order to connect me to the fulfillment blueprint of my Divine Intention. It was the return walk back to love that exposed our free will choice. The blueprint had been casted, it would be my choice of free will to follow and return. It felt like it was for my own purpose, and for that of humanity as an example of breaking through the limitations imposed by the human condition. Breaking through the illusion that has blinded the collective along the experience of life. The beautiful walk to the Heavens provided me the spiritual strength, courage, and love needed as the experiences of my reality crumbled away with the force of my faith, shining light onto the darkness within and around me. I knew there would be a return to the Heavens, so that meant I had to endure the physical experience that needed to play out in order for it to occur.

Once my heart and soul were at the purest vibration attainable in my human body, naked in the universe, the light of our infinite energy illuminated how my mind, words, and body language were in contradiction to my truths. It was evident that this would be a process of clearing, aligning and being me in a way that had never before been energetically experienced through this body. It was as if I had to become grounded to the Earth before I could begin the next phase of the journey, and energetically ascend with my body to discover my soul's truths.

It felt like I needed something to soften the blows and parachute me to Earth upon the descent for my final landing. I needed to grow deeper in love in order to become grounded and ascend wholly back to you. I could feel that there was a missing vibration; another vibration of love before I could harmonize with yours. I needed to know my own.

As I tried to settle into everything, my body let me know when it was time to refocus. While alone, tired, and only having the strength to surrender, you sent me an Angel of Love. Another mirror to reflect the parts of me that I could not yet see on my own, a mirror of my own vibration of love. I deeply and dearly welcomed the assistance especially when it embodied every expression of you and your love. It was a trifold of divinity linking everything to the physical reality. You manifested me, I manifested you, then you manifested an Angel of Love since you could not be physically present. I prayed that I had done the same for you when you needed it. I knew I wanted to know your love more deeply and felt you returning to mine.

Just as I was trying to find fluidity in the experiences, calling for you through our collective human heart, your Angel of Love appeared from the silent existence within my physical world orb. I knew you sent me another light being so I could grow deeper into my truths. Although my heart smiled in the awareness that a meta-physical trinity was forming in the physical, a mirror of its energetic power, I was very much unaware of many details as they unfolded. All of my senses, physical and meta-physical alike, were hypersensitive and on alert. I was not so much surprised yet startled by the intensity and curious of what the navigation would look like.

There was a force bringing me, my dear friend who gave me the Hildegard books, and another co-worker into a tight group of raw and vulnerable humanness. Organically and authentically, we were unknowingly connecting in both realms of existence creating a powerful and magnetic trifecta; a superhuman triforce across both realms. Just as I knew the love flowing from your heart and into mine was bridging spiritual love from the Heavens to experience on Earth, I knew our trifecta now manifested was healing through our now collective love. I brought you with me every time I showed up since you were at the source of my powerful love.

As we grew into our similar and powerful abilities, we all tried to balance into our own humanness. None of us understood ourselves fully until we allowed ourselves to be seen. I could clearly see my friends; I was just unable to see myself. And as with you, when I looked at them, I saw myself. All I could sense was that the sentiments and actions that fueled the force was the choice for us each to expose the raw and vulnerable quagmires of the heart, making sense of our purpose for living. This was when I started to experience the meta-physical make its way into the physical in a sustainable and healing way. Through nurturing the new trifecta, we were each exposed to the unedited and unfiltered selves. This was so important for me on the journey back to wholeness. It turned out to be equally as important for them, and in their own way; life-saving ways.

I had not been able to stand firmly in my own love. This trifecta grew me into that strength merely by letting me be me; however, and whatever that looked like. I knew my dear friend and I were soul sisters, yet integrating a new person was overwhelming. My heart could not keep bouncing and acclimating and healing and longing. I knew I had requested something to grow me into your love, yet I did not have anything to give. Thankfully, that was the purpose. It was time to surrender to the love being sent to me so my love could heal. Something I was not yet able to do when our human beings met. It was exposed that I had tried to show up as a healer when we met; a healer sent to heal your broken love just as you were healing my broken love. Love was teaching me through the trifecta that only once I was healed would my love organically heal those encountered. I did not have to do anything except love. It was clearly not time for me to show up as a healer, it was time for me to be healed. It was time to practice the surrenderance to love in the physical realm and let love heal me.

While I continued to surrender to love, a year and a half passed before I experienced another platelet crash. In August 2019, I was able to mitigate a critical situation with backup rescue medications my doctors agreed to prescribe over the prior years of instability. This was the arsenal that I knew I had on hand if ever I needed to start treatment immediately. In this particular instance, I started the treatment at home on a Friday evening, and after 24 hours passed with no sign of improvement, I drove myself to the emergency room. I knew that I did not have time to wait until Monday to see my doctor.

It was the first time in all my experiences that I had to drive myself to the hospital. I was so far beyond my comfort zone yet knew it was an instrumental step in standing on, in, and for my own, in addition to the emergent state of my body. I had an intense headache that had potential to cause an aneurysm, petechia were still appearing in new areas on my body, I was in a significant amount of pain, and I was incredibly nervous. Life and death on the brink of a breath. Generally, I could feel when the medication would stop the destruction while counts restored. Since symptoms were not improving and I was unable to discern if the medication was working, I knew I needed assistance and fast.

I had already decided on the way to the hospital that if my counts were over twenty thousand, I would return home. I just needed lab work to confirm. When the lab results came back and my counts were twenty-four thousand, I thanked the staff and discharged myself. Although still extremely low, I knew they had been much lower just hours before the test. I knew I would see my doctor in one day when their office re-opened from the weekend and a treatment plan would be initiated. I went home, waited to coordinate with my doctor, and after my visit continued the steroid medication.

My doctor was very eager to get me off the steroids as quickly as possible because he was starting to see the impacts of the twenty-year regimen was having on my body. Once my counts were at safe levels within a couple of months, the usual weaning process began. During this time, our trifecta took advantage of serendipitous work opportunities for us to get together and spend time unedited. It felt like none of us had ever held the time and space, nor felt the right support to allow it.

For me, the expressions of love felt fleeting and unsustainable, which was in complete opposition to what my heart wanted to do. It felt like my physical body needed to be held in love. It felt like my body needed to feel the vibration of love on the outside so it could sync with the vibration of love emitted from my heart, joining forces in the cells of my body. It felt like my physical body needed to be taught that spiritual love was sustainable in the physical reality, bringing the Heavens to the Earth and grounding your love into this life experience. It felt like my heart needed to know that my love was enough to do that.

One evening when we were unexpectedly all together, I was explaining to my dear friend the most recent energetic experiences endured. Or at least trying. Although unapologetic in my expression, I did acknowledge that this is what me and my friend would normally talk about, and our new friend was welcomed to join in if they had anything to contribute. We welcomed new perspectives especially as it related to energy and the cosmos, and he had previously demonstrated his knowledge about both.

As the evening of cooking, talking, and laughing unfolded, our new relatively quiet friend began slowly reiterating the same expressions I had shared yet in a different language. I had struggled to find my own words and had sloppily used words of vibration, light, universal energy, intentions, and manifestations, yet he effortlessly spoke in terms of molecules and photons. While I sat across from him as he spoke in a language of quantum physics, all me rejoiced as I heard the language I had longed to hear. Very similar to the experience at the table when I met my Earth Angel. I knew you sent him to teach me. I knew he was your Angel of Love. Especially when I saw a glimpse of a tattoo and inquired about its meaning. It was one word in a different language. The word was love. When I looked at the tattoo closer, it reminded me of the many tongues and versions of love being spoken in modern times. The tattoo somehow bridged an eternity old love to the stories of love in my heart in the unfolding. Tears fell steadily from my eyes as I felt wisdom unlock from within me, even though my mind could not process quickly enough. As usual, my soul danced as the trifecta was forcefully on display around me.

Just as I began marveling in the truth that there was a language for my experiences, he stopped speaking only to later find out that it was because he thought my tears were tears of sadness. I myself was still earning that more often than not my tears were shed when standing before and experiencing magical perfection as it unfolds within and around me, not because I am sad. As my body integrated the brief scientific explanations into my energetic experiences, I discovered truths that almost instantly put self-inquiries to ease. The experiences, the sensitivities, the visions, the sounds, everything made sense. Just like your love clarified everything about my meta-physical being, his words were unlocking truths about my physical being.

Amidst the same moments, and during what felt like the blink of an eye, I learned that I am a multi-dimensional traveler, and capable of astral projections across spacetime. I unearthed the truth that for all my adult life I have been traveling through spacetime, charged by spirit and energy of the collective all the while energetically ungrounded in my human body. Although I was not sure why, it made sense. I had felt deep protection during the realization that my unawareness meant I had done so unsafely and unprotected, collecting cosmic energy that further compromised my human vessel's ability to embody the energy meant to be expressed in this life. I had too much energy, more than my body could contain. The Global Wave of Healing Energy had served it purpose. I somehow struggled with knowing that I had to reduce and funnel my energy back into my body. It felt like I was cutting off and stifling my potential.

Even so, everything was finally finding their home to rest. The images in my mind, the visions I had experienced, the memories I held, the lives I lived, the vibrations of my body, the heat my body generated from all the energetic processes underway, the entanglement of my human heart and feeling your love so deeply, and the experience of words my soul longed to hear, were all syncing and intensifying into stillness. My own tears of peace were washing my energy clean.

After spending an evening laughing, crying, and crying from laughing so hard. I woke up with bruises around my eyes from the constant wiping of tears; the same way the ailment manifested decades earlier when first discovered. I knew something was impending when we woke up for work and I had black eyes. Although it indicated low platelets, I was at peace since they were caused from the purest love and joy. It had been a very long time since I had held such emotion, perhaps since my ITP was diagnosed. I had to acknowledge that during the same timeframe, unexpected occurrences transpired in the workplace impacting my role in stressful ways; ways that my body was unable to escape even though my mind was able to see through them. This only exacerbated my already weary state of being. There was poetic irony that it manifested in the same way; the start and ending to a journey without you. Just as your love was making full circle, I knew these beautiful souls were a part of my physical world love until the end. This was my tribe. My Trifecta. The trinity that would ground me through the process and beyond.

New to the storyline of my blood, our new trifecta friend shared that his father was a microbiologist and has spent his life studying human blood. He encouraged me to meet his father to see if he had anything to add about how to achieve balance. I was apprehensive at first but then leaned into any expansion of love for self and what an experience may yield. So, one day I called, introduced myself, and asked if we could visit.

By the time of our visit, I was not feeling well, and my body was very achy. Even so, I attributed it to a game room mural I had been commissioned to paint as a Christmas gift. Although planning to only stay for an hour, we casually visited at his dining room table. I noticed my bodily aches and my headache slowly drifted out of my awareness the more we spoke about my blood, nationalities and cultures, experiences that mold us, purpose in life, mindfulness, happiness, and choices. Four hours later we ended the conversations, and before leaving I asked if he would be willing to review prior years of blood work records and advise if there is an untold story. It felt like there was more than what my oncologist was sharing. It felt like my oncologist was only seeing me for my platelet count, and not all of my being. I did not realize how much I needed another perspective in order to trust myself.

Once I left and was in the silence of my vehicle, all my bodily senses returned, and I could feel my body calling out in discomfort. Every cell in my body ached, and I could feel every pulse of my heart within the confines of my head. I could not wait to get into my bed. Time was slowing down as the ten-minute drive felt like an hour. Although I was still on medication, it was clear that my response to steroid treatment was waning. I was unable to sustain the balance and my platelets drastically dropped again. I senses this is what was meant when I was advised that I was leaving my body behind. It was as if I left my body in the vehicle while my soul went for a visit. When I returned to my body my senses flushed back.

This all proved to be too much. I wondered how to keep my body with me when I did not even realize I was leaving it behind. Once again, I found myself at home alone and rescuing my body from a rapidly decreasing platelet count. It was evident that my physical world experience was responding and aligning to the meta-physical shifts occurring within. This was how my body had always responded to the meta-physical realm and coupled with the work stress, my physical body was once again overwhelmed. I prayed deeply that I would figure all this out. I could not continue like this anymore.

My humanness had to experience the shifts since I was still using the physical world to teach me about the meta-physical world. I could feel the cusp of an energetic barrier that I was about to break through knowing it would shift me into using the meta-physical world to explain the physical experience; a space that felt more in accordance with my authentic being. It was not something I could fake or pretend to achieve. Although the voice within was always wise and knowing, my body could not keep up, exposing every false truth it was programmed to believe. I knew this was the final stretch of the journey. My vibration balanced with each meta-physical discovery made and the physical world alignment demonstrated the meta-physical journey underway. I was starting to get the hang of my multiverse and was more capable of discerning within which dimension I needed to be present. At first, I always thought it was in the physical reality. The distortion of time and space taught me otherwise.

While present in the physical, two days before Christmas, there I was again, driving myself to the emergency room in the middle of the night after the growing intensity of my headache as the indicator I may not have much time. My headache was getting progressively worse just as quickly as the petechia were spreading. My rescue medications were not working, and I could not reverse the direction of my falling counts fast enough. I remember shaking as I tried to take the medication.

Although considerably less nervous, I was still very timid in my self-navigation. I checked myself into the emergency room and waited for my turn for triage assessments and admittance. Once I was assigned an assessment room and lab work performed, it was evident that my counts were too critical at four thousand platelets. I needed further treatment and fast. While doctors sought out the guidance from my oncologist and the treatment to administer, I was admitted into the hospital.

By morning time, on high levels of steroids pending further treatment, I waited for my doctor to arrive. I contemplated much of the same; how I felt, how my body looked from its failing platelets, how do I sustain health, and how to live beyond surviving. Although the timing was as it used to be, it was true, the last occurrence almost two years prior was indeed the last of its kind.

My doctor entered my room and calmly stated that they would not be able to treat me. He explained that the immunoglobulin therapy that was normally given was on nationwide shortage. As a result, I was not included in the priority recipient list for treatment. I was humbled by the truth that there were others who needed the medication to sustain breath as well. I felt uncomfortable in the truth that someone, somewhere was making the decision that my life was not valuable enough to receive the medication that had proven to save me. I wondered if it was the consequential balance for choosing to take the journey of my soul which likely caused the crash.

A platelet infusion was recommended as the only means to increase counts quickly, even with the knowingness that my body would destroy them just as quickly as they were infused. With no other viable means to increase counts quickly, I agreed and was able to rest knowing that it was in my best interest. I thanked the donors that would be saving me. After the orders were placed, my doctor kindly stated that since they were going to have to treat me with a pill medication, after the infusion I could go home. He did also state that if I was uncomfortable going home with such low platelets, I could stay at the hospital. I graciously opted to leave once complete the transfusion was complete which led to a discharge in the late afternoon on Christmas Eve. With only ten thousand platelets, covered in petechiae, and praying deeply that I would wake up the next day to the rising sun, I drove myself home and wrapped last minute gifts for my three sons. It felt like a celebration of a joint birth into Christmas morning, again. The cycle of birth, death, and rebirth continued.

It was not until after I was back home that my friend shared that his father was concerned about my health and advised him to stay close. He indicated that he was not surprised that I ended up in the hospital and admittingly had noticed my diminished color and drained appearance during our visit. The next six weeks were a blur as my body tried to balance unassisted into comfort. With prednisone as the only therapy, I suffered tremendously behind the walls of my home, praying for peace in both realms alike.

I begged for the suffering to be over if it was indeed my time, and if not, I asked for clarity how to navigate back to health. It felt familiar in how it felt in my youth, and even a year prior when I was navigating the divorce, finding a new home, and ensuring our children adapted well by using love, communication, and attention as the guide. Even so, it was completely new, I was completely new, with an energetic connection in my heart, and being pulled through the abyss by yours.

Receiving your Angel of Love felt like the final round of lessons before the journey of wholeness would be complete. I was completely closed off. It was as if you sent this Angel to help grow me into your love more slowly, balanced, and pure. My heart found your love in the universal abyss and as I returned to Earth, I felt my heart close and restrict every expression of my love, which in turn prevented your love from reaching me. I felt every aspect of my heart close the more my energy funneled into my body. The closer and more grounded I came to Earth, and embodied, a shield around my heart grew more dense. I could not understand what and how it happened, even angry with myself for not being able to sustain the vibration of love.

At times I wondered if I would ever be able hold my heart open. And then suddenly, I would feel a surge of your love flush fear and doubt out of my body and restore knowingness, expanding the energetic field beyond my body. It felt like together we were redefining my energetic boundaries, pulling them from within the depths of my heart now exposed and encompassing all my body, restoring my soul shield. It did not make logical sense, yet my body was telling me it was occurring and needed it in order to complete the journey. Albeit saddened by my own inability to keep my heart wide open, I accepted that I would do my best to reopen my heart and walk back to you with every pulse of our hearts now beating as one.

Within our trifecta, it was clear that we were all spiritually connected to energy and trying to make sense of our unique experiences. It was also clear that my dear friend represented the higher vibrational energy and navigated through her heart, while our new friend held the lower vibrations and navigated through his mind. I was the one transitioning from the mind and returning to the heart, so they both held a unique mirror to my journey. This was all amplified when I experienced the divine energy flowing through our trifecta. It helped me understand all the energetic experiences I had endured. It was as if I had met you in the future and knew of all the things I would have acquired along the way. I was confused because I knew I did not have them and felt deeply that you were delivering them to me. And you were, just not in the material form I had envisioned. I started to feel once again that I was walking backwards in life. This time to collect the new elements of you in the discovery.

Similar to the experience of my youth, I was left with my infinite potential trying to funnel into a finite state of existence in my body and to discover how to navigate. It seemed like everyone else was walking a gradual walk of ascension, not descending from above. It created a perception of traveling back in time while advancing into the future. All I really knew in the moments was that collectively within the trifecta we were able to hold a safe space for each other to navigate and express our unique meta-physical sensing. They appeared to just live in their truths whereas I was acutely aware of my navigation. This interestingly enough led to us practicing how to take physical world action in response to our meta-physical sensing. This also allowed me to see and appreciate how we each connected and sensed energy differently through the lens of our unique humanness, yet it always proved to be connected and manifested in some way amongst us. It allowed me to practice our powerful love.

There was a tremendous amount of inherent and easy trust that flowed through our trifecta connection. During a couple of months of discovering how powerful our joint force really is, the surges of energy were overwhelming at times. I had discovered that creating art was the easiest means by which I could release the energy, as an expression of the vibration of love stabilized within me. I was overjoyed because creating art has always been a part of who I am but always experienced the ungrounded nature of my creations while in process. It felt like I was being connected to my artistic dreams through the source of its inspiration. Even so, there was more to the purpose of my artistic expressions that were acting as a segue for release. They bridged the meta-physical experiences into my physical. They were the means to find my words.

I recall asking my friend to talk to me in the language of quantum physics as he had done before when my humanness was awakened to a scientific language. My body longed for a language to process my truths. Instead of receiving his words, my humanness struggled with how to integrate the wisdom of my old soul into expression of this body. I still could not read the sacred books of Hildegard von Bingen, nor the Bible, and it seemed as those deeply connected to my soul were silenced in some way by their own journey of purpose. I did not know how to integrate the ancient truths of healing energy, natural remedies, and the vibrational truths in everything. I was not sure how to incorporate the journey of my soul and the vibrational healing tools available as a gift to unwrap. I needed to allow for all the experiences, the truths, and your love, to settle into my being and transform my physical reality. All I knew to do was hold your love close and envision my body wrapped in love and light. I prayed for you, or your Angel of Love, whichever was in my best interest. One of you always showed up.

Although a telecommunications network engineer responsible for lighting up dark fiber, he had already exposed through his silent demeanor and intentional disposition that universal wisdom rested within. It was so incredibly clear that he was living the physical manifestation of lighting up the dark, just as I was doing in the meta-physical realm. We were both lighting up the dark so others could find their way; me in the meta-physical realm enduring the expansion into my quantum state of being to lead the way for a quantum existence, and him in the physical realm engineering fiber connections to construct networks designed to connect, exchange, and evolve into quantum computing. Our spiritual love held the contract of light that joined us in unity. A balance between realms of existence in the making; a quantum existence.

It felt like I was a meta-physical energetic being, and he was the physical manifestation of me in the human experiences fueled by your love in my heart. When I looked at him, I saw me. Just as your reflected absolutely everything about my meta-physical and spiritual being, he reflected every human expression of my physical being. We were identical in our humanness; how our bodies operated, how we processed information, how we integrated experiences, our sensitivity to energy, and how we navigated life. We were same in our service to acts of love. I could see that he was my physical world twin, just as you were my spiritual world twin. Between the two of you, I saw my completeness.

Despite my requests, he never spoke of quantum physics again in the way my heart yearned. As with your silence I knew it was because I had to find my own voice. It felt like he knew that too yet proclaimed it was because he was a self-taught physicist, a past time interest of sorts, and believed he did not have the language to have such a dialogue. His reasoning being was that he did not know the language of mathematics. I noticed a resemblance to the human limitations that Einstein himself struggled with as a result of his genius. I knew he was guiding me to my own words yet felt lost in the abyss. I then asked that if I drew what I was seeing if he would assist putting words to the images. He questioned my intentions when he realized I was suggesting that I was going to draw quantum physics. I assured him that if that is what he was calling the process, then yes, yes I was. It felt like it was my only hope to get it out and find my words.

Once the holiday season was over, I knew I could not go back to work. I knew I could not return in the same capacity as before, and once I had stepped away I did not want to return in any capacity. I knew I had to make choices to change my circumstances. I knew I had to take action, yet my body was so weak, I was fatigued, I was aching and nauseated while bound to my bed. It felt like I was taking my last breaths. I desperately requested to be complete with the journey; within either realm would have been acceptable. If it was to be alive and on Earth, then I felt a desperate need to gain sustainable control over my body.

For once, I just wanted to feel good in my body. And if it was my time, I felt content with what I had learned and where my heart landed, connected to yours. I celebrated that for the first time ever I was at peace with my body failing. I welcomed knowing you fully in the meta-physical realm where we met. I even asked to end the suffering if it was only going to get worse. When I spoke the words that it felt like I was dying and communed with your love, I knew it was not my time. I understood that I would continue to be a work in progress, and by seeing you in your fullest potential I was able to know my own. I had to stay the course.

Instead, I learned when it would be my time, in the future over a decade out yet not more than two. There was a strange sense of relief; as if I could releasee the uncertainty of when my death would occur, especially since I danced with death so frequently. I knew that any dance between now and then would not end my human existence. I felt my body relax into life like never before. I did also learn that when the time does come, my awareness will ascend with my energy, leaving my consciousness watching the vessel that ceased breath as I float above. It was my exit path and I saw it clearly.

Mirrored in the physical world, I clearly saw my exit path from the workplace which represented everything about the old way of living. I knew it was up to me to act accordingly. I was not expecting to experience what that would mean to my heart. I found myself struggling to surrender to being labeled as disabled when I had lived a life proving my ability, primarily to myself. I was aware of my limitations. I lived with them every day. I knew how to manage myself physically. I had made it thus far and trusted that I could keep my body alive, not realizing I was not honoring what it needed. I was focused and striving for what I wanted. As I grew into the uncomfortable expansion of self, I filed for short term disability and began exhausting my paid time off. It turned out that once short-term disability was approved, I never went back to that place of employment. I never went back to the older versions of self I was choosing to leave behind. I was walking towards love while filling myself up with light.

With the help of my children, I made it through January and knew there was more to the journey ahead in both realms. I began discussing treatment options with my doctor since continued prednisone use was no longer a viable option. I knew I needed something to assist my body in remembering how to balance into healthy platelets, despite my soul's truth in knowing the Earth has what is needed to heal. Torn between an ancient wisdom yearning for expression in the times of today, and the need of modern medicine to assist in the dance.

My doctor, as he and others had done throughout the decade prior, tried to convince me to take a pill medication that had been scientifically proven to increase platelet counts. Although many could not understand my explanation as to why I would not take the medication, it was clear to me, as it had always been. I knew enough to prevent going against my truths, and my truths were that my body made enough platelets, yet my immune system was destroying them just as quickly. We all knew this truth. Science reflected this truth in the hundreds of lab results acquired over the years.

Even so, illogical rationale was constantly pushed upon me, and I was encouraged to agree to a medication that was designed to increase production and would thereby make me feel better. I agreed my counts would increase yet make me feel better was not likely. It did not seem to concern anyone that it would only increase my counts by forcing my body to over produce platelets so that the destruction appeared less, masking the true ailment from science. It felt like a request to sacrifice how I felt in order for science to appear correct. I felt so tired of people telling me that my feelings did not matter and that I was too sensitive. I tried to express these sentiments, yet it felt unheard and misunderstood. It was not emotional sensitivity. On the contrary I had spent most of my life longing to feel emotions. These were different feelings. The way my body felt was critical to my survival. The way I felt was not the way others were interpreting my feelings. I had to find better words.

Reluctant to medicate with falsehoods, I knowingly aligned with my own spiritual science, yet I remained nervously stubborn in my treatment. I quietly honored the meta-physical experiences underway noting the more I learned about the depths of my soul, the more my physical world realigned and gained balance. My platelets would be an indicator of my success. I had no other choice than to trust that I would find a treatment designed to heal and restore balance to my platelets; a medication for me and my body.

Unbeknown to me and my medical team, there was a pharmaceutical company that had recently received FDA approval for treatment of adults with chronic ITP who had an insufficient response to previous treatment. Approval was granted in April 2018, the same month and year that I had made the choice to move out and pursue a divorce petition, ultimately setting my heart and body free to evolve. This company had manufactured a medicine designed to treat the very nature of my immune system and its platelet self-destruction. The medication was designed to target the very system that the other medication was proposed to mask and overwork. The moment my research revealed its existence, I knew this was the medication for me. It felt like the great reveal of a sacred gift from my Angels. My heart was full of gratitude.

Adamant and persistent, my doctor agreed to oversee the treatment and we prepared to forge a path as the first patient to try this medication in his practice. Although my focus was more on sustaining my own health, I also saw how it could help others with self-attacking immune systems. I knew that as I long as I healed myself, I would heal the world around me. I kept that in focus as we began the regimen. Heal myself and I would in turn heal the world. I finally felt that truth a year later when I learned that another patient was also achieving balance with the same medication.

As the first recipient in the local practice, I coordinated with my doctor and the manufacturer to arrange for a trial therapeutic dispense of the medication while trying not to be overwhelmed that the annual cost of the medicine was more than I earn in a year, albeit only one third of the cost for a life-saving round of immunoglobulin treatment. I encountered the support team of the manufacturer which turned out to be an entire team ready to secure access to the medication. I was repeatedly encouraged to rest and take care of myself while they worked to dispense a two-month gratis supply, secure coverage with my insurance company and establish long term treatment. I cried in gratitude on the phone many times in awe that they were designed and so willing to assist patients such as myself and worked hard to ensure access to medication.

My doctor agreed to my request to begin with the lowest dose and titrate up, versus his recommendation to start with a high dose and titrate down. My body could not handle the foreign substances of anything, even a lot of foods. My body was sensitive to everything, and I knew it needed to be as pure as possible. In agreement, I was prescribed the lowest does recommended by the manufacturer. Trusting it would work out, and my insurance would cover the expense, I continued on medical leave focused on the new treatment and the meta-physical experiences leading me to health.

I was even aware of my contradicting request to have the insurance company cover the medication albeit the insurance was through the company I desired to leave. I could feel myself suspended between the pull from both sides. It was easier to just ride the waves to the shorelines of peace. While we awaited the response from the insurance company, we waited to see how my body would respond.

All was well for about three weeks. I was able to rest and trust that the meta-physical experiences were healing my body to the extent that it could, leaving the remaining balance to be achieve with this team and the medication they have created. I felt an unfamiliar sense of relief overcome my being as I awaited once again on others to determine what is in my best interest, knowing that my meta-physical truths would supersede. Then the tables started to turn. Unbeknown and hard to see at the time, the circumstances were turning and in my favor.

You were nowhere to be found in my physical experience other than nestled in my heart and flowing through my trifecta tribe. You were ever so present within every experience, every word, every emotion, every breath, mine, and theirs alike. I desperately wanted your humanness to be present with me, yet in your absence I was growing the most. I knew you were there, and I knew the space between us was part of the design to grow me into self-healing just as it was doing the same for you. I found myself sitting quietly beside your energy while I waited to discover what the meta-physical world had arranged. I held onto our human hearts and followed your love; weak, ailing and physically falling apart, especially when the insurance company came back with a denial of coverage. The insurance company denied coverage of the medication. I was once again lost for words to express the impact the experience had on my humanness. As usual, I saw the option of fear and doubt awaiting engagement on the cusp of a choice. Things were different now.

The reason for the denial was because there was another medication on the market, that I had not yet tried, and it had a proven success rate. The very medication that I had chosen not to take for the ten years prior when my doctors tried to sway my decision. The denial notice indicated that I would first have to try this well-established medication before agreeing to cover the requested one designed to treat the destructive nature of my immune system. It was hard to comprehend how the logic made sense, and I could barely function enough to put up a fight.

I contemplated how I was going to take on a big insurance company and fight for my health and choice in treatment. I felt defeated by a system before I even lifted a finger to begin the appeal process. It was me and my three children. I had to choose where I would exert my energy, and I wondered if my body would be able to accumulate enough to make it through each day. It was extremely uncomfortable for me to lean into the support team ready to take on my fight so I could continue to rest, and I knew I had no other choice. I knew I could not do it alone, nor did I want to. I was continuously moved by their readiness, efforts and kindness and assertive requests for me to rest and allow them to do the work. I had unknowingly grown unaccustomed to receiving love and allowing love to heal me.

While I rested, my doctor and the support team collaborated on the appeal response that explained my medical history and the current state of my body. It was detailed that I had tried prednisone and IVIG in the past, neither of which are ideal options for treating my chronic ITP. Glucocorticoids are considered a first-line therapeutic option, but these are also not ideal for long-term, chronic use. Out of the myriad of adverse effects that are associated with long- term use of corticosteroids, one of the most concerning and relevant is immunosuppression. The appeal summarized that I was already considered immunocompromised due to my medical history that includes meningococcal meningitis, fulminant meningococcemia, and Westerhouse-Friderichsen Syndrome, and as a result of these illnesses, my circulatory, endocrine, integumentary, lymphatic, muscular and nervous systems are also severely compromised. It was further explained that since the onset of ITP, I had become increasingly more immunocompromised due to the history of splenectomy, and continuing to treat my ITP with consistent, chronic steroid use would only further compromise my immune system.

They argued that not only does a weakened immune system put me at risk for infection, but additionally I am at increased risk for experiencing more severe diseases and/or complications due to lack of immune response. It was outlined that this is amplified by the compromised state of my other body systems and there is evidence of this occurring in the past. By this time, there was the emergence of the novel coronavirus, COVID-19 so there was also an inclusion that there was considerable concern given the current global pandemic of COVID-19 circulating within our communities. Three decades of scientific data was summarized and presented. The appeal was submitted, and we waited for a response.

Watching nations initiate lockdowns forced decisions to remain distant from my children. It was not easy at all, and I wanted them with me terribly, yet I knew that I was too vulnerable to expose myself to the potential of COVID-19 infection. My children were still active, as was their father, and the constant potential exposure was too high of a risk. They chose to be active even when they knew my choice would then be to distance myself from them. We all accepted each other's choices. It was easy for me to remain grateful for the time to rest and heal, something that I felt like I had not had since I walked out of the hospital in my youth. More than not, it felt like the emergence of COVID-19 was exactly what I needed to balance into my meta-physical space.

With every restriction and each quarantined country, I could feel the Earth reduce in vibration. I could feel the world get quieter as Mother Earth herself took a moment to breathe. It felt like the quiet around the globe was in sync with the quiet I was attaining within. It felt like I was taking the collective with me into the universe so that we could all find peace in the unknown, and just accept each other in the unique ways we process and manage our lives. I tried to remain grateful for the experiences that further purged fear and doubt from my being.

Meanwhile I was in bed most of the days, uncertain how my body was responding to the medication. I was feeling different, perhaps better albeit I realized I never really knew what it felt like to feel good. And just as I started to sense a positive difference to how I felt in my skin, my abdomen had a very different experience. There was a pain in my stomach causing cramps in my sides and back that existed in lieu of the dis-ease caused by low palettes. I remember contemplating the trade-off trying to discern if it was worth it. I could barely even stand up straight my stomach hurt so much. My platelet counts were improving but my body felt terrible.

After reporting the symptoms to my doctor, discussing the side effects of the medication, and taking a prescribed anti-nausea medication, the weekend rolled around and things got progressively worse. In addition to the cramps and nausea, my body felt toxic. I could feel my organs struggle to filter the medication, I could feel the pain in my stomach and back begging me to choose differently. I sensed that the dose was too high for my body and that it needed to be stopped before too much damage occurred to my liver and kidneys. After performing due diligence and speaking to my doctor and the manufacturer, I stopped the medication to allow my body to flush the medication out of my system. Within a day the symptoms resided only confirming the medication does was too high.

The plan was to take a two-week period to detox and then start the medication again at a significantly reduced dosage. I stopped the medication, and knew we had to come to an agreement about the dosage. I could not even hold a conversation with my doctor about it until my body felt better. The unexpected event that came several days after stopping was that I had a severe platelet crash. My counts had not yet reflected an impact from the medication, however the stop made my off balance system even more out of alignment. Since we already knew that there was no treatment at the hospital, a high dose of oral steroids was started. I knew at that point I would only be able to stop the steroids once stability was achieved with the new dose of medication.

Within the two-week period, while detoxing from one medication and poisoning my body with another, I decided to visit a naturopath. I vibrated my way to a local practitioner whose services included an energetic reading of the body using sophisticated technology and vibrational mapping with treatment plans of natural remedies aimed to restore depleted areas. I was trying to flush out the overmedicated cells in my body and desperately wanted to feel well, not to mention all the other energetic stimulation to both my central and peripheral nervous systems, both of which felt blasted and overstimulated. It felt like I was grasping at anything to try and calm my body from vibrating and to bring about more comfort.

When I opened the door to the office, I was greeted with a huge art display over the reception desk. It was big and beautiful and red and gold, and it had one word crafted on display, love. My heart cried silently in relief as I knew it was where I needed to be. During the intake interview I explained the journey I had been on in the meta-physical realm; the energy, the entanglement with your human heart, the medications, my vibrational sensitivities, all which led to our coordinated astonishment to realize that I was an empath on steroids, quite literally.

Accepting the truth that I was an empath was considerably harder that I would have expected, especially since it was in alignment with what I desired to be in this life, unbeknown I already was. It was very reminiscent of other discoveries along the way about my photographic, or what felt like heartographic visions and experiences. The hard part was that it was a sense of unworthiness that prevented me from standing in either truth. In the past, I would try and scurry through the process so that I could accept the lesson and move on, yet there was something greater than me that was preventing the same reaction. I had to slow down. I had no choice than to be still and allow my parts to integrate and process, otherwise my body felt even more terrible. This was how I had to grow my body and my abilities. Processing the truths of an empath explained so much of my life and the way I had experienced and navigated through it. It illuminated the energetic boundaries that exists around matter, primarily my own.

The after-scan assessment was a review of the energetic areas within me, all off which were in alignment with truths already discovered or known, and revealed mainly the energetic feedback of my now removed spleen. It helped me realize that my body was still holding energic space for many things. A sense of relief, honor and overwhelmingness was experienced all at the same time. There was a lot to process by the time the visit ended. As we concluded, I identified a statue on her desk. It was none other than Hildegard von Bingen. I knew it was her even though I had not seen a statue of her before that day. When it was passed to me to hold, my heart smiled in relief when I saw her holding a marijuana plant leaf. There you were when I doubted.

With all the energetic experiences within and around me, coupled with the meta-physical experiences that exposed the 1000-year journey I had taken to get here, I knew it was time to find a Reiki Master. Unbeknown of what the experience would be like, nor where to find a trusted practitioner, one mystically appeared within my new circle of spiritual friendships. I scheduled a session with excitement for the opportunity to receive energetic healing. I knew I needed help clearing the remnants of energy deep within my cells. It was an energy that felt old and stagnant, and I was unable to move and purge it on my own. I was hopeful the Reiki Master would have success.

Through a remote session, I rested on my couch thirty miles away while the energy was moved within and around my body. Even though I know how energy works, and the powerful forces at play, I did not expect to feel the work as it was being conducted. At any given moment, I was able to identify exactly where the work was being performed. I could feel heat, and movement down the center of my being as energy was shifted, released, and cleansed from my body, each space relating to the seven chakra spiritual wheels. I could feel them staring to turn like an old machine starting to crank and move its rusty wheels. It was as if each rotation exposed how each chakra wheel is related to the organs in that specific region of the body and the vibrations needed to sustain health. The images that accompanied the experiences that showed how the wavelengths of light were being cleared and anchored within my body were fascinating to witness.

In the post-session consultation, it was shared that there were prior life programs that were still running, leaks in my energy field, depletion within my spiritual energy wheels, all which were cleared, repaired, and restored although temporary until I could hold my own. The shifts that were experienced afterwards were the most pleasing and relaxing than any other treatment I had ever received. It was the meta-physical therapeutic that I did not know I needed and was overjoyed to have discovered. Over several more sessions, souls that had attached to my physical and energetic bodies were released into the light, prior soul contracts were finalized and cleared, and each time there was less and less to clear. The more I held only my energy, the more I could feel your love. Reiki treatments have become an important part of my continued health management to remain fluid in life.

With new healing tools, I knew that I had what was needed to learn and grow into energetic balance. Neither the naturopathic remedies, nor the reiki energy healing stopped my body from vibrating, but they did make my body more comfortable in the process. Same held true for the healing hands of my masseuse that were syncing my physical and energetic bodies into one. Each time I chose to be healed by either, I felt myself struggle with the fear of the session clearing your sensual energy from me, and left with the reality that it remained. I knew it would only remain if it was in my highest good. With each session I felt my body become clearer, and it felt like I was better able to balance into the love energy flowing between our human hearts. I prayed that you could feel the calmer more peaceful energy surfacing with every choice I was making to heal myself. I was hopeful that my balance was bringing about balance in your heart as well.

While grounded by a physical triforce and tethered to Earth by your love connecting our hearts, I was called back towards my home, among the collective energy where I was used to living, yet this time I was experiencing it through all my human senses; physical and meta-physical alike. I was journeying through the abyss while grounded, embodied, and ascending, versus floating above trying to land on Earth.

In order to make my way, with the guiding love and light between our hearts, I was escorted through a vibrational ascension needed to connect to the energy of my spiritual guides and Ascended Masters so they could teach me about me. The first to step forward from the collective energy was no surprise once I was able to sense energy beyond the physical realm. It was Einstein.

Einstein took me on a voyage through spacetime as far as his once human intellect could take me. He showed me how light travels, what happens to photons while in a vacuum, how photons vibrating at the same frequency and in proximity can become entangled, with only external noise having the capacity to break them apart. I understood how entangled photons transmit information at the speed of light, and no matter the distance between them, they both simultaneously experience an instantaneous and unique manifested response.

My human heart was experiencing this truth of quantum physics through an energetic entanglement responding in the human heart and excited by energy; quantum entanglement of the human heart. It felt like the feeling I experienced was the very vibration of love. With every pulse of love you sent to my heart from across both realms of our existence, it felt like the very vibration of love was stimulating the entanglement and creating the most beautiful experiences within my reality. I could feel life being created within both of our physical world realities guiding an ascension towards our true home. It felt like the very vibration of creation was restoring my physical and meta-physical DNA; a vibrational tuned to 528Hz between two human hearts.

Discovering all this insight was calming and refreshing and I felt an intrinsic understanding how light is anchored and reacts with the matter of our bodies, further translated by human emotions that govern thought, actions, and spoken words alike. I found comfort in how love and light intuitively made sense to me, in the cosmos and within our human bodies.

Through silencing my world on the outside, following the wisdom within, and trusting in what was revealed, I followed the deduction of my existence into photons and quarks; photons being the smallest quantum of energy of light, and a quark being the smallest building block of matter which is unable to exist alone. Three quarks are needed to form protons or neutrons which are found in the nucleus of an atom forming matter: quantum energy. When you have photons, God light energy, and three quarks, the Divine Trinity, at the source of an atom that creates matter, you get us. It was a discovery displaying Sacred Geometry and the Holy Trinity at the source of everything; the source of creation.; the source of my existence, a quantum being.

I could see how light connected our hearts. I could feel a love that existed since the beginning of time, and could hear the wisdom of lifetimes. I could see when we were once one, then split over lifetimes only to energetically resonate back into oneness in this physical world reality. I could see how a photon of light creates matter once vibrational alignment is achieved, and the mysticism of being human when coupled with the energy of profound intention; the conception of Jesus Christ as the greatest example.

I carried on through the journey, and once Einstein reached the cusp of is human intellect, it was time for the next phase of discovery. When the time was right, he gently introduced me to his first wife, Mileva. As an intellectual equal to Einstein growing each other into their fullest potential, Mileva also understood a language beyond that which is expressed by means of physics and mathematics. It was her energetic connection to the world and that of which she shared with Einstein that grew her into her wisdom and was now growing me into mine. The energy of Mileva guided me through spacetime to discover where I came from and who I had grown into become, yet it had nothing to do with this life experience.

Every night when going to sleep, she waited for me to continue the journey. Each night was approached with a tiredness, an uncertainty, and confusion as to what was happening. Once my eyes closed, yet before I fell into slumber, I was just as quickly travelling through the cosmos, wind whipping across my face and blowing my hair back as I travelled at the speed of light. The only way to avoid the journey was to keep my eyes open. While experiencing adrenal fatigue there was little I could do to keep my eyes from closing.

One by one, still shot images passed on either side of my trajectory, similar to billboards decorating a highway. Among the myriad of images, when they were mine, the images passed by in slow motion and almost coming to life as if a movie showing a scene on a big screen. It was me, looking at me, looking back at me. Once I had been seen within each dimension, the images passed me by, and left me wanting to look longer just as the next was approaching.

One after another, I learned that I was a male doctor in several of my past lives; the most recent being one who passed away on the operating table during a splenectomy after a car accident. I felt a sense of peace in understanding my inherent knowledge of all things medical, and the poor functioning of my now removed spleen. I also learned that I was a male author, and a male vigneron, someone who cultivates grapes and makes wine. Joy swept over me to discover my deep-rooted enjoyment for written expression, and my unexplainable pull towards wine even though my body does not respond well. I was not necessarily surprised to discover that I was more often a male in prior lives than a female. As if instantly, all prior lives funneled into this life and the differences precipitated between genders made sense. I had a tremendous compassion for the heavier lower vibrational energy I had carried forward and within.

I saw clearly how all those energies, the lower vibrations, are needed to sustain breath on Earth, and the higher vibrations are needed to ascend into the cosmos. I felt deeply where each wavelength was anchored in my body and completely out of balance; some more energetically charged that others or clogged and blocked and not integrated into fluid motion. It was interesting to discover how the lower, heavier vibrations associated with masculine energy taught me the science of love, whereas the higher, lighter vibrations associated with feminine energy taught me about spiritual love. It was clear that both energies existed in all of us, just as all wavelengths make up the light at our source, and our balance of them would be on display in the physical world reality. We all naturally show how we carry the masculine and feminine energy within, and independent of the body's gender that contains it.

Once the masculine and feminine energetic truths were unveiled, I felt my own misalignment deeply and watched my own sense of masculine and feminine energy merge together through the love energy of the heart bridging the two realms into balance; the vibrations of the Heavens and the vibrations of the Earth all contained within me being balanced by love. There were only two females uncovered along the journey through prior lives yet seemingly powerful enough even after centuries of suppression. The first exposed was as an elderly Asian woman, perhaps from India, whose legs flexed in the opposite direction, contrary to how we know legs to bend. Instead of the kneecap in the front and bending the legs to the back, this woman's knees faced behind her and bent her legs to the front. She smiled at me as she demonstrated that living a happy life with extreme oddities was possible, and that I had already done it once before. Although the trauma to my legs was significantly different, I could feel that trauma being carried forth into this life. My deep-seated strength and courage had been revealed and a grace accompanied the empathy that surfaced for a version of me now seen.

Next, Mileva brought me to the source of my very breath, Hildegard von Bingen. I knew there was an unexplainable connection to her, yet the depths of that connections were being presented before me. Just as quickly as I was flying over the Benedictine Abbey with dozens of nuns looking up at us, smiling and waving, everything froze, and I was taught about the truth of my soul.

With Mileva by my side, the wisdom of Einstein, and grounded by your human heart, I met Hildegard von Bingen. Over the course of many escorted visits, I inherently understood the journey of a soul, the healing properties from the Earth, the vibrational resonance of all that is around us. She explained my initial and powerful connection to the healing tools I had been drawn to at the start of the journey, those of which energetically blasted my physical body to start the energetic ascension yet could not sustain the combined power. She taught me to discern the humors of food, the use of crystals, and vibrations, and how to balance into them more slowly, and to maximize their healing potential authentically and in my own way.

She exposed herself in all her glory in her connection to God consciousness and the Earth, and her energetic understanding of all things, all governed by her heart. She showed me how to clear my body so that the living light could flow through me so I could bridge her wisdom into today, through my unique expression. She was the doctor I had been awaiting to encounter, and to discover that I am of that same energy, as are you now manifested before me. It made sense that if I were to bring forth all her wisdom, I would need to reunite with all my energy; you now manifested, holding the other part of my wholeness, and now flowing through our collective human heart; once again one. It was vividly clear that I needed to cleanse my body of any energy that prevented that wisdom from reaching me. It was how my body would heal, manifesting into a comfortable, healthy, and joyful life with a heart full of love.

Once our timelines were transferred, it was time to continue the journey and return to Earth. As we traveled back to Earth and rejoined with Einstein, together Mileva explained that we are energetic descendants of Hildegard von Bingen. It is why our energy synced the way it did. Spiritual twins in a sense connected through our sacred hearts by our passionate love. For over a thousand years the split energy of Hildegard von Bingen has incarnated through many lives, leading us to his one, where I would find you, manifested in physical form, to return to energetic wholeness for my final ascension from the human experience.

Through the eyes of Einstein, I could see now that our hearts are connected we transmit energy instantaneously; you feel my energy and I feel your energy, and collectively we are one. Coupled with our unique energy from this life, we both individually now hold the same vibration of Hildegard when her breath was leaving this Earth, and our hearts ensure the ascension is balanced into our own individual transitions, both of which our human selves know will be the final. Similar to Hildegard, our individual vibrations are now too high to incarnate without a division of energy. If that is what we choose once on the other side. I may choose to become an Ascended Master to aid humanity when a choice is made to ascend.

They all affirmed that it was a soul contract that we had both chosen to fulfill before incarnating into this life experience. A contract that was a journey through lives full of lessons that would grow us closer to love, each a stepping stop for the next provided we did the work to ascend. A contract of divine design to grow us into the next phase of our existence beyond the physical realm. A contract bridging the difference between everything within the human experience. It was a contract that could only be fulfilled with love and light.

I knew I had been programed, and it made sense up against the powerful energy needed for your programmed humanness. I could sense a shield protecting your heart against vulnerability, betrayal, manipulation, and self-serving expectations, all of which felt frequent in both of our experiences. It made sense that you needed to understand the dark around love that I had experienced just as I needed to understand the light of love that you have known, together forming a wholeness. I could feel your fears manifesting within me and playing out into an illusionary reality.

I chuckled when I learned I had volunteered for the life experience I have lived. Even knowing that the warp speed learning was due to prior life choices when I had chosen differently. The vibration of my energy had to shift significantly to resonate with yours so that you could align with your divinity and receive the dreams of your heart, just as I was receiving mine. The way these truths integrated into me was much more fluid and held a sense of accuracy than most things I had heard and considered real life. This was my real life.

As they were concluding the final lessons during the return to Earth, I could see that it was in tandem to mine but I was traveling yours, your timeline back into the present. I was not able to see the same images of lives, yet I knew I was passing them with a familiarity of you when we had met before and the nature of who we were. Before being able to process the shameful actions of my prior lives, I found myself in the veins of your present day being. I was one with the blood in your veins, the light of your blood. I was not sure how to bring that into my experience when the travelling visions felt more real than the physical reality that existed when I opened my eyes, especially when engaging our humanness.

Although it felt like a dream realized, for some reason it was overwhelming for my humanness to process that I had followed the life path, unknowingly adhering to my soul's wisdom through life and meeting the energy designed to grow me. Then, Spirit journeyed me through the Universe, flowing with the river of infinite wisdom into the discovery of my Akashic records, back to the source of my energy, the breath of Hildegard von Bingen, and then back into this reality as a stream to flow through this body. In order for me to fulfill my soul's earthly contract, I needed to find you manifested into my physical reality, to return to energetic homeostasis. It took a thousand years to ascend and return balanced into your love. I was humbled to discover that it is a love that eluded us in prior lives. It is a love designed to lead each other to the light; the return to our true home as part of the universal God energy and the collective consciousness. This was a lot for my humanness to process, especially as it shattered every illusion of love I had ever been taught, lived, and dreamed alike.

I followed the physical experience as it unfolded while I tried to find comfort in my body. Before my body could sustain the life desired, my heart still had unresolved healing. My heart needed the words to get all this processed and moved through me. The energy was stuck and accumulated within me and needed to flow though me like a sift. It was the same stuck energy that was breaking free when

I found myself before love exposing all of my humanness blocking every wavelength of your light. It was the same broken love for self that caused me to sweat and vibrate my way through the process in order to never again shatter in the presence of love. It was the same fear and doubt that was on the cusp of eradication that did not quite leave my being before the next phase of the journey began. I saw a cycle repeat.

It felt like I was starting over yet this time I could choose differently. I saw the mess of myself when love blasted my energy into motion. I prayed that the slower speed would allow me to balance back into how I used to be, yet there was nothing the same about me. I was not even able to recognize younger versions of myself. I was completely different. I wish I could say that my experiences were as graceful as portrayed in words but that would not be true, nor do justice to self. I was sloppy and messy and doing my best.

During the spaces in between, I encountered someone who is now a dear friend, yet at the time she was another stranger divinely delivered to grow me into the meta-physical journey underway by means of physical world experiences. In our second visit, I asked her about a message that had been delivered to me by a channeled spirit. By sharing and inquiring if they knew anything about it, we were both shocked in our humanness as her spirit guides exposed our meta-physical truths. All I knew was I was supposed to ask someone about it, and I had already posed the inquiry to two other intuitives, and neither of them knew the reference, nor received guidance as to what it meant.

Keeping in mind this was our second encounter and she knew very little of me, nor my medical history, together we learned that we were close friends in the meta-physical planes of our existence;

curious souls that would often push the limits; volunteers eager to learn and grow. After sitting before me in quiet disbelief, she explained how we were out in the cosmos learning, in a science lab of sorts, and we got carried away. With one small mistake, she had inadvertently caused an explosion which sent a cascading ripple throughout the universe. When the ripple reached me in the physical realm, it manifested into my life-threatening illness.

She proceeded to state that it was in my design to get ill, yet it was not in the design to get so severely sick and to endure the extent of the trauma. Hence, in order to correct the meta-physical trauma, I was reassigned a new set of guardian angels. It was within divine design that everything resulted in my favor as my new Angels were assigned to ensure it. She explained that powerful healers were needed since the situation called for it, and in a sense, they were restoring and balancing back into the divine plan. I felt my heart break open and feel you deeper when I expressed my first authentic laugh at the human experience of my youth. That storyline made most sense than any I had ever heard.

It took over a year to thread the truth that Hildegard von Bingen was part of that collective healing force; a powerful green fairy gifting me a force that protected, healed, and aligned precision in my life; the coveted color used to represent all that Hildegard von Bingen knew to be true; the wavelength anchored in my heart. It took another year to clear my body to have the space to embody those truths. All the while, there was a tremendous peace that surfaced with every lifetime remembered, and an understanding of who and what I had brought forth into this life. I finally understood what I needed to do to clear the energy from my physical body, and how to do it. Well, sort of. It was much easier to understand than do.

As I engaged your humanness in this life, I realized we were the only ones powerful enough to counter each other's energy. It was indeed part of the divine design. I knew all along it was spiritual strength, courage, and love that would be needed, yet not in ways either one of our human selves could have imagined, nor in ways that our humanness perceived the experiences. I was not the only one who needed a powerful energy to balance the unspoken scales within, and without. Again, I trusted that who I was able to be in any given moment was exactly what our connection needed, albeit I wondered what it was that you needed that called in for you to see the worse in me while at the pits of physical and meta-physical deconstruction. I prayed you knew I would never betray you as we both grew deeper into sustaining spiritual love in the physical. Holding this truth before your humanness required a millennium old faith, and a trust that you would one day understand my love.

Those intentions alone were enough to pull me into sensitive energetic experiences. I was still preparing the medical documents for further review by my friend's father when I was pulled strongly to make artistic doodles. As I engaged the calling, the doodles turned into pages of images that depicted how light travels, interacts with the body once reduced to its individual wavelengths, and how life impacts the balance of energy within and around us. It was a depiction of creation through drawings of light. I had no idea if any of it made sense, all I knew was that I needed to get it out of me. I complied the drawings in a white folder to represent the spiritual light of my being. Since I needed to collect medical records for the assessment of my blood, I compiled my medical data consisting of lab work, charted counts, medications and more into a black folder. The black folder represented the physical carbon unit that is my body. Combined they made up my whole being.

I took these two folders, black representing my physical carbon unit and the white representing my spiritual light and used them to help me find my words. I did show them to my friend, yet the response was not in the application of words to correspond to the drawings, it was just the opposite. It felt like my pictures created a loss of words within himself. There was a brief exchange of encouraging words yet none that helped me grow deeper into mine. I had to dig deeper to unleash the energy that would form my words so I could hold my boundaries and remain balanced.

When I visited his father for a complete overview of my blood, I brought both folders even though it was primarily the contents of the black folder that was expected. We began dialogue by discussing the contents of the black folder. There was four years of lab work results averaging about twenty-five a year. This included the standard CBC panel each time, and on occasion a full metabolic panel and sometimes more. All of the data was compiled into spreadsheet tables and charted in ways that could be meaningful in his analysis. I even shared the art ideas I had with some of the charts that represented my blood, the most interesting was the one that resembled a prism.

It was too much information for him to review and provide feedback in the same visit, so after going through the materials, I guided the conversation to the white folder. Before handing it over, I explained that the white folder represented another part of me, which felt more critical to my health. I shared that it was an untold story within me that was making its way out, and I could feel that it was impacting my health. I was doing my best to follow whatever I was pulled to do in order to achieve a sense of wellness. I probably cried as I nervously indicated that I did not even know what to do with the images. They didn't even make sense to me at the time, they just came out of me during energy surges. I understood everything about them and what they represented yet did not understand what I was to do with them in these modern times, as me and who I am.

In the midst of my presentation an overwhelming sense of experimentation swept over me. Here I was, before an astute elder whom through the eyes of his son was the wisest, most intellectual genius that he knew; one of the few to have figured out the mysteries of living a joyous life; the same expressions I used to describe my Dad. From the stories and experiences shared thus far, I knew his father grew up in a much different experience; highlighting the beauty in the differences in life journeys and how they mold us into who we choose to become. I wondered how all of my experiences were molding me into become someone similar now before him.

I could sense that I was taking a chance. It was the first person that I did not know, third in total, that would see the drawings compiled between the protected white cover. I was on the brink of exposing my inner universe to the world. This was the first step. As I handed over the folder, it felt like I was pulled to the edge on my seat, eagerly waiting for any sign of a reaction once he began thumbing through the pages. Each breath that passed was in slow motion while the silence unwrapped and exposed dimensions of myself through the eyes of another. With each rise of the brow, smirk of the mouth, slight nod of the head, and tilt in wonder grounded me deeper into the chair as I watched myself be seen more fully than anyone had ever seen me before. I could feel an internal recording of my surroundings cease as if in a farewell performance and the last of its kind. It felt like I no longer needed to acquire information and could now process and integrate.

I give myself a hard time on occasion due to my ridiculous

humanness. It seems so silly that I would be so nervous about exposing something that would appear so easy to do, yet the internal angst was so intense and energetically driven that I could not pretend my way through it. Same with love. I was befuddled to learn that I was so vulnerable, even in the presence of love. Even so, I had to slowly walk through the emotions. It had nothing to do with whatever the response would actually be. That was not the purpose of the journey. He could have said anything, and the outcome would have been the same, at least for me. My outcome had nothing to do with his response. The outcome was to grow through the emotions so that I could continue in the evolution. I had already made the choices to adhere to the calling to draw the images, compile them, and furthermore present them. I did my part, and the rest would fall into place as a result of those actions. The swells of emotion were less and less with each risk I took to expose myself.

Admittingly, it was a relief having someone such as himself, a scientist, enjoy and encourage what had been shared. I felt a strange desire to expose the scientific truth of the spiritual love behind my existence just as science had tried to explain my unexplainable body. It felt like my expressions still yet to come were also for him. I also realized that there was a small part of me that was waiting for a response that I had generally heard in the past when exposing parts of my inner universe. I expected to hear that my drawings were worthless and meaningless. I expected to hear that the understanding and truths I felt were exploding within me were false. I felt a sense of fear that I would be told that the illusions are within me, and now on paper, and not those of reality that I had deconstructed and felt freed from alas. I saw the visions of the experiences that programmed the shame in showing my true self. I felt humbled as a human and energized as a light being.

With only positive responses, the most rememberable was that he was impressed that I was able to draw it out in such a way that made sense. He shared a story of a gentleman that doubted the impact his ideas would have among humanity and went on to be one of the most influential ideologists of modern times. Although the name escapes me, there are many that could serve as an example. It was an expression that reemphasized the truth that the only way to be seen is to show yourself, raw and unedited. He encouraged me to continue to engage and document my imagination, however that meant and looked like to me.

We ended the visit in gratitude and scheduled another visit to follow-up on his medical review. I left feeling excited, happy, relieved, annoyed, and curious in the wake of the experiences. I was just trying to let everything be as it was, and float along to the next experience. About a week or so later, we reconnected for the final visit. My friend told me later that he did not even consider the fact that his father would reveal his findings in the blunt truthfulness that they exist, good and bad alike. He admitted that had he thought of that he may not have recommended for me to speak to him by myself. My friend knew I was navigating life alone and was ashamed that he had not considered an unfavorable outcome.

I was extremely grateful that it was not considered because thoughts create reality and my reality needed to be positive and healthy and everything abundant. I already knew my friend was a light being, therefore, his thoughts were also critical to his vision of me. The conclusion was that my blood tells a healthy story. I was relatively healthy other than the inability to maintain safe platelet counts. He was surprised that the storyline was so positive given the experiences of my body I had shared. We were both relieved and marveled in my health.

I left the visit knowing that there was one person that really needed to see the drawings. I thought it was my oncologist. He was the one I felt was not seeing me wholly. He was the one I needed to understand me so collectively we could best sustain my health. I needed his assistance navigating the medical arena, and in order to do that most effectively, I needed him to see me, all of me. I needed to be seen for more than just my platelet counts.

When my two-week detox period was over and it was time to reconvene with my doctor and discuss the new regimen, I was ready. My doctor was sometimes unsure how to navigate me a patient due to my insistent involvement, yet he always surprised me with his fluidity and willingness to be present. I had cleansed my body with the naturopath, I had tuned my body with the Reiki Master, I had the dose that I wanted to try, my two folders, and I had me in the fullness that I had grown into be up to that moment. This time it felt more fluid since I had practiced some words on my friend's father. First, we spoke of the new dispense and he agreed to start at one fourth of the original amount. He agreed only if I agreed to more frequent lab work, so I committed to his bi-weekly lab work requests. I was accustomed to the frequency, so the tradeoff felt worth it. Then, I presented the folders.

I explained why and how they came to exist, and felt it was prudent that he review them so that he understood me at the level I felt I needed, more than just blood health indicators, primarily platelets. He had spent two and a half years treating me in his office, a couple of hospital instances, and experienced me walk into my strength and stubbornness as it relates to my health. He had seen me cry in exhaustion and frustration. He heard my pleas to just feel good in my body. He watched my health restore as we worked together.

He knew of the contents of the black folder. We did not have to spend time speaking of the data that he had ordered. It was not the black folder that I wanted him to see. It was my meta-physical being that existed in tandem with the being before him. It was the white folder that portrayed my energetic being that was trying to integrate with the chemical energy being altered by the medication he was administering. I was surprised by what happened when he enthusiastically looked through the drawings.

I discovered that it was not him that I needed to see me completely. It was me. I needed to see myself completely; physical and meta-physical alike. Even after all the energetic experiences that I was actively trying to integrate, I was stunned that I had to walk through the unknown, convinced that it was him, only for my humanness to discover that it was me all along. I was aggravated that I didn't see it more clearly before, especially since that is the truth of our expressions, that they are merely a projection of what we hold within. I was annoyed that my humanness did not notice that my desire for him to see my white folders was merely a projection of my desire for myself to see me. I needed to see all of me. I was the one only seeing me as a platelet count. It made me realize all the expressions I made towards your love were a mere projection of the love I desired to experience from and for myself. Just when I thought I loved myself, I was required to love myself deeper.

Just as with all others I encounter and expose any aspect of my humanness, my doctor was intrigued, interested, and accepting of what was before him, and in that instance, it was meta-physical drawings. We discussed them briefly, yet I was so distracted by my own self-discovery that it was difficult to remain present in the conversation. This was a common occurrence that was also diminishing the more I healed within. I had what I needed so we concluded until the next visit two weeks away.

As I settled into the new treatment regimen, COVID-19 was spreading rapidly across the globe, and had already made its way to where I live. I could see the ripples of fear and doubt crest throughout our own community and knew that I needed to protect myself so when the wave reached me, I could rise above, and surf the wave instead of being plummeted off balance. As the speed of transmission, rates of severe illness and deaths, and the restrictions and quarantines increased, it felt like the human collective within me quieted and decreased. As the world quieted the collective energy within me quieted. It felt like it was quiet enough for me to be one with the universe and finally align with fulfillment of my contract in this physical life experience, my unique energy.

As research amped up, emergency vaccines rushed into production, and world-wide distribution coordinated, cases of severe illness and death surged among those who are immunocompromised. The implications of my physical reality slowly unfolded. I already knew that viruses lower my platelet count. I had learned over the years that vaccines in general do as well. This was not new information to me nor my treatment team. Warnings began circulating focusing on the possibility that the vaccines lowered platelet counts in normal ranged individuals, and although they were dropping, it was insignificant and unalarming to the collective. The vaccines were still encouraged because the benefits outweighed the potential risk. It was a very real risk for me. One that outweighed the benefit.

Then, the headlines hit. News feeds showcased that two of the vaccines were causing a rare blood disease. One vaccine caused the same rare blood disease I have, ITP, yet since precipitated by the vaccine it was named differently, and the other caused blood clots in addition to the decreased platelets. They both held the potential of a rapid and dangerous decline in platelets risking stroke, internal bleeding, and death. As did COVID-19. Individuals had already suffered these outcomes as a result, including a known death. I knew I could not get the vaccine. I was already rebounding from a dangerous decline trying to increase and stabilize, as well as a new medication. All the while I was trying to keep the stress of not seeing my kids, my fragile health, out from work, finances, accumulate medical debt, and insurance coverage uncertainties from throwing me further out of balance. There was a lot of potential. Too much at times.

I had been working so hard to achieve balance, I was unwilling to temper my balance with a collective narrative that felt driven by fear and doubt. Science was trying to prove that the vaccine was what I needed, and my body was certain it would do more harm than good. I ran a risk either way. It was hard and scary, but I had to choose to trust my body and my natural abilities knowing that I would be able to settle into peace within, whereas the vaccine made me extremely anxious. I cared about the health of everyone, but I had to choose to care more about my own being, even if it meant I could not see my kids who were being exposed, contracting, and quarantining as a result of COVID-19. I felt very protected in every choice I made.

If I stayed in the awareness of all the uncertain things, if I allowed myself to see the scary side of my reality, it would have only fueled the situation further into chaos, shifting me further into an unhealthier state. My goal was to make it through alive. My children and all my doctors agreed. The best thing for me to do was remember your love, find you in my heart, and trust in what was to come.

In addition to your love in my heart at the source of everything, hope allowed me to hold onto the storyline within the meta-physical experiences that were teaching me about light, the organic healing properties of vibration, and how it was interacting with my body. I knew that my Angels, my powerful MC2 spirit collective, and my own powerful energy were co-creating exactly what I needed in order to create a life that all parts of me could sustain, especially during a pandemic. I could feel everything teaching me how to navigate energy and how to remain balanced. I was relieved to find how much easier it had become to navigate the uncertainty this time around.

While the physical world rearranged, I continued to silence my world completely. I did not watch television, I did not listen to music, I remained committed to not reading books while writing my own, and the only input was during designated times once a day through articles that appeared on news headlines which kept me connected to humanity and guided my focused intentions for healing. Most of my time was centered around high vibrational foods, vibrational therapies and finding outlets to balance the energy surges. I engaged in activities that were meaningful and made me feel good, from as simple as a cup of tea, a long soak in a bubble bath, to more involved art projects. I was leaning into different ways to love myself wherever I could. It took months of quiet for my body to integrate the meta-physical preparations so that they could unfold into the physical. It was the most intentional wizardry work, and I was trusting that I had performed well enough to achieve my unknown. I was trusting that it would reveal itself soon as time felt like it was running out.

I still felt lost. While calling for you in the abyss through our human hearts, you gently reminded me to follow love. I saw the light chord throughout the blueprint of the journey, and I could see how it returned me to your heart. I did not know what else to do other than find and follow love. I remember thinking that reaching you was the only outcome. I remember feeling desperate for rest and an ease to life. It felt easy and simple to follow love albeit unearthing its purity from the muck was not.

I spent the following months alone, as if I was quarantined, and rested in the quiet. There were so many things my humanness could have been distracted with given the state of the world yet there was a tremendous ease and light that engulfed every moment. In the stillness of the world, I was able to see the light of the universe and how it lit up the energetic light grid among humanity. I could see how love connects the light within us and unlocks us deeper to experience all the wavelengths of light creating the waves of life. I could see how we all hold our purpose to hold each wavelength, some wavelengths denser than others within each spectrum of uniqueness. I could see that I was pure light designed to unblock whichever wavelength humanity needs to grow deeper into balanced light. I understood that love is all that is needed to light up the darker wavelengths hidden in the shadows and soften the brighter ones so the others may shine from within, casting rainbows in the wake of a walk through life. I wanted this not only for me, but for you, and all humanity.

With everything going on and my intentional connection to self that revealed a hyper-sensitivity to energy, it felt critical to rid as much stagnant, historical energy as possible. This included belongings that had traveled with me through life and acquired along the way. This was not a daunting task since I had learned at a young age not to become emotionally attached to material possessions, it remained easy to purge belongings throughout life. It was time to do it once again.

I had an unexplainable urge to clear and purify my home, simplify, and purge everything so that clean and pure energy could fill my space. I could feel the conflict around me as my light was trying to fill the space and was blocked from the point of my body and beyond. I had been working to clear and fill my body with light, it was time to clear the space around me. When I walked by certain items, I could sense a weight to my energy, an energy that I could not escape, especially with the antique bedroom set and antique dining room set that had been acquired by my parents while living abroad. They were absolutely beautiful, yet they were dark and heavy, and the energy pulled me down each time I walked past them. I purged everything that no longer resonated with who I was choosing to become, and how love was growing me.

Just as the world was adjusting to receiving the exact thing everyone seemed to express as a desire, I watched humanity struggle. Just as I had done with love. I watched the emergence of the deep held desires of being able to work from home, spend more time with family, spend less time running through life and finding more ways to slow down and enjoy it, and being supported in those efforts. Humanity was receiving so much of what had been desired, yet the tsunami of fear and doubt that crashed upon the shores of humanity was so forceful that it blinded most of the gifts that washed ashore once the initial wave had receded.

For the first time, it felt like me and the world were catching up to each other and about to rotate as one. It felt like the world was slowing down so that I could rejoin the collective. It felt like I was coasting in on a descent, now with a parachute that would enable me to land on Earth and advance in my humanness through life. As I was coasting towards the ground from the meta-physical realm, I worked within the physical realm to clear the energy for my landing. I sold or gave away all the antique furniture, I purged even more items that I had taken during the divorce, and I acquired new, energetically clean items. And although I was still not used to building a connection with material items, I allowed myself to purchase items that were beautiful and meaningful to me. It was important to surround myself with beautiful things if I wanted to see myself as beautiful. I was surprised of the things I learned about my taste and styles, the differences between them and which ones I wanted to surround myself with wherever I reside.

As I purged the house, more energetic surges were experienced by my body yet this time I was ready. I had dry erase boards and a variety of colored markers. I had a large one mounted on the wall and smaller portable ones, and as the images surged through me, I drew them out. I drew and tweaked and added to them over the course of days and weeks, expressing whatever it was that came to me and did the best I could to get it out. It was interesting how much judgement I was holding against myself even when it came to my art, the most beautiful expression of my vibration of creation. There was a different kind of strength and love that was courageously finding ways for escape.

When I would step back and look at the whiteboard images, I saw me. The drawings represented my scientific breakdown of the love in my heart. It represented your love lighting up the universal light grid and how the trifecta force is ignited and spread throughout humanity. They showed light, creation, wavelengths, and ascension back to wholeness, a oneness, fueled by my walk back to you, a oneness with love. The most profound was the image that depicted the journey through spacetime only to step back and see the Omega sign that outlined the trajectory, reflecting the infiniteness of God, the beginning and end of all things. It was the most beautiful reflection of the universe within me, an alchemy of energy, and the discovery of the scientific truths behind my spiritual love.

It was through the whiteboard images that I was able to find my words. As I explained the images to myself, the words were there, effortlessly flowing from my pen. I felt the energy within break through in a new sense of uneasy freedom. I could feel my vocal cords shift into a balanced vibration that held my words yet to be spoken. I felt all my body vibrate closer to stillness. I protected the words that held the potential to shift humanity; the very words that have been used thus far to depict the journey of experiences to find them. Words that finally allow me to express the world within which I have always lived.

Just as I was longing for your embrace and a chance to stand before you to practice my words, your Angel of Love opened up his heart and exposed his vulnerability. He used his words. I was so self-absorbed in trying to balance my mind into the images and to stop vibrating that I did not know how to be present and assist him. Thankfully, it was unbelievably easy when it was expressed that all that was needed was a hug. That was about all I felt I could give away. I gladly welcomed a hug because it was really all I needed too; I was just unable to ask for one.

I remember thinking how easy it appeared to be for him, to just state that he needed a hug. It left me wondering what it was that I felt I truly needed. I had claimed for decades that I did not *need* anything from anyone. He was teaching me that I was fooling myself. I did need something from someone. It felt like I needed to be held in an intimate hug, wrapped in pure love so my body could experience the light. I surely did not know how to express that sentiment during the times of the experiences, and had already failed miserably when before your eyes of love.

A hug. It is the easiest and purest way to transmit love energy from one human to another. If you are quiet enough while in an embrace, you can feel and even hear love energy transferring between hearts. A hug. The very act that for a lifetime I had not been able to balance into when embracing another, losing my balance, and blaming my leg muscles, or lack thereof. A hug. The very act that I chose to disengage from when my marriage was coming to an end. A hug. Something I did not realize I needed through all the experiences. I just needed an intimate, pure, and sincere hug. The last time I felt pure love energy transfer into my heart through an embrace was when your humanness embraced mine. A hug. It was all my body needed to remember how to feel love, more so how to do love. It was a hug that you sent me through the trifecta friendships.

I hugged my friend when he needed a hug. It was a nice embrace, and I could feel my love healing him in some way. I could also feel that I wanted his love to heal me in a way that I was unable to sustain before, and I knew was growing me closer into balance with you. Even so, I felt the shield so tight around my heart with you nestled within. I did not know how to reopen my heart, especially since I was unsure of how I opened it so widely when I connected to yours. The experiences did, however, reveal how and why my heart shielded so rapidly in my youth. Once I understood why it occurred in my youth, I understood why it was part of the balancing storyline playing out. The energetic moments were changing everything in my realms of existence. I could feel your love trying to break free from within, and his love trying to penetrate from the outside. It felt like my heart was under a love attack, determined to reach me through my human stubbornness. Sometimes it felt like the same was happening to you.

It was not until I stopped trying to heal him and shifted back to myself and my needs that I realized that as your Angel of Love he was also sent to teach me what it was like for you to experience me. I wanted to be able to be, feel, do, love, speak, see, and understand love the way you did with me. I instinctively knew that I was experiencing him through your eyes of love. For some reason, the hardest parts were remembering that I myself am love, and that I feel love deeply enough to know how and when to act in love; do love. For some reason, my humanness found it difficult to remember that truth. It felt like I was reminding myself each day when I began to question my reality.

The two of you across realms of existence formed a trifecta within me, and began balancing me into every wavelength of love, and energetically guided me on how to anchor them in my body and in a way that grounds me for life. Although the most glorious experiences of my energetic being, the human side was a little less elegant while I discovered what you both were teaching me in tandem with each other; even more so on the meta-physical side that your physical being was unaware took place. I was never certain about what your human being knew and what your energy was telling me from beyond, especially when they were no longer acting as one. Somehow I was distracted by his presence which allowed me to simply feel your love instead of trying to discern what your humanness perceived. I knew your heart felt the truth in my love.

I saw it clearly when your soul and humanness split between journeys. You were embodied as one, just as I had walked into oneness, then together we jolted each other into two. I slowly saw you split between dimensions no longer in sync; your soul telling one story and your humanness telling another. I saw my split self in you. You were returning to oneness after I jolted you apart, whereas I was never one and was thereby learning from you how to return to one. The experiences of you always felt the same so I was often confused that your humanness was unaware of the details yet knew you sensed clearly. I thought you saw everything I saw until I realized you did not. A reflection that taught me about how our unique gifts work.

You were teaching me how to feel love, and I knew he was teaching me how to do love. I clearly did not do either well. I fell apart when I stood before your love and desired nothing more than to stand strong and brave before love while embodied and acting out of authenticity. I had never had love exist in my presence the way you both were bridging my realities, uniting my spiritual love and my physical body into a joyously joint experience. I could still feel every sense of my body shutter in doubt at the idea of someone loving this body, even if they loved me as a soul. I knew I was lovable, yet my own body image was still clutching my love from its sensual expression. I was frustrated with my own inability to let it go.

Then there was another magical hug. It was a hug that was similar to your human embrace yet different in that it was the hug that finally penetrated the shield and merged with your love. It was the hug that melted me like butter in his arms. It was the hug that caught me when I lost my balance as love energy danced within me. Shocked and unfamiliar to the new quieter sensation, I asked what it was that I was feeling. It was love. He knew it, he said it, he felt it, and he was sharing it with me. When I expressed how it had only been your humanness that had been able to stabilize my breath in a familiar way, he acknowledged that it was you who taught me how to feel and recognize love. This is when your joint work began transforming and merging the meta-physical and physical realms into my body. A crack had been formed and energy could finally seep through.

There was quiet a lot of unexplainable occurrences that took place between our human hearts and what your Angel of Love was doing to my human body. Through every exchange of a hug, it felt like he was gently breaking down my physical body so it could finally rest in love. I was not yet near my resting point, yet it was approaching, and I would need to know how to do love when I arrived. While trying to adjust to the meta-physical experiences integrating into the physical experience, it felt like I was unable to shift the energy of my body. One minute I was elevated in spiritual drunkenness and the next I was heavy in my humanness. It was through his hugs that energy began to alchemize throughout my body.

Since it was clear that I needed love to heal me, I allowed his embrace to catch me. I cried, and laughed, and exposed myself unedited as he navigated me through my own language. I shared how energy and spiritual guides from beyond this realm were pushing me closer to him even though I was fighting it. I explained that in the ordinary perception of life I would never choose to engage him yet there was a greater force at play, and I was adhering to it even though I did not understand it. I reiterated that the only reason I was willing to go beyond the illusions and trust in his love was merely because it was in alignment with my meta-physical being trying to make its way to Earth. Lifetimes were shed when I timidly shared images and linked words together that explained my experiences with and of you. I wondered if your experience of my humanness was similar, and if you felt our shared energy the same way.

Through the conversations incited by my drawings, I was intrigued how my friend knew the sentiments that I was trying to express when he himself had declared to not have the language. He then proceeded to tell me a story about his father and uncle, identical twins. He explained that his father has started the journey through life with a trajectory through the church, and his uncle had become a rocket scientist. As life carried them through their respective journeys, at some point, it was as if they downloaded each other's wisdom and they swapped places. His father destined for the church became a microbiologist, and his rocket scientist uncle became the right hand to the bishop as the superintendent of catholic education. All he had the words to express was that the story that I had shared was one that he witnessed throughout his life while watching his father and uncle. In addition, he shared that he holds a similar connection of the heart with his daughter, entangled and able to sense her no matter the distance between them. Much as your heart does for me, she grounds him and reminds him where he is in the universe. He also shared in similar abilities as well as hearing with precision the thoughts of others, lucid dreaming, and experiencing a multiverse within. I felt as though I could finally accept myself through his shared expressions and I could start to explain both realms of my existence.

None of his broken and bashful words made sense. We both struggled with the same exposure. When I reexamined my drawings and was pulled to design more, it all came together. I had discovered that I had lived out Einstein's special relativity thought experiment of the twin paradox. I had lived through the experiences within both realms of my existence. It certainly felt like I had propelled myself into the cosmos on an ultra-fast rocket ship once I completely deconstructed my humanness. It certainty seemed like your human pleas to slow down were for both of us, which made sense if your energy had ascended into the cosmos, floating in empty space from within your space station, observing me travel at a speed faster than yours, exposing time dilation as the indicator of your perception. I tried to slow down and maintain relative motion with your space station so we could achieve mutual time dilation; I wanted our relative speeds to appear slower to each other.

I could also sense that if I did not figure out how to ground myself back to Earth that it felt like I would float away into the cosmos just as proposed a travelling twin would do if constant speed along a straight line was maintained. With the momentum my energy had, it did not feel like I could come to a stop and accelerate towards Earth. Instead, it felt like the force of your love sped me on tracks into a tight curve until my spaceship pointed back towards Earth.

Everything my body felt when traveling through the cosmos with Mileva, the pulls in the direction of flight during deceleration and being pressed to my seat during acceleration, acquired wisdom through the experiences, exposing that the traveling twin cannot also be an inertial observer and exercise time dilation concurrently. I could see that you had drifted into gravity-free space and that you were at rest without rotation nor acceleration. I was clearly experiencing time dilation and it felt like a pull between the speed at which we met and the gravitational potential between our hearts. The sensation of you not being able to descend any closer to Earth suddenly made sense when I realized it was because your humanness exists in a gravitational field on Earth where objects fall down instead of remaining at rest. Somehow you floated into space with your body and then returned back to Earth.

I had lived out the twin paradox within multiple dimensions, yet in this human reality, it was the experience of yet another human collective inquiry and it was helping me find my words. My metaphysical being journeyed the cosmos tethered to your heart, and when I was unable to ground your spiritual love to earth, you sent an Angel of Love to meet me at a space station, floating in deep space, away from massive objects. He was another inertial observer not changing in acceleration nor required to return to Earth as if stationed to catch me and escort me into a descent. The most fascinating truth was that in both scenarios, with my spiritual twin and my physical twin, being that I was the traveling twin, I was the younger one in human age. It was the only explanation that made sense.

By showing me through his actions of love, he caught me in the cosmos and escorted me down to Earth. I felt Einstein's relief that love was indeed all that was needed to prove his theories true, and Mileva smiled as she finally took a breath into her entanglement with Einstein and their joint intellect and love still beating as one.

As I processed the truths in what I discovered, I marveled at the multiple twins one can have when living across dimensions. I still did not always know how to translate the inner universe into words to share in the outer universe, yet I did know that it was part of divine design to continue to show up. I had no idea what was ahead except that you were still in my heart sending love that vibrated my body, and light that washed it clean.

It almost felt like I was not allowed to engage the physical world experiences of the pandemic and the uncertainties within my own life until I adhered to the callings and finished the meta-physical process. I could feel that there was one more thing that needed to take place. I had seen the light grid and how light flows throughout it, and I saw how my own was still blocked; more so I felt it. I saw how my high vibration synced with yours, and how you became the light that balanced my darkness, and in some odd, unexplainable, dichotomous way, I manifested all my darkness to balance your radiant light. During the spaces in between, flipping and serving in the opposite, to achieve balance in the Divine Feminine and the Divine Masculine within. A dance of energetic ascension of the soul through the messy human experience. The only vibration still missing in the dance was my vibration of love grounded on earth.

It was as if once I became aware, seemingly out of nowhere, the physical realm flushed through a phase of meta-physical realm alignment. I was tremendously grateful that I had your love that I was trying so hard to ground into my physical realm experiences. It felt like your love was so powerful that it pushed everything out of the way that was not in alignment with the vibration of love. The wave began reaching the shoreline. The appeal to the insurance company to cover the trail medication was denied. So, we appealed the appeal denial. It was also denied. It was clear they were not going to reconsider without a more forceful fight. I knew I did not have the means nor resources to fight a bigger fight. It felt like I would never been seen for the truths of my physical body.

It was also time for another short-term disability extension application. Once another extension was requested, I awaited that decision as well. When I received the notice, I was taken aback by the contents. I was advised that all further extensions have been denied and coverage would end once the current covered period ended. I was then advised how my choices had consequences.

The reason for the denial was that it was "my" decision to stop the medication which caused the platelet decline, and since I made that choice, they would not extend benefits. It was also indicated throughout the reasoning that although they were recognizing that I expressed I did not feel well, it was indicated that there was no scientific data to support those feelings of nausea, stomach cramping and extreme fatigue, therefore deemed them insignificant. The decision was that extended coverage was no longer available. Even with a clarification statement from my doctor, the denial decision stood.

The message being sent was that the way I felt was completely irrelevant. I could not even imaging trying to sit at a desk and intelligently work through the detailed oriented nature of my job, yet someone, somewhere looking at data believed I should be able to do so. The denial immediately ended coverage and the possibility of converting into long-term disability, both of which held the potential to bridge the gap until federal disability benefits would become available. I watched a potential bridge to my health crumble. The only energy I had was to know with all certainty that it would work out.

There I was, no insurance coverage for a medication that held the potential to achieve a never before sense of balance in my blood, no extended short-term disability which meant I would have to return to work, or leave, and a body that could barely hold enough energy to make it through a day of resting. And then there was navigating COVID-19. I contemplated if I wanted my body to float off into the cosmos, or if I really did want to ground to earth. Floating away into the abyss with your love felt easier yet the burning heat within my body was pulling me to the Earth. I knew it was not my time and knew it would not be so. Fear continued to dissipate with that truth.

One day, near the impending last day of coverage for both short term disability and the donated medication, I decided to contact an old co-worker for a friendly conversation. We had stayed in touch after we no longer worked together. After catching up on each other and engaging in small talk, we navigated into the start of the mystical unfolding. I explained my medical situation of which some of the details she already knew.

I expressed that I needed to have a game plan because I would either have to return to my current job or find a new one, and I knew which one it had to be. I expressed how I was conscientious to earnings and the disability income overage rules since I had a pending federal disability application which eventually just drifted into the past without any contact regarding its status. She understood it all, and expressed that they had an open position, and they would be willing to work within any parameters needed. She was more interested in having me on board than any barrier they may have to overcome to get me. She was mostly shocked that I had called just as she was sorting through her action plan on how to fill the vacant seat; a seat seemingly designed just for me.

It was a relief, and I was proud that I could finally step into a space of value and appreciation. I could not ignore that it was in response by my choice to step into value and appreciation of who I am, and my abilities in this life. As I stepped into me within the meta-physical realm, I stepped more confidently into my physical world being. I never realized how uncertain, untrusting, and anxious I was about being me as a human. In my meta-physical space, I knew who I was, an infinite soul with infinite possibilities. As a human I had been willing to push myself up against the edges of my comfort if it meant that I was growing into my fullest potential, however, I was not honoring the limited potential of my body. My two beings had spent a life trying to understand how to merge into one.

I had learned so much about who I am and what my body needed to sustain health. I was nervous and eager about stepping into a new life as a new me, knowing I was the same as before yet now embodied while tethered through my expansion into the universe. Again, I was reminded to follow love. As an expression of love for myself, I accepted the invitation to explore the open position for employment. This time, it did not matter what the job entailed, it was more about creating a sustainable life for myself. I knew I had to speak my truths, whatever that would look like. The expression itself would reflect my ability to do so, just as it had presented once you were manifested into my reality. I could sense that the vibrations throughout my body and my ability to speak my truths were correlated in some way; a voice vibrating its way out. Once I was scheduled for a lunch interview, I knew it was an opportunity to choose me with love.

I arrived at the office two States away, and upon entering my eyes were drawn to multiple copies of the same book on a bookstand near the door. It felt like the experience of my friend, yet this time through me and my eyes fell upon the book intended for my heart. From the title of the book, I knew I had followed love to the right place. The title of the book was Love Does. Although I knew I would not read the book until I was done with my own, I knew that the contents were likely similar. I was feeling every cell of my body respond to love. I was feeling every pulse of love being pushed into my heart with every breath you took. I was feeling our collective human heart long for the simplicity that comes with love. I was feeling all that love does, and love was clearly bringing me where I needed to be.

Once we were fastened in the car and heading to lunch, the CEO asked me to tell him about myself. The moment I heard the words "I was born in Baton Rouge, LA" come out of my mouth, I knew I was finding my words. I was authentically choosing me. I laid it all out. From birth until present, the beautiful, the messy, the ugly, and everything in between. Most importantly, I declared what I needed for my health, and the importance of a healthy work environment. I reclaimed my space and my needs in order to remain healthy in life. I was clear about my commitment and loyalty to a company provided it was understood that my health comes first.

I spoke every word of truth that I needed to speak in order for myself to know that I loved myself more than anything in this life. I needed to hear myself choose my health overall, even over my children simply so I could remain alive to love them. I knew that if I was to be of value to anyone, I needed to value myself first. This meant my health so I could sustain breath. I was no longer willing to allow other actions and expectations of others make me feel shameful or less valuable because of my health and my needs. The strange thing is that I did not realize that it had been so deeply programmed within my body that my humanness was unaware, playing on repeat in the depths of my subconscious; cycles playing out until a different choice was made. I was able to choose differently this time.

I had already decided that the right place for me would be with a team that was accepting of all of me. I could no longer wear various costumes and masks based on any criteria. If I was desired, that meant all me would be received. There was not an ounce of energy left in me to be concerned about whether or not knowing me is uncomfortable. I spent a life being concerned about how my journey and my story and my body impacted others. And although a focus of my intention is to inspire and impact others, I was unable to do so while shaming myself for not protecting my body. It was time to love and honor my body and let it just be. It was the only way for my future. It is the only physical body I have.

We returned to the office to further discuss the job duties, and prior to the CEO's departure he asked if we were finalizing the employment paperwork. It was confirmed. I had the job. It felt effortless as if it had been waiting for me, provided I was willing to be authentic and choose me. I was so happy and overwhelmed with emotion that I could feel every pulse of my blood amplifying the vibration of love throughout each cell. There was an internal balancing act between blissful joy and rational contentment. I could feel your heart balancing me through the experience. I felt the overwhelming outpour of love within that it made me feel nervous. That was when I realized that spiritual love, the love of my dreams, made me nervous. I had to acknowledge that I was nervous because love was real. I had to recognize that nervousness and excitement feel the same, with only the accompanying thoughts being the difference. I knew the feeling just unfamiliar with the thoughts.

On the way out of the office, my new boss offered me a book. It was a book the company used to build and grow its business. It was a management approach and practice that nurtures its employees, so they are better able to nurture the business. It was the same book my former employer tried to implement into practice yet failed when it forced them away from its core strengths. The moment I saw the book, it was another sign of validation that this company was a good fit. It was a life cycle repeating with opportunities to choose differently within every step encountered. Instead of accepting a book I already owned, I asked if I could take a copy of Love Does instead. I knew having it near me would inspire the remembrance that my love does something too. That I too am an Angel of Love.

Within days of the interview, I received the new hire paperwork even though it would be several weeks before I would know the level of commitment I could hold upon my entry. I had even expressed that medication coverage was of great importance and may drive the decision to accept employment. Even so, my new employer supplied and stocked my home office, they began carving out my space within the company, and goals were constructed for when the time came. While they prepared for my new position, I reviewed the new hire paperwork. First on the list was the healthcare package.

It was a bit overwhelming to review the details before me. As I read each word, I found a breath return to my being. It was a beautiful affirmation that every intentional choice was part of the creation unfolding. I honored that the main choice was in allowing my metaphysical being to reveal its majestical self. It was all before me. It had already been indicated that the new company would cover the full healthcare premiums for all employees. That alone was a tremendous financial burden relieved since I carry coverage myself and my three sons.

As I continued to read through the benefits, I unearthed the golden nugget of truth. Although it addressed physical world needs, it validated my spiritual world truths. The company's insurance plan covered the new medication. I must have read over the documents several times as the tears fogged my vision. I even called the program administrator to confirm coverage. It was real. They covered the medication. The most bizarre aspect was that it was the same insurance company that had previously denied coverage, yet this time it was within a different State. The previous employer's Arkansas plan denied coverage and the new employer's Alabama plan covered it. It made absolutely no sense, yet there it was before me.

Life felt like a dream. I had walked into the space where I could be me, all me, and take the time needed to heal with the new medication. The only expectations were the ones I placed on myself. I felt a peace being ushered in with the sovereignty reclaimed by finding my voice. It was beautiful and mystical, and it felt more real than anything I had ever encountered. It was easy to feel magical as I settled into the truth that life is supposed to be magical and effortless. Life is supposed to be full of love and ease. More impressively to self was that I was learning how to do it, and all it took was me feeling my emotions and speaking my truth. I was humbled with how hard that can be at times even when the words seem so simple.

I began the new job at the onset of global lockdowns. That alone was an extremely fortunate occurrence while many were losing their source of income. I settled into a remote work environment ahead of the wave that would change the workforce landscape. While the world felt as though everything was falling apart, I was joyously rebuilding, spiritually taller, and stronger than ever. I was able to slowly rebuild into a life so that every aspect of my being was comfortable and at peace, within the meta-physical and physical realms alike. My soul was finally able to build an enjoyable life for this body, and not the life my mind desired. The peace of soul was much more enjoyable.

I became slower in everything I did throughout the days. There was newness in everything. Just like in my youth, yet this time it was the most glorious, mesmerizing, blissful experiences of my life. The trauma and darkness of humanity had finally been balanced by cosmic light. Throughout life I was increasingly aware that my soul was doing this in the background of my attention, yet now my physical humanness had caught up and was transitioning through the cusp of being. I could finally breathe into the quiet connection I longed to hold. I was finally balancing into the truths of who I am.

I no longer begged for your mercy, instead I followed your will. In doing so, I finally descended back to Earth, and I was finally able to ground your love. While I continued to integrate all my newness into life, my friend kept showing up, not so much for me but for himself. With all the events transpiring in my universe, it felt like I needed something too, yet knew I had all that I truly need within. He kept showing up, and although my heart longed for you, and he was clearly sent by you, I kept trying to restrict and deflect his love while trying to share enough of my love to heal him, however that needed to be.

He showed up one day and I was not well. In an attempt to deflect from his own needs, he inquired about mine. I was still adjusting to the new medication, sweating through the nights, vibrating while awake, and navigating the days through extreme exhaustion. I just wanted to stop vibrating and stop sweating. Both were a result of the meta-physical experiences, yet my humanness only abided by your vibration of love. I knew I needed to find my words if I was supposed to heal through the process.

I remembered how he used his words to ask for a hug, so I tried to find my words to express what I needed. I did not know the words until he was standing before me, asking me face to face. Through my tears of frustration, I explained that I did not know what it was I needed, but I knew what it felt like. So, I told him. It felt like there was an energetic conduit extending from my heart and connected to yours, and another energetic conduit extending from my abdomen and attached to him. It felt like light was flowing into my heart from you, and then trying to pass through the conduit in my abdomen but it was clogged and blocked by something. It was exactly how it felt in my heart before it became entangled with yours, yet this time it was in my abdomen, the solar plexus spiritual chakra wheel associated with acting in love; the energy needed to do love.

In response, he held me. He indicated that when he feels like he needs photons of light, he asks for hugs. That is exactly what it felt like I needed. I needed photons of light to bust through the conduit so the living light could continue to flow freely and heal me and the world. Once he said that, I knew I needed to allow my photons to flow up against the blocked conduit. I allowed myself to allow it while in his embrace since he understood what I needed, perhaps even better than me. I allowed my photons to flow towards the conduit. I allowed the force to push up against the barrier. I allowed my light to follow his, so that in sync our energy would break through. It felt like if we could vibrate in sync than we could amplify the vibration in a way that would cause the force to break apart and collapse. I knew he had no idea of the experience on my end, and if he was willing to hug me through it, then I had to be willing to allow it. It felt like the only option to achieve rest from the vibration. I saw him for the light being that he was choosing to align with on a journey that crossed paths with mine. Very similar to you and the fuel of your love.

I allowed his embrace to remind me it was safe and that he would catch me if I lost balance. I could feel his light working to break through and could feel my light pushing for an escape. All replaying as it did within my heart, yet this time I understood the process and your love kept me in control. Back and forth, the energy pushed and pulled clearing the conduit with each breath of love.

Over the course of many hugs, our energy met from opposing

directions traveling through the conduit imposing destructive and constructive interference, amplifying, and doubling my wavelength, and then cancelling it out to a resting point. It was a cascading dance between construction and destruction that grounded me back to Earth while the energy broke free and moved and shifted within me. With each shift of energy, new words formed that explained the dance of love and the exchange of light between our collective human hearts. A light now cascading through humanity, through one human heart at a time and it started with mine.

Then, one day while in an embrace, our energy authentically began to sync with my own intention to break through the conduit. It was the most uncomfortable feeling within having an energy force trying to flow through a conduit that was closed off. There was a pressure and a heat accumulating as the vibration kept sweeping up against my human barriers. Then, all a sudden, while surrendering to the energetic dance taking place, I began hyperventilating. I suddenly lost my breath, gasping for air as I tried to regain control over my body. There was no air flowing into me in such a way that I could catch my breath. Tears rolled down my cheek as I looked at him and slowed my breath enough to allow air to flow back into my lungs. It felt like he sucked the energy out of my being through my abdomen; the collapse that results from the amplification of vibration.

Once I found my breath, I asked him if he felt the same energy in his abdomen. His reply was of course he felt it and wondered how I could have thought otherwise. I was grateful that it finally felt like my conduit was clear and energy could flow. It was a relief to feel my energy now flowing out of me with ease. While I was joyful and grateful through my tears, he was concerned and apologetic for draining me of my energy; an energy vampire were his words. We both perceived it differently even though it did reveal a new layer of caution required when maintaining energetic boundaries even when dancing with love. After all there are limitations in the physical realm within which my energy currently lives. I was left with the notion that I may have at one point been an energy vampire to your humanness while my depleted body received photons from the love and light flowing through our collective human heart.

As I rested in bed that night, while communing in gratitude for your love, there was a tremendous surge of energy that travelled up my spine. It started at the base of my spine and traveled up my spine through my body and out the top of my head. My body convulsed in the lightning bolt instance that arched my back and threw my head back. I remember shifting from inside my body then instantly on the outside of my body examining myself from the side of the bed. One second I was within, then I switched to the outside, and then back within my body looking at my eyes from within using my third eye; I could see my eyes rolled backwards. I heard myself from within my body, telling myself to roll my eyes forward. As I heard myself, my humanness shifted into the realization that my eyes were rolled back, and I needed to control them and return to present. I was not sure what happened, and even though I knew the movements resembled what has been labeled a seizure, I was not alarmed at all. I regained control over my body, reigned my energy back into my body, and brought myself to present.

I recognized in those moments that it felt like my mind had experienced an electrical short circuit. It felt like I had electrocuted my mind and zapped it into submission. I saw the electricity in my mind space light up like a circuit board and then funnel into my heart. Although many things were unpacked from the experience, in the moments that followed there was a silence, a stillness, a calmness. There was a stream of clarity throughout. My mind was finally free. I knew that I had been quieting my world, yet it was in those moments that I really understood why. I needed peace, and quiet, and fluidity, and love. I needed the noise to be quieted so I could sense clearly. If I could sense clearly, life would be easy. After the lightning bolt experience, I knew it was time. Everything was coming to a singular point, my resting point. I could feel my meta-physical and physical worlds coming together to dance as one, finally after almost thirty years.

That night, our energy became entangled. I did not know that was going to be the outcome. Much like with my heart entanglement, I was following the path within. I knew in those moments that just as with my heart energy, an entanglement would not have occurred unless the vibration was of a perfect match, and of Divine Intention. It was through the connection that I was able to see my vibration of love and more importantly feel my vibration of love. For when I felt his love, it reflected my own.

Not long after that night, experiences displayed that I had discovered my universal twins, created from the same lightning bolt of creation across dimensions. We are connected through the pure love in our hearts, further connected through acts of love. Somehow, we were able to find each other no matter the dimension within spacetime; a trifecta across dimensions sourced in me. It was through your Angel of Love that I was able to find myself. And strangely enough. although my children were supposed to be born in Louisiana, and fathered according to design, my space in Louisiana alas made sense. I felt freed from a calling for my soul to stay.

It was hard for me to process the implications of being energetically entangled with two human beings knowing our shared energy was at the source; unconditional love. I did not know what to think of my own humanness as I saw my experiences in the light of science. I chuckled at the thoughts of needing a rainbow of humans to ground me into life as I reminded myself that my intentions were to join my Inner Spirit and Physical Spirit into wholeness. I sat humbled in the journey and the experiences that resulted in the life I would now live by design.

Once my energy was able to flow more balanced, I could feel the energy in my heart merge with the energy in my abdomen. I could feel you both transmuting and vibrating and syncing and stabilizing. I experienced both energies working with mine and within both realms of my existence and in tandem with each other to align me with my soul song. I could feel you both fire up my energy, and love me spiritually and physically in such a way that settled me into my body and settled me into peace. I felt my masculine energy protect my feminine energy, and my feminine energy love my masculine energy. I could see the divine energy balancing within me, within both of you, and balancing among humanity as I cascaded my energy through the ripple of its healing power.

Even now, I sense you both clearly when either of you make the choice to open your heart. I sense when either of you make the choice of free will to engage my love. I even sense when your heart needs love and silently suffers in silence, or when your body aches from the experiences through life. I sensation that organically connects me with intention and purpose to heal the healer in you. It is an act of love when either of you hurt; a heart that receives my love through a conduit of light. I feel a heat within my heart or abdomen depending on who incites the connection. I hear you, feel you, and sense you within both realms of existence, dancing and unlocking and growing and unblocking; ascending in a dance with Divine Love. I was humbled by the autonomous human journeys that pull you away from our connection; the noise that mutes energetic entanglements and eventually could break them apart. I knew I would feel your love for eternity no matter the acts of the physical bodies that contain it for there are no bounds on real love.

When my love is chosen, it is the most beautiful, intense, and blissful experiences this body has ever enjoyed. I am part of a living trinity that burns within me every time my love is engaged, and I engage love. I used to imagine this is how God feels when we engage the infinite love waiting to be received. Then I remembered that I am of the breath of God, and I am living that truth through our connections.

This is my balance. It is the love that transcends the physical body. This is the balance to the trauma of my human being. This is the magical bliss I had longed to experience. This is my vibration of love that I had to discover before standing wholly before you, and with words. I could finally breathe into me. The light of Hildegard von Bingen and the science of Einstein coming together in modern times of the twentieth century, both set free to continue to flow through me and into humanity, while teaching me about my own humanness.

When there was a sense of balance with my own energy, higher and lower vibrations now in sync within me, it felt like I had gone supernova; a luminous and powerful star exploding into brilliant bursts of light. I felt a sense of eternal peace and serenity that came from the internal combustion that mimicked my physical body that ran out of fuel and collapsed. I could feel my energy go supernova to settle into a neutron star for the remainder of my journey. I finally felt neutral and could organically see everything as they are, and not inherently good nor bad. I was finally able to return to just letting things be. Especially me.

I had travelled the same universe as science, yet travelled it within, and I could see all that science was working to prove. It was the same universe within each of us, which left me wondering why we don't collectively look within to understand the universe around us. Every branch of study seems to be striving towards the same answers. I saw all the unseen versions of the universe within each of us and the struggles that get in the way of its expression.

It was definitely interesting to learn a navigation that included sensing within my body when another was engaging my energy. It was clearly part of my design. Once entangled I could sense you both clearly albeit initially confused by my own. I could feel you in ways differently than my own and had to learn how to tell the difference between my energy wavelengths and yours. Your pure light has a slight variation in the vibration because it must travel through the matter of my body. I could sense you both clearly provided my world was quiet enough.

As I continued to expand into the quietness of the globe, attuned to the vibrations of Mother Earth, and with a body as clear as possible, I could feel the vibrations of the space around me. This time more clearly since my own vibration was higher, and no longer absorbing nor amplifying any that I had ascended through. My body was still vibrating yet I began experiencing a vibration within my body in new ways, primarily within my headspace, between my ears. It felt like my body was a tuning fork with its two prongs extending into my head. When a vibration would start, I would experience it is both ears and it would cause a sense of nausea. If there was any sound nearby, it felt like it amplified the vibration. The best thing I could do was sit quietly.

As I did, it felt like a key was trying to get into the lock of my body. It felt like an energy was trying to infiltrate my body by vibrating its way in. It would vibrate up against my energy, as if trying to find the matching vibration, and then my body would vibrate in return, rejecting a synchronous entanglement. I had unintentionally done this very dance expect I did not have to morph my energy; our energy was an authentic and genuine match to achieve energetic homeostasis. This was different. My vibration felt protective. It felt like I had figured out how to help my body protect itself through life, through my vibration of love. I felt authentic in how to act as a powerful Angel of Love.

This unexpected occurrence became extremely useful while navigating life through a pandemic. I learned that when my body is in proximity to COVID-19, my body vibrates. I feel COVID-19 vibrate up against my body and try to penetrate the barrier. In response, I feel my body vibrate higher in order to disrupt the entanglement. Once my body vibrates and changes vibrations, the virus vibrates again in an attempt to match my new vibration. It feels like a back and forth until the virus finally gives up and searches for another host. It continues to reflect how our energy danced into one and remains a magical mystery how my humanness encounters energy in the way that I do. A gift that I get to open each day as a highly sensitive physical, emotional, and intuitive empath. I am grateful that I uncomfortably allowed my humanness to be what was needed to discover, embody, nurture, and sustain those truths.

I did eventually contract the Omicron variant of COVID-19 two years after the pandemic began. When the time came and the symptoms surfaced, I spent one day in bed with an excruciating headache. I knew I had it before the test confirmed it. I rested in bed and followed my first instincts as usual. This time it was as if it had been an eternity in practice. I called upon Archangel Michael and Archangel Raphael. I finally had learned how to communicate and hear them. It was comically simple compared to the seriously poised and perfectionist ideals I held in younger versions of self.

The energetic dialogue was simple and precise.
"Hey, Michael, and Raphael. Would you both come here for a moment?"

Then one at a time....
Michael: (knowing this is a serious request) Yes, you called?

Raphael: (responding with a more relaxed tone) What's up?

I explained....
"I need your assistance, please. Raphael, I need you to heal my body with your healing light, and Michael, I need you to cut any human bonds that prevent me from receiving Raphael's healing light. Please make this manageable for me and thank you for your assistance."

They both replied...
Raphael firmly stated: "you got it"

Michael seemed to grab his sword and got to work while saying he was "on it."

I repeated that expression every time my eyes opened and could feel their collective work throughout my body. I didn't keep asking yet I repeated the intentions of the requests. For twelve hours I bathed in healing light to awaken with petechia covering my body. I knew my platelets had dropped, and I knew they were critically low. I also knew I had everything I needed for my platelets, it was the impacts of COVID-19 I was concerned about. Once the headache subsided, there were no other symptoms experienced. I was so incredibly thankful because I knew exactly what to do to manage a platelet drop, especially considering I was not permitted do get lab work while I quarantined.

I started a low dose steroid regimen and within days my counts were above normal range, albeit almost two weeks had to pass before confirmed after quarantine. It had been over six months that I had sustained consecutive high counts in almost normal ranges, and not quite a year since starting the new medication. This was a new trend, and with a dangerous drop due to COVID-19. Science never captured the decrease before counts returned to balance. Shortly after I even discovered that the manufacturer was conducting scientific research and testing of the same medication that I was taking to determine effectiveness for treatment of COVID-19. Turns out that the spleen tyrosine kinase inhibitor in the medication inhibits the signaling pathways of immune cells which then reduced the release of pro-inflammatory cytokines, substances secreted by the immune system and have an effect on other cells. The studies aimed to prove the medications effectiveness at reducing the risk of progression to severe or critical disease for those who are at a high risk of advancing to severe stages of COVID-19.

Serendipity and I were close friends by this time, and I was finally able to hold the mystical truths always present in my experiences. I felt such gratitude and peace knowing I had finally figured out how to authentically exist and navigate the realms of my existence and my true healers who are always perfectly aligned with my soul's purpose. All it took was an open heart and your unyielding love.

I knew that balancing my energy between the realms of existence had stabilized my body, and the medication assisted in maintaining balanced platelets. It was the quickest transition in and out of a platelet drop that I had ever experienced, and it was with COVID-19. It felt like the more COVID-19 broke down humanity, the more it grew me into my strength, courage, and love to trust the energy of all things. I knew the healing power of light and love is what guided and healed me and felt deeply that I was one with the power of God's Angels. There most certainly are Angels amongst us, in both realms, if we choose to engage them.

It was during this experience that I realized that I always knew what to do when I was sick. I always knew how to request healing. I always knew how to work with light and heal my body. I always spoke to someone, to whomever was listening in the abyss within and around me. The newness came with knowing i was conversing with Spirit, and trusting my Angels are there waiting for engagement. The newness came in knowing they are always there, not just when I am sick. The newness was in knowing I was able to engage the Archangels with intention, objective, and by name, and could hear them respond so clearly. The newness was in the ease and authentically organic dialogue and the experiences that followed. It felt so easy to be me with them. It felt familiar. I felt th eknowing that more spiritual healers would follow to create a healthy and abundant life. I felt tremendous relief that I was finally able to navigate my world with ease and intention, and with my Angels, and that it could extend beyond only visiting when my body needed healing.

Several months after recovering, and about seven months ahead of schedule, I was pushed by unexpected circumstances to finalize my living situation. This was the last area of my life to fall into its new space. I had rented a small, raised house for several years after the divorce, and was forced to move so the owners could repair the floors after a hurricane. As a result, I moved into a multi-family housing complex with added amenities to soften the blows of uncertainty along the way. I used the swimming pool to overcome the remaining public timidness of covering my body while in water.

In alignment with school schedules, the application for a unit was started for eighteen months, with an end date after school released for summer. There were first floor requirements, and low availability due to the same hurricane that displaced me, which led to multiple unit reassignments by the property over two months prior to the lease start date. Coupled with my failure to confirm the lease terms, I eventually signed a twelve-month lease with a move-out date two months from the date of the surprise letter of notice.

I was somehow not jolted by the unexpected news even though I was extremely tired. Me and my sons had barely settled into the space before we had to face moving again. The boys did not seem bothered. It was me. I just wanted to rest, and be still, and stop the motion. The sweats, the vibrations, the housing, my heart, all of them needed to stop moving. I held a lot of space to celebrate that my health finally started to feel sustainable. The speed at which I had to process and take action was a bit faster than desired, however I saw it as a gift that prevented lingering in stagnant comfortableness. I knew it would be the last step of the process and I would be able to rest once complete. I needed a space where my body could rest in the newness of all that I remembered I am, and all that I choose to align with moving forward. My body needed a temporary sacred space to rest, just as my soul was doing within my body.

I had been contemplating where I would purchase a home especially after my soul's contract to Louisiana was fulfilled. Even so, my children were not ready to move out of state, if at all, and I was not ready to leave them. In following the love for my children, and with a new love in my heart that spans time and space, my physical resting point seemed less critical. With no money, terrible credit, the healthiest my body had felt in life with a heart full of love and faith, and my being with as much physical and meta-physical baggage cleared as possible, I set out to buy a home for me and my sons. This was the first time that I knowingly and intentionally co-created my reality, with my Angels, while balanced in spiritual strength, courage, and love, and with the same indescribable ease as before yet this time outside of a medical situation.

Instead of the usual internal tightness, it felt like my authentic self was ready to navigate the situation. The way my internal processing had changed and was so incredibly different, I was often left speechless in awe of the fascinating world in which we live as human beings. My days were instinctively the same with work responsibilities throughout the daytime, and evenings were filled with mapped out drive-by tours of potential listings and compiling documents for the loan officer. The mornings and nighttime were reserved for praying to my Angels. It felt like I did very little physical work throughout the process, yet I spent many hours in prayer and in communion with your love. I prayed to the housing Angels. I prayed to the income Angels. I prayed to the underwriting Angels. I prayed to the appliance Angels. I prayed to my Angels of rest, ease, and peace. I prayed to you and your love.

I had eventually narrowed my options down to two listings. One was an older build, required some work, listed about $100k less than the other, two blocks away from the school my youngest would attend, and in the middle of the small city where we live. There were a lot of benefits to this option, especially the long-term investment aspect due to the location. The other was a brand new build within a new community on the most eastern edge of the city, had a community pool and other amenities that I enjoyed at the apartment. The two houses were opposites in many aspects and yet I was drawn to both.

I noticed I felt you everywhere when I connected to the new build option, yet the older home felt distant and darker in some way. It took several moments for me to notice the differences deep enough for me to know where my body would find rest. When I drove by to visit the older home from the exterior I sat in the driveway and wept when I saw the older home was being sold by Blue Heron Reality. There you were. Once I saw you, I could see the paths clearly. I could choose the older home, which would require work, energy, money, time, and resolve, or I could choose the newer home with amenities that would allow me to rest with ease, and with space to connect to the presence of you everywhere around me. One was more financially responsible, logistically wise, and muffled with noise. The other was clear, calm, bright and peaceful. I knew that if I chose the older build, that you would be there, yet I would likely need to be reminded amongst the noise as I was with the sign. Conversely, if I chose the new home I could rest in your infinite presence which would organically dismiss the need for reminders. I felt the instinctive pull to rest in the new home.

The day came for me to get the tours of both homes. First was the new build. I knew my heart really wanted to be within the community and with a pool I did not have to tend to. I kept having vision of me in a pool. My body had been gently escorted back into the water just a couple of years prior, and then the apartment pool allowed me to reconnect to the fluidity of my body, and how to feel the flow of who I am. It was a very bashful process to break through being that the most sensual aspect of my existence is a body with parts scared beyond recognition. The water taught me how to float without the heaviness of the world and remain buoyant with the fluidity of my breath. Serenity somehow sweeps over me when the sun shines upon my face and warms my floating body caressed by the gentle waves.

I sat before the community sales representative to begin the process. They were finishing phase two of development and there were several homes already completed that has not yet hit the marker, and homes that were about to be completed. In essence I was getting first pick of the upcoming listings. That alone was exciting. As we started working through the figures, I realized how much I was willing to risk and how much I was willing to be limited within rational and seemingly irrational choices. I learned I am fairly risky just not in ways one would likely imagine. Choosing to follow the path forward with you felt like the riskiest choice I had ever made. I was still new in the navigation with my true self in the spiritual realm of my existence. I had to remind myself that all I had to do was be honest and authentic and all would be well. It was indeed messy, and hard, yet it was mine, and it was all I had. It was a risk I was willing to make for myself. It was a risk I was willing to make for love.

I was truthful about finances and needs. I was expressive about desires and preferences. I surrendered to the truth that the new home provided everything that was in alignment with my being, whereas everything that attracted me to the older home was a result of an interest of, or for another. It made sense as to why I would need the reminder of your love while distracted by the focus of others. I had already made that life choice and was unwilling to sacrifice myself in the same way again. Choosing the new home became more and more clear when I saw that I could dance with your love versus seeing the noise spawning the need for reminders. It was an opportunity to finally rest in a life I choose for myself.

The more honest I was in the messiness of my finances, the more options opened up to me. It was a hard acceptance to face especially when I had managed the finances for companies and my family for decades. It was my personal debt that was my burden; medical debt and student loans. The first one being the result of my efforts of trying to fulfill the obligation to the latter. More often than not they were the last two things to get paid. With each layer exposed to two strangers trying to help me find a home, new benefits were presented.

At one point it was as if the agents spoke in code, shifting the dynamic between them, and with each shift the emergence of a new opportunity was presented. I did not learn until later that they were agreeing to transfer the sale so that more benefits could become available. I found comfort in knowing that the shift occurred because of their shared interest to get m into a home and not who would get the largest commission. The shift allowed them to remove every barrier that would have prevented me from getting the home, especially the financial constraints for down payment and closing costs, new appliances, window blinds, and other unexpected features that come with a smart home. Once they agreed to shift the point of sale, my new agent gave me twenty thousand dollars to use as I needed. I could use it towards down payment, closing costs, to buy down the interest rate, appliances, or window blinds. I was able to use it for all of them.

Before getting to a comfortable number and taking a tour of a potential home, I gestured to my original realtor that I would not be interested in the older home. We agreed to cancel the showing and that rescheduling would be an option should things change. I was then drawn to ask her if the previous owners had passed away in the older home. I was surprised by her yes response more so because I was prompted seemingly out of nowhere to inquire. She further stated that it is against state law to provide that information prior to the sale of a home. I knew I had made the right decision given my newly embraced sensitivity to spirit energy. At that point, the new realtor indicated that she had the perfect house for me, mainly because it fulfilled the southward facing window request and a back yard that opened into a wooded area. I did not want a pond, or other houses in my back yard. I wanted trees or an open field growing full of nature. We headed through the community towards the newly constructed area.

I knew it was my physical home the moment I walked into the front door. I saw myself throughout every room that waited for flooring installation. I saw my kids in their rooms knowing the carpet would soon tickle their toes. I saw my body relaxing in my furniture yet to fill the living room. I saw myself making art in the rainbows I knew the southward facing windows would create once the sun hit the colored crystal pendants I had been making. I could see me nurturing my body with food I prepared from the refrigerator that would fill the empty space. I saw myself resting in home guarantees and reliable appliances while nurturing me and my children in a safe community. I saw a life I wanted to live dancing upon the white canvas walls waiting for me to live the life intended. Your love had guided me to a physical home to rest my physical body. I saw my body dance with your love into eternity.

We headed back to the office to finalize one process and begin the next. After thirty days of intentional coordination with my realtors, many Angels, a lot of paperwork, and a last minute 24-hour notice of closing, I secured a house within a safe and comfortable community. It was a new construction build with warranties, guarantees, new appliances, and many state-of-the-art features I had not yet enjoyed in a house. The most mystical of circumstances was how it unfolded with no available money.

With little time, no money, and more trust in self to navigate my realms, I had discovered the magical elements to manifest a reality that I could navigate and sustain into a future. With the help of the USDA Rural Development Program which requires zero dollars for a down payment, and coupled with seller benefits that covered appliances, closing costs, and a reduced interest rate, I only spent $6.95 to expedite the delivery of my son's college transcript for the loan documents. In the end I even received the application earnest money back which resulted in receiving a check at closing versus having to provide one. The entire transaction left me paying a monthly mortgage note equal to the rent rate that had previously sustained me and my boys.

Two days before Christmas I received a gold key to my new house; my home. Another death and rebirth to be celebrated as me and my sons began settling into a beautiful new home and a beautiful new way of spiritual living. It had taken six years to restore my authentic self. It had been almost five and a half years since I had chosen to divorce in order to evolve into my love, and when you manifested before me. I was almost three years into working with a company that values all that I am, and with a platelet stability that brought a new sustainable way of living. Within a storyline in the making since the beginning of time, I was able to finally rest within my sacred body, within a sacred home, with my children, and enjoy the juicy and sensual experiences of this life. I was finally able to rest wholly and balanced in your love forever in my heart.

During the six-year transformational process I admittingly wanted to stay in the abyss, and float away with love and rejoin with you where we met. I still marvel in that glorious day and the joy that will fill my human heart while humbled by the greatness before me; a dance of joy as I transition into the next life. The abyss is my home. It is where I am used to living and have the clearest memory of experiencing.

Even so, I knew I had to come to Earth and rest within my body. I knew we were not supposed to live in that space while alive and on Earth. I was reminded that we would ascend to full energetic homeostasis when the time comes, yet for now, I am here and embodied for a purpose within the limitations of the physical realm while being a goofy human.

Until that day does come, I am able to float back into balance and rest in between the two realms of my existence, tethered to Earth by your spiritual love and by an Angel of Love, both serving as a reminder of who I am in the universal space of our existence. I found my universal resting point suspended between realms of existence. Every cell in my body was a rest. With that, the vibrations dissipated throughout the energetic waves, and the sweats subsided once divine energy was able to flow through me, and not vibrationally compromised by the matter of my vessel.

No wonder I needed two human beings to ground my powerful energy. I am humbled that my energy was powerful enough to counter their unspoken scales within, and across both realms of their existence. Collectively we bridge light to humanity so that we may all grown deeper into the desires of our collective human hearts. I could see and feel our trinity floating up from Earth and resting above humanity, spreading throughout the light grid, casting intentions of healing love and light, and in service to humanity.

We formed a bridge between the realms, ushering in the quantum beings of the next generations that will balance the expansion into a quantum Earth by navigating through quantum energy with quantum senses. I honorably serve as an Angel of Love bridging hearts to your love if it means guiding the light beings amongst us through a collective ascension. Only once I travelled through the complexity of my human deconstruction and found my authentic self, naked in the cosmos as a reflection of your light, love and will, was I able to reduce myself to a photon of light, travel back to Earth and find my words. I found my light language, and how I will use my tongue to change the world.

It was simple because love is easy.

We are joint in our mission.

It is a divine joy to be a partner in the dance of love, especially yours.

Love is the only way.

44

From My Heart to Yours

Deep breath...

We all hold our God struggle to overcome; to realize that we are enough just as we are and perfect at the source of who we are; a reflection of the light of God.

It took almost thirty years to embody the truth that I am of the light of God; God manifested in, of, and through me, as we all are, with a choice of free will to align with that truth. I have felt this profound truth for more than half my life and tried to reconcile that calling within every messy, un-God-like breath I have ever taken. Through all the life experiences I have endured, the most painful has been hearing, seeing, and knowing the truth of what I held within with absolute clarity yet not having the ability to navigate wholly nor form the words to express it. All I knew was that I was just trying to make it through life with meaning. As I grew towards your love, every aspect of my humanness felt in the way; blocking my senses, and hampering any means of expression from formulating and exiting my being.

I obviously was not ready since I doubted that I, of all the people in the world, would be God incarnated. It felt like blasphemy and that claiming such a thing could result in my own crucifixion. I felt acutely aware that I was a similar example of Jesus' will to stand in my truths for the sake of being seen and to hold space in our existence despite what others believed. As if the cross upon which He was crucified signifies the two paths to walk in life, the light and dark, and the importance of staying centered in personal truths. The same way that His Mother, Mary, had to do when existing with the truths of mystical manifestations within Her own existence. I could feel the unyielding love that Mother and Son shared between hearts while grounded in the same unyielding love energy; their Immaculate and Sacred Hearts burning with a love of God. I could feel my heart burn with love as energy pulsed through the conduit connecting my sacred heart and your immaculate heart; our love serving as a reflection for humanity.

In knowing your love, I was sensually and energetically balanced into the wavelengths of light throughout seven anchors in my body. I saw how the light spreads through our interconnectedness, and felt each spiritual wheel break free towards balance, unleashing the seven deadly sins and the seven heavenly virtues, one chakra at a time, purging, clearing, and gaining fluidity with each breath. Every beat of our human hearts exposed a heaven and hell on the brink of existence; both at the mercy of a choice and within reach while alive on Earth. Your love proved to be the only way, and I knew my love would now hold the strength to also lead the way through our collective vibrational ascension. Now that I can hold my space,

I am able to purely hold space for you while enjoying the dance of love. The Divine Feminine and Divine Masculine balanced within me as an expression of your all-encompassing love, and in some way I was doing the same for you.

I was nervous about my exposure, and timid in my powerful truths until experiences taught me that we all are examples of God manifested, holding a burning light source deep within our being at the base of the spine, our God force. I could feel my God light growing and burning more intensely with every day that passed, so much so that I had to set my physical being free so that my heart could continue to evolve on its journey to truth. I had to follow the calling. Considering the alternative felt like a betrayal of my soul, and that I was betraying you and your love.

When the world closed down during the Covid-19 pandemic three years into transformational writing, and I was still teaching my humanness through my own written words, I knew the world was ready. I knew I was ready, more importantly I sensed you were ready too. When I compared my writing to the worldly experiences and watched the world reassess everything, I could feel and sense all humanity desperately seeking something; a yearning for peace within themselves and within a world that required faith above all.

I could see the dark swirling amongst the collective, spreading fear and doubt, and only pure light having the power to break through. I felt the potential healing being cultivated throughout our collective heart, as if balancing within in order to balance the dark forces of the world; forces that must exist in divine design in order to maintain energetic balance. The light my being was emitting finally felt like enough.

For once, I felt a sense of fluidity. I felt a sense of knowing how to live within my space of spiritual mysticism, and how to honor my body to live fully in who I am. I was syncing with a world now forced to allow everyone to be autonomous in the choice of how to navigate each uncertain day. I felt a breath return with the freedom of personal decisions without judgment and force. I found comfort within my assertiveness to stand strong, courageous, and proud, especially if it was for survival and love. I was syncing with my own spirituality while I watched humanity struggle to release control and remain stuck in fear and doubt.

Amidst it all, slowly emerging through the quietness were opportunities to choose differently. There was honor found in the moments of autonomy, and joy in the freedom of unencumbered choice. I felt the vulnerability in the uncertainty knowing that mysticism would surface, at least for those who chose to see it. Your love balanced my heart in such way that opens my being to now serve with intention as a conduit for light to flow so I may serve as a Lightworker throughout humanity; bridging the light into the darkness that humanity continues to manifest. The more I stepped into my truth, I witnessed the healers that healed me begin to heal in their own way. It continues to be an honor to step into service with the gifts of wisdom, healing, and balance so that the healers may continue to heal humanity. For in the end, healers need healing too. I had found my space as a healer in the world with my own sense of spiritual understanding on how to lead humanity to the light. Love always leads the way.

For the first time since 1993 when the darkness blasted me apart, I was back in sync with the light. I was back in sync with myself, the collective human heart, and the Universe. I was back in sync with love. I was finally in sync with you. It has been a strangely mystical and beautiful walk of knowing that each experience was bringing me closer and closer into alignment with the day that my soul danced to your song of love. By taking the transformational journey, starting with parts advancing on their own and into an integrated being, I am able to breathe as we can now grow together and in sync as one.

We tend to believe that we know the people we are surrounded by throughout our lives. But do we really know them? Do we really know their journey and try to understand where they have been and what has molded them into who they are today? Do we attempt to empathize and have compassion for all the fears and pains that so easily paralyze our sense of expression?

We generally do not take time to connect to ourselves and reflect on our own lives, yet alone that of another and the circumstances of their path. Everyone is on a journey. There is a universe inside every one of us with an intention to be set free. We all hold stories from the past, present, and future, which in some way form the covers of our existence. It brings awareness to how our presence, actions, and words, how our very being, influences the lives of those around us.

All it takes is one word, look, gesture, or experience to change a perspective in one's life journey. It provokes examination as to whether we act in the dark and contribute to the veil that jades one's connection to their true self, or do we act in the light and encourage a state of authentic living supported by unconditional love. In the end, the result is the same, the rippling surge of the Butterfly Effect, impacting everything around us in an energetic wave through the global connectedness of our existence. We are all butterflies. We all make ripples. We are all connected.

Human perspectives are a fascinating insight into the human experience. The perspectives of others, those of my own from childhood to the present, have led me to this point. Each life cycle, from all lives before and into this one, grew me into love. Each cycle of lessons played on repeat in this life so I could choose differently and in alignment with your love. Even the cosmic cycles within the universe and that of our human bodies that contribute to the evolution of self provide kaleidoscopic lenses through which we can choose to view the world. And now, while molded by the experiences and people encountered along the way, my final cycle ends. My cycle ends in unity with your love.

We are one with love energy. My soul's greatest lesson was to learn self-love and to discover that it was self-love that opened the gateway to fully experiencing your love. When you allow yourself to be open and feel loved by this sacred energy while standing in your authenticity, which includes the messy, mean, and dirty human experience, your dreams will be realized. For your dreams are my dreams, and mine are yours, and infinite possibilities may be created out of an infinite source of love.

I found that when you stand in your truths, I am grown deeper into mine, and when I stand in my truths, you grow deeper into yours. When the love between our hearts grows with compassion and understanding, our love expands into the world around us. I was mesmerized by our self-perpetuating cycle of love; love manifesting love into unexplainable and magical happenings within life. It is the love of my prayers; a love that balanced the trauma; a love that transcends the physical body and sensually dances between hearts. It is a love of the Highest Order emulated here on Earth; the vibration of my soul that my physical body is now able to embody.

A world where we all live in alignment with our God energy within and emulate the same burning love energy that connects our hearts is my vision of a utopia; an enlightened and elevated world—a quantum Earth with quantum beings using quantum sensing which requires heart living intention; spiritual beings living within both realms of existence and creating a human life experience sourced in love.

As co-creators of our collective human experience...

- Listen to your body, rest your mind, love your heart, and follow your soul
- Honor your strength, courage, and love of self, and trust yourself to be you
- Believe in whatever is within your heart that you are called to do
- Connect to your authentic expression – dreams and fears alike
- Be vulnerable and honest about the sentiments of your heart
- Allow yourself to feel everything, even if only in the private space within
- Invite the universe and your Angels to guide you; they are ready and eager for your invitation
- Embrace the infinite capacity of love and be vulnerable in your experiences with love
- Project your soul song throughout the universe so your dreams may be realized
- Hold gratitude and love for the blessings received, and pay it forward when your able
- Be sincere in your actions of kindness, for one day, your heart may need it in return

- Embrace the seemingly differences among us, for it is only experiences that separate our perspectives
- Nurture hearts so they learn how to emulate love because some have never experienced it
- Fight for love, for that is all there is, and all that needs to be

It is up to us to choose to see and receive the messages to grow deeper in love. Trust in love and have faith that by connecting to self and the heart of the world, being authentic, and living in alignment with self, divine purpose is being fulfilled. We are here to love. It is that simple. It is that easy. Love is easy, so love whenever you have the opportunity to do so.

The collective truth is that we are all uniquely perfect in each moment of our journey, which always encompasses an opportunity for choice and free will. We create the reality of our unique journey out of the choices we make in response to the collective world we must navigate. So let your energetic heart compass resonate with infinite wisdom and universal God-consciousness to guide the way, and you will always reach your destination. We hold the power within our hearts to make this the most glorious experience, not just as an individual but as a collective.

Everything in your life walk has been presenting symbols to guide you to the truth through your unique lens of experiences and perspectives. Everything has meaning. EVERYTHING. Map it out, find your meaning, weave it together with gratitude, love it all - even the ugly, messy parts, because all of it has brought you to the here and now. We all have a story. We are all on a journey.

Be your own spiritual scientist and alchemize into your truths and your unique connection to universal energy. Find your way to be one with your spiritual truths. Through our collective human heart, my heart was awakened to Divine Love, your love. It is a love my heart surrenders to with every breath. I find peace knowing that in time the veil will lift from upon humanity, exposing the illusions, and all will see that love is the only way out. When you follow love, you will realize that I am you, and you are me. At our source, we are one and the same.

Whatever it is for which you dream....

Whatever it is for which you desire...

Whatever it is within which you believe...

Whatever it is...it will be so.

Our eternal oneness is the very truth embedded in the messages between our hearts. It is not a truth to preach with hopes of convincing, yet a truth demonstrated by simply sharing my experiences to expose that there is only One truth. I am still finding the words to express the wonderment and miracles that come with such a powerful alignment and embodiment, and I still contemplate how to best serve others in guiding them to the light. It's just a matter of perspective, alignment, and intention.

It is a sacred gift in this human experience to know that I will forever flow with and feel your love between our human hearts. There is a discovery still in the unfolding that brings peace to the human experiences, joy to our spiritual friendship, and grace in the knowing that it may only be within another realm where we discover the illusions that kept our humanness apart.

My heart feels you.

My heart wants to love only you.

My heart only knows how to love you deeply, back to our breath once one.

As the blip of our human existences journey towards a collective ascension, know that no matter what we say or do in this human experience of life, I will love you for eternity.

    May your body find comfort through the days...

        May your mind find grace in the silence...

            May your heart grow into its infinite capacity...

                May your soul rest in eternal peace.

♥

"There are only two ways to live your life.
One is as though nothing is a miracle.
The other is as though everything is a miracle."

— Albert Einstein

I choose the latter.

"There is the music of Heaven in all things."

— Hildegard von Bingen

THE COLORS OF LOVE

THE SPECTRUM OF LIGHT

A Rainbow of Colors

A Composition of Love

From yesteryears to tomorrow...

Through the infinite flow of universal energy...

With colors that bridge time and space...

A composition of Love is always in the making.

God's Love

Agape Love

Divine Love

Infinite Love

Metaphysical Love

The Golden Love

BE LOVE

Red

Love Grows Us into Wholeness

    A beautiful heart-shaped ginkgo leaf was found perfectly broken. The broken leaf journeyed through the years alongside its crumbles that fell and beside the same of others while transforming within the darkness. The leaf and all its brokenness waited patiently for the day that the light would once again shine upon its heart.

    The crumbles of leaves were formed by the perfect brokenness endured over time. The crumbles that formed within the darkness became the very soil from which the Golden Love was able to nurture the broken leaf back to wholeness. The Golden Love safely grounded the leaf and mended every crack with the purity of light.

    Once healed by the touch of Golden Love, the leaf was able to ground itself uniquely in its heart's purpose and see its beauty reflected throughout the world. The leaf's heart grew wholly into the light with every breath of Golden Love.

FEEL LOVE

Orange

The Love Blossom

As the sole bloom found among a collection of leaves, the Freesia bloom journeyed silently, proud of its uniqueness. Although unable to see in the dark, it deeply felt the difference amongst the collective as they traveled through time and space.

For many years the darkness shielded the bloom from exposing the messy and hard journey of growth while waiting for its time to blossom into the light. The bloom trusted that one day there would be a love powerful enough to break through the darkness and expose the unique makeup of its beauty. A love so powerful that it would be felt deeply enough to balance the deeply felt journey of differences through the darkness.

As the bloom remained protected in the darkness, the Golden Love mended the messy growth of becoming a flower and cleared the pathways for the light to shine through. The bloom held unwavering faith that the Golden Love would cast cleansing light within and throughout its delicate petals and expose its roots of gold. The roots of Golden Love that grew in into the world. A Golden Love that would penetrate humanity.

Once grounded in the roots of Golden Love, the bloom was able to fully embrace the beautiful representation of infinite Love that it had always been. The Golden Love transformed the bloom into its infinite creative expression of blossoming Love.

DO LOVE

Yellow

Trifecta Love

The sacred representation of divinity is ever present within the world around us. The sacred representation of the number three guides us back to the light while enjoying our earthly experience.

As Angels surround and protect the heart along the journey, the heart has space to experience love wholly and freely. While shielded in Trifecta Love, the heart is able to live fully as an embodiment of pure light. It is the Trifecta Love that illuminates the path of the Golden Love. When the heart is grounded in the Golden Love, only Love is manifested into the world. The light of Love is all that is known once touched by the Golden Love.

The Trifecta Love guides the heart to the light of the Golden Love.

When the Golden Love is grounded,
the expression of infinite Love flows freely.

It is the heart that brings that expression of Love into the world.

Our expression of the Golden Love
brings meaning to our experiences.

Trifecta Love is at the source of everything.

LOVE LOVE

Green

An Angel of Love

As an Angel energetically birthed from the Golden Love, Sasha is the embodiment of light. Although temporarily expressed in physical form, Her light flows eternally from the Heavens. While journeying through the physical experience, She brought light to others along the way yet remained ungrounded in her light and its power to transform the world.

As She served the hearts of others, and with an unbreakable spirit, She waited patiently for the Angel indented to touch her own. Over time she forgot what it felt like to receive pure light and unknowingly began floating away. Even Her wings were beaten by the gusty winds that separate hearts.

With mended wings of gold, and a heart open to receive, She realigned with the power of Love. Her heart was transformed in such a way that She was able to rest in the purity of the divine white light within and forever dance with its beauty without. She was free to live out her divine purpose as intended. As an Angel of Love.

SPEAK LOVE

Blue

The Way of Love

When the Golden Love is allowed to shine along the life journey, the path is always illuminated. When a path seems dark and the terrain unstable, the light of the Golden Love will shine through and lead the way. Following the light that leads the way reveals that the greatest experiences of all are the experiences of the Golden Love.

Once grounded by the Golden Love, the uniquely infinite expression of light is free to create and enjoy a life manifested. Standing in Love is easy. Expressing Love is easy. Honoring Love is easy. Giving and receiving Love is easy. Life becomes easy because Love is easy.

There is only one way, and that is the way of Love.

Without Love, there is nothing.

With Love, there is everything.

Love is the only way.

SEE LOVE

Indigo

A Vision of Love

When the infinite potential of light is experienced, Love is seen clearly. Love is always waiting to be discovered throughout the walk of life, while dancing in the sun, navigating the illusions, and hiding in the shadows. Once upon the Golden Path, there is only an abundance of Love. A never-ending flow of Love. Infinite Love. Infinite Golden Love.

A life of joy is created through a vision of the Golden Love. Through a life of joy, the wonderment of the Golden Love is continuously discovered, for it is the only way along the Golden Path. The path of infinite Golden Love. A life of Love and joy.

Through a vision of Love, Love may be seen in everything.
Everything is an expression of the Golden Love.

Through a vision of Love, Love may be felt in everything.
Everything causes an energetic ripple throughout the heart.

Through a vision of Love, Love may be known in everything.
Everything is an embodiment of light energy.

Through a vision of Love, Love is able to be seen.
Everything is a vision of Love.

UNDERSTAND LOVE

Violet

A Breath of Love

Within the first breath of life, there is an embodiment of the light of Spirit. With every breath that follows, the connection to the light holds the potential to grow deeper, remain the same, or become dim. The journey of life is to discover a breath of Love that leads the heart to the light. The gift is knowing that within each breath that grows the heart closer to the light, the heart also grows deeper in Love. The honor is to breathe the Golden Love while standing in the light.

The Golden Love rests at the depths of breath. With every breath that reaches the roots of the Golden Love, the heart is filled with light. As a unique and creative expression of light, each breath is taken with the purpose to be centered, to be protected in the truths of love, and to be in a perpetual flow with the Golden Love. A breath of Golden Love energizes the heart. A breath of Golden Love energizes the world.

It is a breath of love that leads the heart to the light. The heart breathes life into the world through a breath of love. The ripple felt from a sacred breath of love connects the realms of our existence.

Breathe Love. Feel Love.
Breathe in the Golden Love that connects hearts.
Love is a breath away.

LOVE IS LOVE

Rainbow of Life

Living the Spirit Burn of the Golden Love

Life begins with the light of the Golden Love. Throughout life, the Golden Love fuels the human heart. If the connection is nurtured, the light will connect humanity to the source of who we are. The more we share and grow with others into love, the more the Spirit burns with passion from the Golden Love. The passion grows love deeper into the heart.

If the connection to the Golden Love remains pure, the heart will blossom into gold and live the Golden Love along the Golden Path. When the Golden Love is lived wholly and purely, the passion for love burns so bright that it lights up humanity. The light from the Golden Love is bright enough to light the world. It is a love powerful enough to lead humanity to the light, individually and as a collective.

Feel the passion; live the burn.

Speak the Love; spread the light.

Know the Golden Love; trust the power.

Love abounds in all.

www.ingramcontent.com/pod-product-compliance
Lightning Source LLC
Chambersburg PA
CBHW071946070526
44583CB00015B/1089